The Easy Guide to OSCEs for
SPECIALTIES

A step-by-step guide to OSCE success

MUHAMMED AKUNJEE
GP Vocational Training Scheme, London

SYED JALALI
Foundation Year Doctor, Cardiff

and

SHOAIB SIDDIQUI
Foundation Year Doctor, Brighton

Illustrations drawn by
MUHAMMED AKUNJEE

Foreword by
GRAHAM BOSWELL
AND STEVE RILEY

Radcliffe Publishing
Oxford • New York

Radcliffe Publishing Ltd
18 Marcham Road
Abingdon
Oxon OX14 1AA
United Kingdom

www.radcliffe-oxford.com
Electronic catalogue and worldwide online ordering facility.

© 2009 Muhammed Akunjee, Syed Jalali and Shoaib Siddiqui
Reprinted 2009, 2010, 2011

Muhammed Akunjee, Syed Jalali and Shoaib Siddiqui have asserted their right under the
Copyright, Designs and Patents Act 1998 to be identified as the authors of this work.

All rights reserved. No part of this publication may be reproduced, stored in a retrieval system or
transmitted, in any form or by any means, electronic, mechanical, photocopying, recording or
otherwise, without the prior permission of the copyright owner.

The information provided in this textbook has been collated by the authors and has been checked
against the most up-to-date and relevant hospital guidelines. Although great effort has been
made to verify and check all aspects, the authors, editors and publishers take no responsibility
for any inaccuracies found in the book or for any medical advances that may affect any aspect of
clinical practice. The authors also stress that the mock marks schemes in the book do not reflect
the practice of any university, medical school or other related official bodies involved in OSCE
examinations. They have been included to aid student OSCE revision and constitute the authors'
own subjective assessments. The authors are in no way responsible for the candidate's performance
in the examinations based upon the mark sheets or information contained in this work.

British Library Cataloguing in Publication Data

A catalogue record for this book is available from the British Library.

ISBN-13 978 184619 250 0

Typeset by Pindar NZ, Auckland, New Zealand
Printed and bound by Hobbs the Printers, Southampton, UK

CONTENTS

PREFACE

Following on from the unprecedented success of *The Easy Guide to OSCEs for Final Year Medical Students,* which was commended in the BMA book competition 2008, we have been inundated with requests from medical students and doctors alike to continue the series. This second book, *The Easy Guide to OSCEs for Specialties,* has drawn from and built upon the strengths of its predecessor and applied it to the diverse nature of medical specialties.

Specialties are playing an increasing role in the medical curriculum following the introduction of the foundation year programme. Junior doctors are now expected to be competent in a wide range of different skills in medical fields including obstetrics, paediatrics, geriatrics, anaesthetics and palliative care. For this reason medical schools are now standardising OSCEs in specialties and making them an essential component for qualifying as a competent junior doctor. Amongst medical students, OSCEs in specialty subjects are notorious for being the most difficult to prepare for due to the lack of a book dedicated to the subject. We have written *The Easy Guide to OSCEs for Specialties* to fill this void and ease the already burdensome workload of medical students.

The Easy Guide to OSCEs for Specialties has been compiled by recently qualified doctors who have experienced the new OSCE system firsthand. Drawing on the success of the first book and taking into account feedback from students and doctors, this book has been written in a fresh style covering over 80 OSCE examination stations in a wide range of different subjects. We have maintained the style and approach of the first book, which was well embraced by medical students and examiners alike.

This book is unique in its own right, covering medical specialties including obstetrics, gynaecology, sexual health, paediatrics, dermatology, rheumatology, orthopaedics, emergency medicine, anaesthetics, geriatrics, patient discharge, palliative care, and the all important communication skills. We have inserted a larger number of time-saving, student-friendly mnemonics, more vivid diagrams and extra clinical conditions to aid the revision process. We have also added end-of-OSCE station case summaries to simulate the information a student would be expected to glean and present to the examiners under exam conditions.

This book, in conjunction with its companion, *The Easy Guide to OSCEs for Final Year Medical Students*, should provide a step-by-step guide to OSCE success. We hope that these books will provide essential reading for medical students of all years and in particular help those who are facing the daunting prospect of OSCE examinations.

Muhammed Akunjee
Syed Jalali
Shoaib Siddiqui
November 2008

End of year OSCE examinations for specialties prove to be a sticking point for a number of medical students. Not least due to the vast array of specialty subjects students need to read, digest and practise but also due to the lack of any single comprehensive text on the subject. *The Easy Guide to OSCEs for Specialties* with its innovative approach, well-researched material and breadth of knowledge provides the student with a firm foundation to tackle the often difficult OSCE scenarios head on.

In keeping with the approach of the popular *The Easy Guide to OSCEs for Final Year Medical Students*, this book maintains and improves on it in many ways. There are an increased number of vibrant illustrations, boxes of facts and differentials in addition to well thought out clinically relevant case summaries.

The book also deals in depth with a wide range of difficult communication skill stations giving students an excellent framework to approach such scenarios in full confidence both under exam conditions and in real life.

We are sure that this book will be rewarding for medical students and examiners alike. We believe that it is essential reading for any student wishing to excel in their exams.

Graham Boswell MBBS FRCP
Consultant Physician
Medical OSCEs and PACES Examiner
Trust Foundation Programme Director, Hywel Dpa Trust

Steve Riley MB BCh MRCP MD Dip Med Ed
Consultant Nephrologist and General Physician
University Hospital of Wales

November 2008

ACKNOWLEDGEMENTS

We would like to thank Jovad Ahmad, A&E staff grade, Brighton and Sussex University Hospitals and Faisal Goni, Foundation Year House Officer, London for their valuable advice and contributions to this work.

For each OSCE station we have defined a set of criteria which can be used when assessing oneself under examination conditions. The figures of 0, 1 and 2 indicate how many marks have been allocated for performing the task defined. Some criteria have been allocated two marks and this indicates that more than one task must be accomplished in those criteria to attain full marks. If only one task is completed then a score of 1 will be attained. A score of 0 is given if the task was omitted completely.

Some OSCE criteria have no marks allocated. This is to reflect that this is not a core competency skill, but that the inclusion of the task illustrates flair and higher achievement.

At the end of each OSCE station are five-point scales. The first indicates the examiner's mark for overall ability and the second five-point scale (in stations where role players are used) is for the role-player's overall assessment. A grade of 0 indicates an extremely poor performance, in which the candidate has not fulfilled any of the OSCE criteria, displayed poor communication skills and a lack of consideration for the role player's feelings. A grade of 3 indicates a fair performance, fulfilling most of the OSCE criteria and one of 5 is given to an exceptional candidate who has fulfilled the OSCE criteria and performed the tasks competently and with confidence.

Obstetrics

OBSTETRICS: **Obstetrics History**

INSTRUCTIONS: You are a foundation year House Officer in an antenatal clinic. Miss Newham has been referred to the GP for antenatal booking. Elicit a full obstetric history. You will be marked on your communication skills and your ability to take the history from the patient.

INTRODUCTION

0 1 2

☐☐☐ **Introduction** Introduce yourself appropriately and establish rapport.

☐☐☐ **Name & Age** Elicit the patient's name and age.

☐☐☐ **Occupation** Enquire about the patient's occupation.

HISTORY

☐☐☐ **Concerns** Elicit all the patient's presenting complaints. Use open questions and explore the patient's health beliefs. For each concern or complaint, elicit the patient's ideas, concerns and expectations.

'Good morning Miss Newham. Congratulations on your pregnancy. I hope everything is going well. How are you feeling today? Do you have any concerns about your pregnancy?'

☐☐☐ **History** For each complaint ascertain the time of onset, presenting features and associated symptoms. Explore each symptom systematically using appropriate mnemonics, e.g. SOCRATES (pain), ONE RESP (shortness of breath).

Questions to Ask in Vaginal Bleeding	
Onset	When did it first begin? How long did you bleed for?
Frequency	How often does it occur? Has it happened in the past? Has it stopped now?
Volume	Did you notice any spotting on your clothes? Did you have to use any tampons, pads or sanitary towels? Were your clothes soaked? Were there any clots?
Pain	Is it associated with any pain (constant, colicky)?
Cause	Common causes of vaginal bleeding:
Early (<24 wks)	Miscarriage, ectopic pregnancy, hydatidiform mole
Late (>24 wks)	(Antepartum haemorrhage) Placental abruption, placenta praevia, uterine rupture

CURRENT PREGNANCY HISTORY

☐☐☐ **Present Preg.** Enquire about the date of her last menstrual period (LMP). Establish the patient's certainty of the date, the regularity of her cycle and the typical cycle length prior to her LMP. Enquire about previous contraceptive use.

Symptoms Note for symptoms of pregnancy including morning sickness, indigestion, urinary frequency and breast tenderness.

☐☐☐ **Gestation** Calculate the number of weeks that the patient is pregnant and the estimated date of delivery. Ask the examiner for an obstetric wheel or use the formula below.

Calculating Estimated Date of Delivery
EDD = LMP – 3 months + 1 year and 7 days + [cycle length – 28]

Complications Ask if there have been any problems with this pregnancy, such as bleeding, spotting, or pain, or whether she is concerned about her blood pressure, her sugar levels or the baby's development. Has she had any recent urine infections or is she known to be anaemic?

☐☐☐ **Tests** Enquire about the tests the patient may have had performed, including ultrasound scans (dating scan, anomaly scan or further scans for complications), Down's syndrome screening (blood test and nuchal scan), chorionic villus sampling and amniocentesis.

Pregnancy screening timeline

Screening tests for pregnant women in chronological order

Down's syndrome blood tests

Chorionic villus sampling

Amniocentesis

Blood test for alpha-FP for NTD

No. of weeks

0 2 4 6 8 10 12 14 16 18 20 22 24 26 28 30 32 34 36 38 40

Ultrasound dating scan

Nuchal translucency scan

Ultrasound anomaly scan

Third trimester ultrasound scan for complications

PAST OBSTETRIC HISTORY

☐☐☐ **Previous Preg.**

Ask the patient if this is her first pregnancy or if she has been pregnant before. If she was pregnant before, ask how many times she has been pregnant and whether she has had any miscarriages, stillbirths or terminations. Enquire about the gestations of previous pregnancies and the mode of delivery, i.e. was it spontaneous or induced, per vaginal (ventouse/forceps) or Caesarean section. If by Caesarean, ascertain the reason for this and whether it was an emergency or an elective procedure. Establish the birth weights of each child and whether there were any complications during the pregnancy or during delivery.

Common Obstetric Definitions

Gravidity	The number of pregnancies in total including any miscarriages or pregnancies lost before 24 weeks
Parity	This is the number of potentially viable pregnancies beyond 24 weeks delivered not including the current pregnancy
Para 3	Three term deliveries
Para 2+1	Two term pregnancies and a miscarriage at 20 weeks
Multiparous	Delivered live or potentially viable babies >24 weeks gestation
Nulliparous	Never delivered a live or potentially viable baby >24 weeks gestation

Rhesus

Enquire about the patient's Rhesus status and whether she has received any Rhesus antibody injections.

Causes of Abdominal Pain during Pregnancy

First Trimester	Ectopic pregnancy (amenorrhoea, colicky and shoulder tip pain)
	Miscarriage (passage of products of conception, uterus normal size)
Second Trimester	Miscarriage
Third Trimester	Labour (contractions between 5–10 min, water breaks)
	False labour (irregular non-persistent contractions)
	Pre-term labour (labour <37 weeks)
	Placental abruption (dark painful blood, woody hard uterus)
	Uterine rupture (scarred uterus)

Other Causes	Appendicitis, cholecystitis, GORD, urinary tract infection (UTI), gastroenteritis
Mnemonic:	**'LARACROFT'**
	Labour, **A**bruption of placenta, **R**upture (ectopic, uterus), **A**bortion, **C**holestatis, **R**ectus sheath haematoma, **O**varian tumour, **F**ibroids, **T**orsion of uterus

ASSOCIATED HISTORY

Gynae. History   Ask about the date and results of her last smear test (if indicated).

□□□ **Medical History**   Has she had any operations or been admitted to hospital in the past? Does she suffer from any medical problems including hypertension, diabetes, epilepsy, DVT or jaundice? Enquire specifically about thalassaemia or sickle cell anaemia.

□□□ **Drug History**   Is she taking any regular medication, prescribed or over-the-counter? Is she taking folic acid supplements and when did she start? (These should be started 3 months prior to conception and continued for 3 months into pregnancy). Does she have any allergies?

Family History   Is there any history of diabetes, high blood pressure or pregnancy-induced hypertension? Are there any congenital illnesses that run in the family? Is there any history of twin births in the family?

□□□ **Social History**   Does she smoke or drink alcohol? Has she ever taken any recreational drug? What type of accommodation does she live in and is anyone at home with her? Is she in a stable relationship? Will there be any help at home with the baby after delivery?

CLOSING

□□□ **Rapport**   Establish and maintain rapport and demonstrate listening skills.

□□□ **Summarise**   Check with patient and deliver an appropriate summary.

'This is Miss Newham, a 23-year old nulliparous woman who is currently 16 weeks pregnant. She is gravidum 2, parity 0 + 1 due to a previous termination of pregnancy at 12 weeks. She is currently happy with her pregnancy with no concerns and has been taking folic acid supplements up until 3 months gestation. She suffers from no relevant medical illnesses or any allergies and is in a stable relationship with her boyfriend. She has no concerns but would like to know how many times she should visit the doctor and midwife.'

EXAMINER'S EVALUATION

0 1 2 3 4 5

☐ ☐ ☐ ☐ ☐ ☐ Overall assessment of taking an obstetric history

☐ ☐ ☐ ☐ ☐ ☐ Role player's score

Total mark out of 26

DIFFERENTIAL DIAGNOSIS

Miscarriages

A miscarriage, or spontaneous abortion, is defined as the loss of a foetus before 24 weeks of gestation. A loss of pregnancy after 24 weeks is considered a stillbirth. Up to 30% of all pregnancies miscarry, with 80% occurring in the first trimester of pregnancy. The frequency of miscarriage decreases with increasing gestational age. It is classified into threatened, inevitable, septic, incomplete, complete and missed miscarriages. Chromosomal abnormalities account for 50% of all spontaneous abortions. Other causes include polycystic ovaries, high BP, diabetes, fibroids, SLE, obesity, caffeine, cocaine and cigarette smoking. Recurrent miscarriage is described as the loss of three or more pregnancies in succession. It affects approximately 1% of all couples and warrants further investigation. Symptoms of a spontaneous abortion include a history of vaginal bleeding with blood clots and severe suprapubic abdominal pain. Vaginal bleeding may be so great as to soak tampons, pads, sanitary towels or even clothes. Contractions and abdominal pain may coexist but tend to resolve in a complete abortion. This is associated with the passage of products of conception and a cessation of vaginal bleeding. A concurrent fever, chills, raised white cell count or peritonitis may suggest a septic abortion and require antibiotics. On examination of a complete miscarriage, the abdomen is soft and the uterus is either normal or small for the dates. A pelvic examination will reveal a closed cervical os with a non-tender cervix and adnexal masses.

Classifications of Miscarriage	
Threatened	Bleeding during pregnancy with a risk of miscarriage. The foetus is alive and uterus normal for dates. Cervical os remains closed. Minor bleeding and pain noted
Inevitable	Foetus may still be alive but is yet to be expelled. Miscarriage is eminent. Bleeding is heavy with significant pain. Cervical os is open
Incomplete	Foetal parts have passed but some remain in utero. Cervical os is open with small-for-date uterus

Complete	Products of conception have been expelled. Bleeding and pain has decreased. Cervical os is closed and uterus has returned to normal size
Septic	Uterine contents become infected causing endometritis. An offensive brownish discharge is noted with a tender bulky uterus. Patient is febrile with abdominal pain
Missed	Foetus has died in utero, but a miscarriage has not yet occurred. The uterus is small for dates with no heart sounds and the cervical os is closed

Ectopic Pregnancy

The term 'ectopic' originates from the Greek word *ektopos*, meaning 'out of place'. It is defined as the implantation of the embryo outside the uterine cavity. It complicates 1% of all pregnancies and represents a major cause of maternal mortality. Risk factors include previous ectopic pregnancies, PID, salpingitis, tubal surgery, intra-uterine device (IUD) and assisted conception. The most common site for implantation is the inside lining of a fallopian tube (97%). Other sites include the cornu, cervix, ovary and peritoneum. As the trophoblast invades and destabilises the thin lining of the fallopian tube, it haemorrhages into the lumen and expels the implantation, resulting in a tubal abortion. If the tube ruptures, it can lead to a massive loss of blood with loss of the patient's life. In unruptured cases the embryo may be shed or absorbed and converted into a tubal mole. An ectopic pregnancy should always be suspected in a sexually active woman who presents with bleeding or abdominal pain. Clinical features include an absence of periods (amenorrhoea) for 4–10 weeks, a sudden onset of colicky lower abdominal pain (later becoming constant) and scanty dark vaginal blood. Intraperitoneal haemorrhage is heralded by syncopal collapse and shoulder-tip pain. On palpation, the patient is found to have a tender abdomen and an enlarged uterus with a closed cervical os. A pelvic examination reveals cervical excitation on movement and a tender adnexal mass.

Placenta Praevia

This is when the placenta implants in the lower segment of the uterus; occurring in approximately one out of two hundred pregnancies. It is usually more common in women who are multiparous, of increasing age and with uterine scarring following previous Caesarean sections. Most cases are discovered on routine ultrasound examination as a 'low lying placenta', but a significant minority present with severe PV haemorrhage. Placenta praevia is classified according to the relationship of the placenta with the internal os. A marginal praevia is when the placenta is near or adjacent to the cervical os. However, if the placenta partially or completely obscures the internal os this is known as major praevia. Such patients present with painless, bright red antepartum haemorrhage that increases in frequency and intensity over a number of weeks. The foetus may present with a transverse lie and breech presentation. A digital vaginal examination must not be performed in case massive bleeding is initiated.

Placental Abruption

This complicates 1% of pregnancies and occurs when part of or the entire placenta separates from the uterine wall before delivery causing significant bleeding. Blood can track its way down the myometrium and presents as a dark, painful antepartum haemorrhage. However, in 20% of cases, visible vaginal blood is absent, known as concealed abruption. On examination, the uterus is found to be tender and contracted, and in severe cases it may be woody and hard. The foetus may be difficult to palpate and foetal monitoring may show signs of compromise. There are a number of risk factors that predispose to abruption, including:

Risk Factors for Placental Abruption	
Mnemonic: PIPES	
Pre-eclampsia	**E**ssential hypertension
Intra-uterine growth restriction	**S**moking
Previous history of abruption	

INSTRUCTIONS: You are meeting Mrs Foster for the first time. She is G4 P1 and is now 37 weeks pregnant. She has had her booking bloods and 20 week ultrasound scan, all of which have been normal. Please carry out an obstetric examination upon the patient and present your findings to the examiner as you go along.

NOTE: In the OSCE setting you may be provided with a dummy instead of a real patient. Ensure that you treat it with the same courtesy and respect as you would a real patient.

EXAMINATION

0 1 2

☐ ☐ ☐ **Introduction**   Introduce yourself. Elicit her name, age and occupation. Establish rapport.

History   Ask her whether she feels any foetal movements. Enquire about when they first started, their frequency and how many times a day she feels them, and whether they have changed in quality and quantity.

Consent   Explain the examination to the patient and seek her consent.

☐ ☐ ☐ **Chaperone**   Inform the patient that you may obtain a chaperone.

Position   Ask the patient to lie flat on the couch. Ensure she is comfortable and expose her abdomen from the xiphisternum to the symphysis.

INSPECTION

☐ ☐ ☐ **General**   Stand and observe the patient from the edge of the bed. Look for signs consistent with pregnancy, scars, skin changes and foetal movements.

Signs to Observe in the Obstetric Examination	
Symmetry	Symmetrical/asymmetrical abdominal distension
Scars	Pfannenstiel scar (low transverse scar from a previous C-section)
	Laparoscopic scar
Skin Changes	Linea nigra (dark pigmented line from xiphisternum to the suprapubic region), striae gravidarum (purplish stretch marks denoting current parity), striae albicans (silver whitish striae denoting previous parity)
Umbilicus	Flattening, eversion (polyhydramnios, multiple pregnancy)
Movements	Foetal movements (occurring after 24 weeks of pregnancy)

PALPATION

□□□ **General**

Enquire about pain before beginning the examination. Gently but firmly palpate the mother's abdomen. Note the uterine size, symphysio-fundal height, liquor volume, foetal movements, lie, presentation and uterine contractions.

□□□ **Uterine Size**

Attempt to palpate the uterus and gauge its size. The uterus is palpable between weeks 12 and 14 and is level with the umbilicus by week 20. By week 36 the uterus is at the level of the xiphisternum.

Amniotic Fluid

Estimate the liquor volume, noting for excessive amounts of fluid (polyhydraminos – gestational diabetes, foetal abnormality, idiopathic), reduced volume (oligohydramnios) or normal volume. Easily palpable foetal parts suggest reduced volume, while difficulty in palpation indicates increased volume.

□□□ **SFH**

Establish the fundus of the uterus before measuring the symphysio-fundal height (SFH). Use the ulnar border of your left hand to find the fundus by repeatedly pressing on the abdomen from the xiphisternum downwards, until firmness is felt. Once the upper limit is established, place a tape measure, blind side up, measuring the distance from the fundus to the pubic symphysis. Turn the tape measure around to reveal the SFH in centimetres.

SFH Proportional to Gestational Age

The SFH provides an approximation of the gestational age in weeks. It is measured in centimetres from the symphysis pubis to the fundus. The margin of error increases with weeks of gestation

Weeks of gestation	Margin of error
20–36 weeks	+/– 2 cm
36–40 weeks	+/– 3 cm
>40 weeks	+/– 4 cm

36 weeks
28 weeks
20 weeks
12 weeks

Uterine size

Fundus is palpable from 12–14th week
Uterus at level of umbilicus at 20th week
Uterus at level of the xiphisternum at 36th week

SFH (Symphysio-fundal height)

From week 20 the fundal height increases by 1cm / week and the SFH in cm approximates to the number of gestational weeks (up to week 36)

Foetuses

Determine the number of foetuses present. Palpation of two foetal heads, a large uterus compared with gestation and auscultation of two separate foetal heartbeats with a variance of 10 bpm suggests the presence of multiple pregnancies.

☐☐☐ **Lie**

Palpate the foetal lie by facing the mother and placing one hand on either side of the uterus. Gently palpate down towards the pelvis. Determine the position of the foetus's back and limbs in order to ascertain its lie. Describe the lie as longitudinal, oblique or transverse in relation to the longitudinal axis of the uterus.

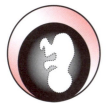
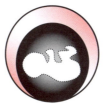
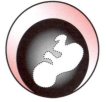

Longitudinal lie
Buttock and head palpable
at opposite ends

Transverse lie
Pelvic inlet remains empty.
Foetal hand maybe
palpable in the flank

Oblique lie
Head or buttock felt in the
iliac fossa

☐☐☐ **Presentation**

Turn and face the mother's feet. Firmly press above the symphysis pubis to determine the presentation. The presentation is the part of the foetus that presents first in relation to the pelvic inlet. Note if it is a cephalic (harder, rounder object on palpation) or breech (broader, softer object) presentation.

☐☐☐ **Engagement**

Engagement represents the amount of foetal head that has entered into the pelvis and is described in fifths of head palpable. It normally occurs after 37 weeks of gestation. It is an approximation of how many finger breadths of the head is palpable above the pelvic inlet. A foetal head that is more than 50% entered into the pelvic brim has only 2/5 of its surface area palpable

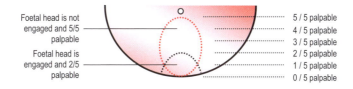

Foetal head is not engaged and 5/5 palpable
Foetal head is engaged and 2/5 palpable

5 / 5 palpable
4 / 5 palpable
3 / 5 palpable
2 / 5 palpable
1 / 5 palpable
0 / 5 palpable

Degree of engagement of the foetal head

abdominally and is engaged. If the foetal head is palpable by three or more finger breadths (i.e. less than 50% of the head has entered the pelvic inlet), it is not engaged.

AUSCULTATION

☐☐☐ **Heartbeat**

Locate the anterior shoulder of the foetus and use a Pinard's stethoscope or sonicaid to listen for a heartbeat. If using the sonicaid, use ultrasound gel and wipe it off afterwards. Note the foetal heartbeat (normal between 110–160).

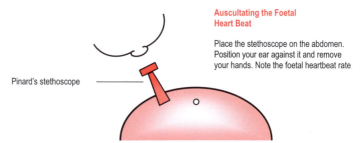

Auscultating the Foetal Heart Beat

Place the stethoscope on the abdomen. Position your ear against it and remove your hands. Note the foetal heartbeat rate

Pinard's stethoscope

CLOSING

☐☐☐ **Oedema**

Check for the presence of ankle or sacral oedema.

☐☐☐ **BP**

Offer to check the mother's blood pressure (pre-eclampsia).

☐☐☐ **Urine**

Offer to check urine for proteinuria (pre-eclampsia) and glucose (gestational diabetes).

Cover

Replace the woman's clothing.

☐☐☐ **Summarise**

Thank the mother. Answer any questions and summarise your findings.

'This is Mrs Foster who is currently 37 weeks pregnant. Her abdomen is consistent with a single uterine pregnancy and her SFH is 36 cm. The foetus is in longitudinal lie and is cephalic in presentation. The head is 5/5 palpable and not engaged. On sonicaid auscultation, the foetal heartbeat is 140 per minute with normal variation.'

EXAMINER'S EVALUATION

0 1 2 3 4 5

☐☐☐☐☐☐ Overall assessment of obstetric examination

Total mark out of 22

DIFFERENTIAL DIAGNOSIS
Abnormal Lie

The foetal lie describes the position of the baby in relation to the longitudinal axis of the uterus. The foetus can be described as having a longitudinal, transverse or oblique lie. If the foetus is in a longitudinal lie, it can either be a breech or cephalic (head palpable in the pelvic inlet) presentation. In the oblique position the foetus's head or buttock can be palpable in either iliac fossa. In the transverse lie, the baby lies across the uterus with the head palpable in the flank and the pelvic inlet remaining empty. An abnormal lie is considered to be any position held by the foetus that is not parallel to the long axis of the uterus. Before 36 weeks an abnormal lie is common and is not predictive of the lie or presentation at the time of labour. On the other hand, an abnormal lie after 36 weeks is more likely to persist at the time of labour. It occurs in 0.5% of all pregnancies and is associated with pre-term labour, multiparity, multiple pregnancies (twins), polyhydramnios and placenta praevia. An abnormal lie is regard as safe before 37 weeks with the baby able to spontaneously progress to a longitudinal lie before labour. Beyond 37 weeks, an ultrasound should be carried out with a view to performing a Caesarean section.

Breech Presentation

The presentation is the part of the foetus that occupies the pelvic inlet. It can be either a cephalic or breech. A cephalic presentation is when the head is presented in the pelvic inlet, while a breech presentation is when the buttock is palpated instead, and the head is noted at the fundus. The incidence of breech presentations dramatically reduces through pregnancy with up to 40% at week 20, falling to 3% at term. It is associated with pre-term labour, multiple pregnancy, fibroids, placenta praevia, polyhydramnios and oligohydramnios. It is categorised as extended (baby's legs extended at the knees and flexed at the hip), flexed (flexed at the knees and hips) or footling (one or both feet found below the level of the buttocks). A breech presentation is only of concern after 37 weeks of gestation. An attempt at external cephalic version may be performed before considering a Caesarean.

Polyhydramnios

The amniotic fluid or liquor bathes the foetus in fluid, cushions it from trauma and promotes lung growth and development. The volume of fluid increases with gestational age, reaching a maximal volume of 1 litre by 34 to 38 weeks of gestation. Polyhydramnios occurs when the amniotic fluid exceeds 2–3 litres. It can be due to impaired swallowing by the foetus or a blockage of the foetus's gastrointestinal tract. There is a strong association with congenital abnormalities such as oesophageal or duodenal atresia, Hirschsprung's disease, anencephaly, spina bifida, and trisomy 21. Other causes include Type 2 maternal diabetes mellitus, multiple pregnancies and macrosomia. Polyhydramnios predisposes to pre-term labour, placental abruption and malpresentation. On examination, the uterus is found to be oversized for the expected dates.

Oligohydramnios

Oligohydramnios is suggested when the amniotic fluid volume is less than 500 mL at 34 weeks of gestation. It can be caused by the inability of the foetus to contribute to the amniotic fluid and produce urine (renal dysgenesis, polycystic kidneys, Potter's syndrome) or a rupture of the amniotic membranes. It can result in the poor development of foetal lung tissue. On examination, the uterus appears to be small for dates with discrepancies in serial fundal height measurements. The foetal parts are also easily palpated through the mother's abdomen.

Multiple Pregnancies

Twins occur in 1 out of 105 pregnancies with triplets occurring once in every 10 000 pregnancies. Predisposing factors include a family history of twins, an increase in maternal age, multiparity, in-vitro fertilisation and induced ovulation. Perinatal mortality increases with multiple pregnancies by a factor of four compared to singleton pregnancies. This can be explained by a higher incidence of miscarriage, pre-term delivery, intra-uterine growth retardation, congenital malformations and malpresentation. On examination, the uterus can be felt to be larger than expected for dates. There may be evidence of polyhydramnios with more than two foetal poles and multiple foetal parts palpable. On auscultation, two distinct foetal heart rates can be heard with a difference of 10 bpm between rates. The diagnosis can be confirmed on ultrasound.

INSTRUCTIONS: Mrs Tomlinson, a 48-year-old woman, is concerned about an abnormality in her breast. Take an appropriate history and carry out a full examination of her breasts. The examiner will ask you for your findings and your interpretation of them.

HISTORY

0 1 2

☐☐☐ **Introduction**	Introduce yourself. Elicit the patient's name, age and occupation. Establish rapport.

★ History of Presenting Complaint

☐☐☐ **Lump**	When and how did you first notice the lump? Has the lump changed in size since then? How many lumps have you noticed? Are the lumps only in one breast or are they in both breasts?
☐☐☐ **Pain**	Is there any pain or tenderness in your breasts (mastalgia)? When did it begin? Is it in only one breast or both? Is it continuous or intermittent? Does anything make the pain better or worse? How severe is the pain? What impact does it have on your life?
☐☐☐ **Discharge**	Is there any discharge from the nipples? Is it from one or both nipples? How much discharge is there? What colour is the discharge (clear, milky, yellow, green, bloody)? Does the discharge come out spontaneously or only on expression?
☐☐☐ **Cyclicity**	Are your symptoms associated with your menstrual cycle?

ASSOCIATED HISTORY

☐☐☐ **Medical History**	Have you previously had any breast disease? Have you had any previous investigations of your breasts (e.g. ultrasound, mammography, biopsy)?
☐☐☐ **Menstrual Hx.**	When was your last period (LMP)? Are they regular? Are they painful? At what age did you start menstruating? At what age was your menopause?

Obstetric Hx.	Do you have any children? How many children do you have? Did you breast-feed your children? Are you pregnant?
□□□ **Drug History**	Are you taking or have you previously taken the oral contraceptive pill or hormone replacement therapy?
□□□ **Family History**	Has anyone in your family suffered from breast disease (parents, grandparents, siblings, children)?
Social History	Do you smoke cigarettes or drink alcohol?
Concerns	Do you have any idea as to what the problem may be? Are you worried that it may be anything in particular?

EXAMINATION

Consent

Explain the examination to the patient and seek her consent.

'You have told me a lot about your breast problem. I would like now to examine your breasts to try and find out what is going on. This will involve undressing to your waist. Are you happy to proceed?'

□□□ **Chaperone**

Inform the patient that you will obtain a chaperone.

Expose

Ask the patient to undress to her waist so that her breasts are adequately exposed. Provide the patient with a blanket to cover herself.

★ Inspection

□□□ **General**

Inspect the breasts with the patient's arms by her side (not elevated). Look for any obvious lumps, skin changes, nipple changes and discharge. Also note any signs of previous surgery or radiotherapy to the breasts (e.g. scars, radiation marks).

Signs to Observe in the Breast Examination

Breast Symmetry	Symmetrical (same level)/asymmetrical
Contour	Shape deformity
Swellings	Breast lumps
Skin Changes:	
Discolouration	Erythema
Puckering	Fixation/tethering of breast lump to overlying skin
Peau d'orange	Orange peel appearance (breast carcinoma)
Scars	Breast augmentation/reduction surgery, previous surgery
Nipple Changes:	
Eczema around Nipple	Paget's disease

Nipple Discharge	Look for discharge on the patient's nipple or on clothes
Retraction/inversion	Nipple facing down and in rather than down and out (carcinoma)

Inspect the breasts with the patient's arms elevated and placed on her head. Look for any indentation or tethering of any swellings (malignancy) and for asymmetrical contour of the breast. Repeat the inspection but with the patient's hands pressed firmly on her hips.

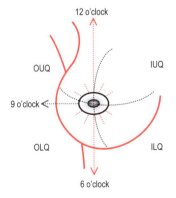

Breast Examination

Inspect the breasts with the patient's arms by her sides, hands placed behind her head and finally against her hips

Next, inspect the axillae for any swellings (enlarged lymph nodes) or the presence of any scars.

★ Palpation

□□□ **Position**

Lie the patient at an angle of 45 degrees. Enquire whether there is any tenderness and ask the patient to point to any lumps that she may have noticed. Start palpation on the side that is normal. Ask the patient to place her ipsilateral hand behind her head.

□□□ **Technique**

Palpate all four quadrants of the breast using the flat of the fingers of one hand, use the other hand to steady the breast. Use a rotary movement of the

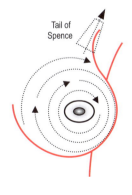

Breast Quadrants

IUQ	– Inner upper quadrant
OUQ	– Outer upper quadrant
ILQ	– Inner lower quadrant
OLQ	– Outer lower quadrant

Breast Examination technique

Palpate the breast using an outwardly spiralling technique. Note any lumps and describe their position in relation to the areola, e.g. 2 o'clock position

fingers when palpating and gently compress the breast tissue against the chest wall to feel for the presence of any lumps. Examine the breast in a concentric ring starting from the nipple and working outwards. Examine the whole breast including its borders and then palpate the tail of Spence with the thumb and the forefinger.

☐☐☐ **Lump**

If a lump is present note any tenderness and establish the site, size, shape, surface, edge and consistency of the lump as well as the colour and temperature of the overlying skin (compare with the surrounding skin). Determine if the lump is fixed or tethered to the overlying skin and to the underlying structures.

Describing a Lump in the Breast

Site	Right/left breast, upper/lower, inner/outer quadrant
Size	Measure dimensions using a ruler
Shape	Circular/irregular
Surface	Smooth/rough
Edge	Well-circumscribed/ill-defined/irregular
Consistency	Firm/rubbery/stony hard/spongy/soft
Temperature	Hot/normal
Mobility	*Move the lump up and down and side to side:* mobile/fixed/tethered

Nipple

Ask the patient to squeeze the nipples to express any discharge. Note the colour of any discharge and then smear and swab for cytology and microbiology.

Types of Discharge from the Nipple

Colour of Discharge	Diagnosis
White	Lactation
Yellow (exudate)	Fibroadenosis, abscess
Green (cellular debris)	Fibroadenosis, duct ectasia
Red (blood)	Duct carcinoma, duct papilloma

☐☐☐ **Lymph Nodes**

Rest the patient's left elbow in your left hand, taking the weight of her forearm. With your right hand, palpate for enlarged lymph nodes in the anterior, posterior, lateral, medial and apical regions of the left axilla. Also feel along the medial aspect of the humerus for enlarged lymph nodes. Repeat the process on the other side. Now palpate both supraclavicular fossae for lymphadenopathy.

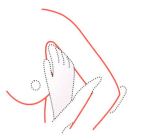

Rest the patient's elbow in your hand while examining the axilla with your spare hand. Note for enlarged lymph nodes

Differential Diagnoses for Breast Lumps

Traumatic	*Fat necrosis*	Hard irregular lump with history of trauma
Infective	*Pyogenic abscess*	Tender lump with pus collecting in the abscess caused by bacterial infection
Physiological	*Fibroadenosis*	Fibrocystic change. Peak incidence above 35 years old
Neoplastic	*Fibroadenoma*	Benign tumour occurring in women below 35 years old
	Carcinoma	Malignant (primary/secondary)
	Phylloides tumour	Rare fibroepithelial tumour
	Duct papilloma	Benign proliferation of epithelium in major ducts with bloody discharge in single nipple and swelling lateral to the areola

☐☐☐ **Repeat**   Repeat the above examination on the other breast.

☐☐☐ **Liver & Lungs**   Palpate the liver edge and the spine for any tenderness and auscultate the lungs.

☐☐☐ **Triple Ax.**   Mention to the examiner that for any detectable breast lump, you would refer the patient for triple assessment.

Components of Triple Assessment

1 Medical history and clinical breast examination
2 Imaging: mammography (<35 yrs) or ultrasound (>35 yrs)
3 Biopsy (fine needle aspiration, cytology and/or core biopsy histology)

☐☐☐ **Summarise**   Thank the patient and cover her. Answer any questions and summarise your findings.

'This is Mrs Tomlinson, a 48-year-old woman who has recently noticed a unilateral right-sided breast lump. There is no pain or discharge. She was previously well and is still having regular periods. She is nulliparous and has never breast-fed. Of note she has taken the oral contraceptive pill for

10 years. There is no family history of breast disease. On examination, there is a 3 cm by 2 cm irregular-shaped nodularity in the 2 o'clock position of the right breast. There is overlying skin tethering with no skin discolouration. There is no associated axillary lymphadenopathy. I would like to refer this patient for urgent triple assessment to exclude potential malignancy.'

EXAMINER'S EVALUATION

0 1 2 3 4 5

☐ ☐ ☐ ☐ ☐ ☐ Overall assessment of breast examination

☐ ☐ ☐ ☐ ☐ ☐ Role player's score

Total mark out of 35

DIFFERENTIAL DIAGNOSIS

Breast Carcinoma

Breast cancer is the most prevalent cancer among women and accounts for one-third of all female cancers in the UK. Risk factors which could lead to the early development of breast cancer include nulliparity, first pregnancy after the age of 30, early menarche, late menopause, hormone replacement therapy (especially when combined), obesity, BRCA genes (family history), not breast-feeding, previous breast cancer and taking the oral contraceptive pill. The age of onset for breast cancer is usually above the age of 35. The characteristics of breast carcinomas are firm, irregular masses that are rarely painful but are often tethered or fixed to the skin. Accompanying features include nipple changes, localised oedema, lymphadenopathy, bloody discharge and symptoms that correlate with metastatic disease (breathlessness, backache, jaundice, malaise and weight loss). It is not uncommon to find a positive family history of breast cancer.

Risk Factors of Breast Cancer	
Mnemonic: 'risk can be assessed by History ALONE'	
History (FH – BRCA genes, PMH), **H**RT	**O**besity, **O**CP
Abortion, **A**ge (>30 yrs)	**N**ulliparity
Late menopause, **L**ack of breast-feeding	**E**arly menarche

Fibroadenoma

Fibroadenomas are the most common benign tumours of the female breast and arise from an overgrowth of fibrous and glandular tissues. They develop at any age but are more common in young women (25–35 years old) and are often mistaken for cancer. Fibroadenomas are rarely painful in nature but may be bilateral and multiple in number. They are smooth in surface, well-circumscribed and rubbery hard in consistency. They are usually small (1–3 cm in size), highly mobile (unlike breast carcinomas) and can occur in any part of the breast. Due to its highly mobile nature it is sometimes termed 'breast mouse'.

Fibroadenosis

Fibroadenosis or fibrocystic disease is the most common cause of breast lumps in women of reproductive age. Their peak incidence is in women between 35 and 50 years of age. They are rare in women younger than 25. Patients usually present with single or multiple lumps in the upper outer quadrant of the breast and associated cyclical breast pain that is greatest premenstrually. The lumps are often smooth and rubbery-firm in texture and are usually bilateral in distribution. Sometimes there is nipple discharge that is clear, white or green in colour.

Fat Necrosis

Fat necrosis is a painless hard irregular-shaped lump that forms in an area of fatty breast tissue that has been exposed to trauma or previous surgery. Due to associated skin and nipple changes, including nipple retraction, dimpling of the skin and tethering, it can often be indistinguishable from breast carcinoma.

Breast Abscess

Breast abscesses usually occur in women of child-bearing age between 18 and 50 years old. They are most often associated with breast-feeding due to the infiltration of trauma-permitting organisms (commonly *Staphylococcus aureus*) that cause an infection and generate an abscess. Associated symptoms include a tender, hot, spherical lump in the breast with erythema and localised oedema and a pus-coloured discharge from the nipple.

Intraductal Papillomas

Intraductal papillomas are benign proliferations of duct epithelial cells within lactiferous ducts, which commonly affect premenopausal women. The patient may notice a small painful lump located near or just behind the areola with a bloodstained discharge from the nipple. It is commonly solitary in nature but multiple swellings in contiguous branches of a ductal system may rarely occur.

Phylloides Tumour

A phylloides tumour (derived from the Greek word for leaf) is a rare fibroepithelial tumour composed of epithelial and stromal elements that arises from the periductal stroma of the breast. They can be classified as benign, borderline or malignant depending on their histology and are commonly confused with fibroadenomas. They occur between the ages of 30 to 50 years and are more common in Latin American and Asian women. They are typically painless, large, bulky, fast-growing masses that are firm, smooth and mobile on palpation.

OBSTETRICS: Urine Dipstick and Blood Pressure

INTRODUCTION

0 1 2

□ □ □ **Introduction** — Introduce yourself. Elicit the patient's name and age. Establish rapport.

DIPSTICK URINALYSIS

★ Explanation

□ □ □ **Fresh Sample** — Explain the importance of providing a fresh sample in the sterile container provided. Generally the urine sample should be no more than 4 hours old.

□ □ □ **Cleaning** — Explain the need to clean the genitalia thoroughly with soap before providing a sample.

□ □ □ **Mid-stream** — Explain to the patient how to deliver a mid-stream urine specimen and the importance of this.

'We need you to provide us with a fresh specimen of urine in this sterile container. So that we do not get any misleading results, it is important for you to clean and wash the area down below well, before taking the sample. Take the specimen bottle and sit as far back on the toilet seat as possible. Start to pass urine for a few seconds and when you are about halfway through, place the pot into the stream of urine and collect enough without overfilling it. Once you have done this please return the bottle to me.'

★ Testing the Urine

□ □ □ **Wear Gloves** — Wash hands and wear a pair of non-sterile gloves.

□ □ □ **Test Strip** — Check the expiry date of the Multistix box and then remove a single testing strip, closing the lid immediately after doing so.

□ □ □ **Dip** — Note the colour (cloudy/debris) and odour (pear drops – ketones, fishy – infection) of the urine. Place the whole stick in the urine for 1 second, ensuring that all testing areas are covered. Tap away any excess urine and hold the strip horizontally.

| | Read the stick correctly after 60 seconds or for the length of time indicated by the box.

□□□ **Results**

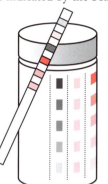

Dipstick Urine

Remove a testing stick, and dip within the urine sample for 1 second. Tap away excess and hold horizontally. Wait 60 seconds before interpretation

□□□ **Disposal**

Dispose of the soiled material and gloves in the yellow bag.

✷ Closing

□□□ **Explain**

Appropriately explain the findings to the patient.

Urine Dipstick Protein Analysis

Trace	Seldom significant
+	Proteinuria may be significant
++ or more	This is significant proteinuria and requires quantification with 24 hours collection

□□□ **Laboratory**

Mild proteinuria may be the result of a urinary tract infection. Even in the absence of nitrates or blood, request to send the specimen to the laboratory to confirm the presence of bacteria.

Check

Confirm that the patient has understood what you have told her.

'I dipsticked your urine and found some protein (+1). Often this may be simply the result of a urinary tract infection and hence I will be sending a sample to the laboratory to confirm this. However, on occasions, in pregnancy this may be due to raised blood pressure. Therefore I would now like to check your blood pressure to make sure it is stable.'

BLOOD PRESSURE

NOTE: It is important to select the appropriate cuff size to determine the patient's blood pressure. Cuffs that are too large for the patient's arm may result in a blood pressure that is lower than expected whilst cuffs that are too small may give a falsely elevated reading. The cuff bladder should have a width equal to at least 40% of the upper arm circumference.

☐☐☐ **Explain**	'Before I check your blood pressure, please could you sit up straight and remove your jumper. I will place a blood pressure cuff around your arm and inflate the cuff. This may feel a little uncomfortable. I will then place my stethoscope on your arm and take your pressure.'
☐☐☐ **Confirm**	Check that the patient has rested for at least 5 minutes.

★ Procedure

☐☐☐ **Cuff**	Choose the appropriate cuff size for the patient.
BP Machine	Check that the cuff is fully deflated and attached correctly.
☐☐☐ **Position**	Correctly position the patient with her arm horizontal and fully extended. Place the BP machine approximately in line with the level of the heart.
☐☐☐ **Placement**	Palpate the brachial artery and place the BP cuff neatly and securely around the arm above the antecubital fossa.
☐☐☐ **Check**	Check the approximate systolic level by palpating the radial or brachial artery once the cuff is inflated.
☐☐☐ **Procedure**	Auscultate over the brachial artery in the antecubital fossa and deflate the cuff slowly by 2–3 mmHg per second, watching the BP reading closely. Confirm the patient's systolic pressure by noting the pressure when the first audible Korotkoff sound can be

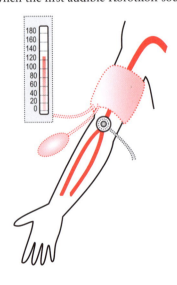

Measuring Blood Pressure

Choose the appropriate sized cuff. Feel for the brachial artery before placing the cuff around the arm. Listen with the stethoscope over the brachial artery while gradually deflating the cuff watching the BP closely

heard. Note the diastolic pressure by the muffling or disappearance of the Korotkoff sound.

☐☐☐ **Repeat**   Take at least two BP measurements.

☐☐☐ **Accuracy**   Ensure that the BP reading is measured to within 2 mmHg of the correct value.

    ★ **Closing**

☐☐☐☐ **Interpreting**   Pre-eclampsia is diagnosed with a blood pressure reading of >140/90 and a 24-hour urinary protein of >0.3 g.

Indication for Hospital Admission

Symptoms	Signs
Headaches	Proteinuria of 1+ or >0.3 g/24 hrs
Blurred vision	Diastolic blood pressure >100 mmHg
Epigastric pain	Suspected foetal compromise

    Concerns   Deal with the patient's concerns appropriately and allay any fears.

☐☐☐☐ **Documents**   Ask for the patient's notes to document the BP reading.

    Questions   Thank the patient and ask if she has any questions.

EXAMINER'S EVALUATION

0   1   2   3   4   5

☐☐☐☐☐☐   Overall assessment of dipstick and BP check

Total mark out of 30

DIFFERENTIAL DIAGNOSIS

Pre-eclampsia

The term 'eclampsia' is derived from the Greek word *Eklampsis*, meaning a 'sudden development' or a 'bolt from the blue'. It refers to convulsions that occur during pregnancy as a complication of pre-eclampsia. Pre-eclampsia is characterised by pregnancy-induced hypertension (>140/90 mmHg), proteinuria (>0.3 g/24 hr) with or without oedema of the face, hands and feet. It usually develops after week 20 of pregnancy and is resolved only by delivery. It affects approximately 7% of all pregnancies and is more common in nulliparous women, those with a previous family history of pre-eclampsia, extremes of age (<20 or >35 years old), obesity, diabetes or hypertension. It is caused by the inability of trophoblastic cells to invade the spiral arteries effectively. Consequently, the arteries fail to dilate sufficiently, leading to under perfusion of the placenta. This is temporarily compensated by elevating the maternal blood pressure and increasing blood flow to the placenta. Such mechanisms lead to the damage of the hepatic (HELLP syndrome: Haemolysis, Elevated Liver enzymes, Low Platelets), renal (proteinuria) and coagulation systems (thrombocytopenia, DIC). Other symptoms may include headaches, nausea and vomiting, epigastric pain and visual disturbances. Complications include eclampsia (grand mal seizures) that occurs in 1% of pre-eclampsia cases. Severe pre-eclampsia is defined as proteinuria, diastolic blood pressure >100 mmHg or maternal complications.

Features of Pre-eclampsia
Mnemonic: 'PRE eclampsia'
Proteinuria (>0.3 g/24 hr)
Rising blood pressure (>140/90 mmHg)
o**E**dema in the legs

Gestational Diabetes

Gestational diabetes is a temporary form of diabetes that affects pregnant women who have never suffered from diabetes before. It describes a transient elevation of glucose levels that disappears after pregnancy. It affects approximately 2% of all pregnant women compared to 0.3% of patients who have pre-existing diabetes. Risk factors include a family history of type 2 diabetes, a previous history of gestational diabetes, increasing maternal age, obesity, ethnicity and smoking. Complications include an increased risk of congenital abnormalities, pre-term labour, polyhydramnios and increased foetal mortality and morbidity. A glucose tolerance test will reveal an elevated sugar level (>9 mmol of glucose) two hours after taking 75 g of glucose. Women who are diagnosed with gestational diabetes have a greater chance of developing diabetes mellitus later in life.

Urinary Tract Infection (UTI) in Pregnancy

Urinary tract infections affect 1 in 25 pregnancies. Women are more susceptible to infections due to the close proximity of the shorter urethra to the anus. As a result, bowel organisms are able to ascend through the urethra (urethritis) and cause infection of the bladder (cystitis). Symptoms include dysuria, frequency, urgency, nocturia, haematuria, suprapubic discomfort and tenderness, and cloudy or foul-smelling urine. A urine culture is often conclusive of a diagnosis but may take several days to process. If the clinical diagnosis is uncertain, a urine dipstick can provide rapid analysis. If nitrite or leucocyte esterase is positive, UTIs are highly likely. Often blood and urine protein are also detected. Up to 20% of untreated infections can lead to a pyelonephritis (fever, rigors, nausea, vomiting, loin pain). Premature labour is also a significant complication.

INSTRUCTIONS: You are a foundation year House Officer in A&E where you have seen to Mrs Nikalou, a nulliparous 24-year-old woman 12 weeks into her first pregnancy. She is very anxious and has noticed blood on her underwear. The ultrasound shows a gestational sac of 70 mm and crown–rump length of 60 mm. No foetal heart sounds were heard. Explain the results to the patient and what will need to be done next.

HISTORY

0 1 2

☐☐☐ **Introduction**   Introduce yourself. Elicit the patient's name, age and occupation. Establish rapport.

History   Take a brief history of the presenting complaint, including when the bleeding started, how much and any associated symptoms, i.e. pain.

☐☐☐ **Ideas**   Ask the patient if she has any idea what may be causing her symptoms.

☐☐☐ **Concerns**   Ask the patient if she has any worries or concerns about her symptoms.

Miscarriages

Symptoms, Signs and Ultrasonic Findings

A miscarriage or spontaneous abortion is defined as the loss of a foetus before 24 weeks of gestation. Up to 20% of all pregnancies miscarry with 80% occurring in first trimester. The frequency of miscarriage decreases with increasing gestational age. Symptoms include a history of vaginal bleeding with blood clots and severe suprapubic abdominal pain. The vaginal bleeding may be significant enough to soak tampons, pads, sanitary towels or even clothes. Contractions and abdominal pain may co-exist but tend to resolve in a complete abortion. This is associated with the passage of products of conception and a cessation of vaginal bleeding. An ultrasound scan is the investigation of choice for suspected cases of miscarriages. Ultrasonic features consistent with a non-viable pregnancy include:

- An embryo with absent heartbeat when the CRL is >5 mm
- Loss of previously observed foetal cardiac activity
- Irregular-edged or collapsed gestational sac
- Abnormal echogenic material within the uterine cavity
- Lack of growth of the sac or foetal pole over a 5-day period

Foetal heart sounds are good markers for a viable pregnancy with the risk of spontaneous abortion decreasing from 50% to 3%. The earliest time they can be detected is by week 5 of gestation or when the crown–rump length is 2 to 4 mm and the gestational sac is 10 mm

✳ Breaking Bad News

☐☐☐ **Ultrasound**   Break the bad news empathetically, using pauses where appropriate. Pace the information and ensure that you use appropriate body language and silence.

'I have the results of your ultrasound. Unfortunately, I have to break some difficult news to you. I am afraid it is more serious than we had expected. Your scan suggests that the baby has stopped growing and I am sorry to have to tell you that you are having a miscarriage.'

MEDICAL ADVICE

☐☐☐ **Miscarriage**   Explain the diagnosis in simple terms the patient understands.

'Firstly, I would like you to know that this is not your fault. Miscarriages occur in about 20% of pregnancies and in most cases it is due to a random event. There is nothing you could have done to prevent it.'

✳ What Will Happen Next

☐☐☐ **Options**   Explain to the patient the available options in relation to her miscarriage. Take care to be sensitive and acknowledge her emotions.

Conservative   'Most women will cope with a miscarriage naturally without any need for us to do anything. This usually takes place over a week. However, if after a week you do not think that you have come to terms with the loss of the pregnancy or if you are still having heavy and painful bleeding, please return to see the gynaecological specialist.'

ERPC   'If you have been bleeding a lot, or if some of the pregnancy still remains in your womb, you may require a simple procedure to help remove it. This is known as an evacuation of retained products of conception (ERPC). This is a simple operation which should only last up to 15 minutes and you will be asleep during it.'

☐☐☐ **Rhesus**   Explain to the patient the need to check her Rhesus status.

'I now need to take some blood from you to check your Rhesus status. This is to determine if there may be a slight reaction between the baby's blood and yours. This reaction will not cause any problems now but may affect future pregnancies. If there is a problem then you may need an injection to prevent any harm in future pregnancies.'

☐☐☐ **Discharge**   Explain to the patient what will happen after discharge.

'On returning home you may continue to bleed for up to 10 days, but the bleeding should not be heavy or painful. Use sanitary towels until the bleeding has stopped and avoid sexual intercourse. You may experience period-like pains, for which you can take simple painkillers. Expect your next period to start within 6 weeks and you can return to work when you feel ready. If you require a medical sick note, we can facilitate this.'

☐☐☐ **Follow-up**   Offer the patient details of support groups and follow-up.

'Having a miscarriage can be a very emotional and lonely time for you. If you feel that you need to talk to someone we can put you in touch with a support group called the Miscarriage Association. This group consists of women who have all experienced miscarriages and will be able to answer any questions or anxieties you may have.'

☐☐☐ **Summarise**   Summarise back to the patient what you have explained so far.

CLOSING

☐☐☐ **Understanding**   Confirm that the patient has understood what you have explained to her.

☐☐☐ **Questions**   Respond appropriately to the patient's questions.

☐☐☐ **Leaflet**   Offer to give her more information in the form of a handout. Advise her that the leaflet contains much of the information you have mentioned.

COMMUNICATION SKILLS

☐☐☐ **Rapport**   Attempt to establish rapport with the patient through the use of appropriate eye contact. Maintain appropriate body language and an open posture throughout.

☐☐☐ **Listening**   Demonstrate interest and concern in what the patient says. Show active listening and listen empathetically.

☐☐☐ **Pauses**   Pace the information and use appropriate pauses. Allow the patient to speak her feelings freely and without interruption.

☐☐☐ **Empathy**   Respond empathetically (offer emotional support and validate her concerns).

☐☐☐ **Verbal Cues**   Use non-verbal and verbal cues, i.e. tone and pace of voice, and nod head where appropriate.

0 1 2 3 4 5

☐ ☐ ☐ ☐ ☐ ☐ Overall assessment of miscarriage counselling

☐ ☐ ☐ ☐ ☐ ☐ Role player's score

Total mark out of 31

INSTRUCTIONS: You are a foundation year House Officer in general practice. Ms Goldsberg, a 21-year-old woman, has done a pregnancy test that has shown that she is pregnant. Her last menstrual period was 7 weeks ago. She is very distressed when you see her today. Elicit her needs and give her appropriate advice and further management options.

HISTORY

0 1 2

☐☐☐ **Introduction**   Introduce yourself. Elicit her name, age and occupation. Establish rapport.

'I understand that your recent pregnancy test was positive and you are feeling quite distressed about this. I am sorry that you are feeling this way. Can you tell me more about this?'

☐☐☐ **Ideas**   Explore her ideas regarding the pregnancy and what she wants to achieve.

'I can see that this is very difficult for you right now. Have you had any ideas or thoughts of whether you would like to keep this pregnancy?'

☐☐☐ **Concerns**   Elicit the concerns the patient has about keeping the pregnancy (its legality, its effect on any future pregnancy).

'I understand that you are considering an abortion. Do you have any particular worries or concerns about this? Have you given this decision much thought? Do you wish to speak to someone before you make a decision?'

☐☐☐ **Sexual History**   Take a brief sexual history including her current relationship, her consent to intercourse, her use of any contraception and contraception failure (condom split). Also enquire about previous pregnancies or terminations.

☐☐☐ **Menstrual Hx.**   Elicit the patient's last menstrual period (LMP). Enquire about the length and regularity of her cycles.

Social History   Enquire about her home situation, including who lives at home, whether she has discussed her decision with her partner and if she wants to include anyone else in the decision-making process.

MEDICAL ADVICE

☐☐☐ **Legality**

Explain to the patient that abortions are legal before the age of 24 weeks.

'I wish to reassure you that as you are only 7-weeks pregnant it is perfectly legal for you to have an abortion, since in the UK the legal cut-off point is 24 weeks.'

The UK's Abortion Law
The UK Abortion Act of 1967
Termination of pregnancy was legalised in the UK under the 1967 Abortion Act. It can be artificially induced up to 24 weeks of pregnancy. In the UK 90% of abortions take place before 12 weeks. Two doctors (e.g. the GP and a gynaecologist) must give their consent, stating that to continue with the pregnancy would:
- **Endanger the life of the mother**
- **Endanger the physical or mental health of the mother**
- **Be a risk to the physical or mental health of the siblings**
- **Risk that the foetus would be born handicapped**

Most abortions in the UK fall under the second category. Patients must be referred for a termination of pregnancy by their GP, family planning centre or private health centre. No doctor is obliged to consent to or participate in an abortion, but all have a duty of care to refer the individual to the correct department. The 1967 Abortion Act does not extend to Northern Ireland, where abortion is still illegal.

Accessibility

State that the service is free under the National Health Service.

☐☐☐ **Confidentiality**

Reassure the patient that the procedure will remain confidential.

Appointments

Explain that she will be given two separate appointments. The first, to assess eligibility and choice of procedure; the second will be the procedure itself. Also mention that the abortion should be completed within 3 weeks of the first contact she has made with the services.

☐☐☐ **Options**

Explain the options available to the patient for the termination of her pregnancy.

Option 1

'I understand that you wish to proceed with the abortion. I would like to explain the different options available. The first option is to abort the pregnancy using tablets. You will be given a tablet called mifepristone which stops the pregnancy hormones from working and makes you have an early miscarriage. A few days after this you will be given another tablet that can be taken by mouth or inserted into the vagina, which will cause the pregnancy to be expelled. This option is 99% successful if used before 8 weeks and must be carried out before the pregnancy has reached 9 weeks.'

Option 2

'The second option is a minor surgical procedure which is usually performed before the pregnancy has reached its 12th week. You will not need to be put to sleep since it will be done under local anaesthetic. A small tube will be passed into the womb and the pregnancy will be removed. This is a fairly quick procedure and should only take 5 minutes.'

Option 3

'After 12 weeks of pregnancy, a more extensive surgical procedure is required. This involves putting you to sleep under general anaesthetic and removing the pregnancy through a tube passed into your womb. You may need to stay overnight in the hospital after the procedure has been carried out.'

☐☐☐ Complications

Explain to the patient potential complications when undertaking a termination of pregnancy, such as infection, heavy bleeding, potential damage to the cervix or womb, minimal chance of affecting fertility and a failure to terminate the pregnancy, requiring further treatment.

☐☐☐ Rhesus Status

Explain to the patient the need to check their Rhesus status and if necessary anti-D injection may need to be administered.

☐☐☐ Screen STDs

Explain to the patient that all women attending for an abortion are screened for chlamydia to reduce the chances of post-operation infection (salpingitis).

☐☐☐ Implications

Discuss with the patient possible implications after having the abortion, such as her fertility not being compromised and possible emotional response.

Fertility

'It is important to appreciate that having a successful abortion will not compromise your future chances of falling pregnant.'

Counsellor

'After having an abortion, some women experience a number of different emotions. You may feel relieved or sad. All of this is perfectly natural. If you are having problems coping with your emotions, I can put you in touch with a counsellor, if you feel you need to talk to someone.'

☐☐☐ Contraception

Discuss with the patient available contraceptive options.

Summarise

Summarise back to the patient what you have explained so far.

CLOSING

☐☐☐ **Understanding**   Confirm that the patient has understood what you have explained to her.

☐☐☐ **Questions**   Respond appropriately to the patient's questions.

Leaflet   Offer to give her more information in the form of a handout. Advise that the leaflet contains much of the information you have mentioned.

COMMUNICATION SKILLS

☐☐☐ **Rapport**   Attempt to establish rapport with the patient through the use of appropriate eye contact. Maintain appropriate body language and an open posture throughout.

☐☐☐ **Listening**   Demonstrate interest and concern in what the patient says. Show active listening and listen empathetically.

☐☐☐ **Pauses**   Pace the information and use appropriate pauses. Allow the patient to speak her feelings freely and without interruption.

☐☐☐ **Empathy**   Demonstrate an empathetic response (offer emotional support and validate the patient's concerns).

☐☐☐ **Verbal Cues**   Use non-verbal and verbal cues, i.e. tone and pace of voice, nod head where appropriate.

EXAMINER'S EVALUATION

0 1 2 3 4 5
☐ ☐ ☐ ☐ ☐ ☐   Overall assessment of abortion counselling
☐ ☐ ☐ ☐ ☐ ☐   Role player's score
Total mark out of 33

INSTRUCTIONS: You are a foundation year House Officer in obstetrics. An 18-year-old woman presents with colicky right iliac fossa pain. She mentions that she has had vaginal bleeding the last 3 days and missed her period 2 months prior. Her pregnancy test is positive and an urgent ultrasound performed by your registrar fails to demonstrate an intrauterine pregnancy. Explain the likely diagnosis and next course of action.

HISTORY

0 1 2

☐☐☐ **Introduction** — Introduce yourself. Elicit the patient's name, age and occupation. Establish rapport.

☐☐☐ **History** — Take a brief history of the presenting complaint, including when the pain started, its location and associated symptoms, i.e. vaginal bleeding, vomiting, fever.

☐☐☐ **Ideas** — Ask the patient if she has any ideas of what may be causing her symptoms.

☐☐☐ **Concerns** — Ask the patient if she has any worries or concerns about her symptoms.

Ectopic Pregnancy

Symptoms, Signs and Investigation findings

Ectopic pregnancy is defined as the implantation of an embryo outside of the uterine cavity. It complicates 1% of all pregnancies and represents a major cause of maternal mortality. The most common site for implantation is the inside lining of a Fallopian tube (97%). Other sites include the cornu, cervix, ovary and peritoneum. Ectopic pregnancy should always be suspected in a sexually active woman who presents with bleeding or abdominal pain. Clinical features include a 4–10 week history of amenorrhoea, sudden onset of colicky lower abdominal pain (later becoming constant) and scanty dark vaginal bleeding. Intraperitoneal haemorrhage is heralded by syncopal collapse and shoulder tip pain. The diagnosis is suggested by an empty uterus on ultrasound with a positive pregnancy test (beta-HCG levels). A confirmed diagnosis is characterised by the presence of a thick, ring-like echogenic centre located outside the uterus, with a gestational sac containing a foetal pole or yolk sac.

★ **Breaking Bad News**

☐☐☐ **Ultrasound** — Break the bad news empathetically, using pauses where appropriate. The information should be paced with a good use of body language and silence.

'I have the results of your ultrasound. Unfortunately, I have to break some difficult news to you. I am afraid it is more serious than we thought. Your scan suggests that the pregnancy is growing outside your womb. This is known as an ectopic pregnancy. The most common place for it to occur is in your Fallopian tubes and this may the reason why you are suffering from pain and bleeding. I'm sorry to have to tell you that your pregnancy is not viable and will have to be removed for your own safety.'

MEDICAL ADVICE

☐☐☐ **Ectopic Preg.**   Explain the diagnosis to patient in simple terms the patient understands.

'Firstly, I would like you to know that this is not your fault and there was nothing that you could have done to prevent this. Ectopic pregnancies can occur for a number of different reasons, such as suffering from infection or inflammation of the tubes, previous surgery and a condition known as endometriosis. However, in most causes no cause is found.'

☐☐☐ **Surgery**   Explain to the patient why a surgical procedure needs to be undertaken in order to remove the pregnancy.

'As we mentioned before, it is likely that the pregnancy is in one of your tubes and not in the womb. Your tubes were not designed to stretch or grow the way your womb would and are at risk of rupturing if the pregnancy continues. For this reason, we will have to remove the pregnancy and maybe your tube as well. It is important to appreciate that if we do not do this, your Fallopian tube may burst, putting your life at serious risk.'

☐☐☐ **Laparoscopy**   Explain to the patient the laparoscopic procedure.

'We will need to keep you in hospital and perform surgery to remove the pregnancy from your tubes. This will be done laparoscopically, which is otherwise known as keyhole surgery. You will be put to sleep and the surgeon will make two small incisions in your tummy. The pregnancy will be identified and removed, making all attempts to leave your tubes intact. In exceptional cases, open surgery may have to be carried out if the keyhole surgery fails.'

☐☐☐ **Alternatives**   Explain alternative methods of managing the ectopic pregnancy.

'In most cases we undertake keyhole surgery to remove the ectopic pregnancy. However, in a minority of cases and depending on your circumstances, there are two alternative options which may be indicated. The first is simply watching and waiting. In some situations the pregnancy stops growing by itself and disappears without consequence. However, you must be fit and well and blood tests for your pregnancy hormone levels should show a drop before this option can be fully considered.

'The second option is to give an injection called methotrexate. This will cause the pregnancy to stop and shrink away. However, we consider this only in women whose pregnancy hormone levels are already very low.'

☐☐☐ **Advice**

Explain to the patient the increased risk of future ectopic pregnancies.

'Normally, we advise women to wait for three normal periods before trying to fall pregnant again. I must inform you that since you have had an ectopic pregnancy you have a small but significant risk of it occurring again (10%). Therefore, we advise you to visit your GP following a positive pregnancy test so that you can have an early ultrasound scan to make sure the pregnancy is in the womb.'

CLOSING
☐☐☐ **Follow-up**

Offer the patient details of support groups and follow-up.

'Having an ectopic pregnancy can be very emotionally draining. If you feel that you need to talk to someone about how you are feeling, we can give you details of some support groups and if need be, we can get you to speak to a counsellor if you would like.'

☐☐☐ **Understanding**

Confirm that the patient has understood what you have explained to her.

☐☐☐ **Questions**

Respond appropriately to the patient's questions.

Leaflet

Offer to give her more information in the form of a handout. Advise that the leaflet contains much of the information you have mentioned.

Summarise

Summarise back to the patient what you have explained so far.

COMMUNICATION SKILLS
☐☐☐ **Rapport**

Attempt to establish rapport with the patient through the use of appropriate eye contact. Maintain appropriate body language and an open posture throughout.

☐☐☐ **Listening**   Demonstrate interest and concern in what the patient says. Show active listening and listen empathetically.

☐☐☐ **Pauses**   Pace the information and use appropriate pauses. Allow the patient to speak her feelings freely and without interruption.

☐☐☐ **Empathy**   Demonstrate an empathetic response (offer emotional support and validate her concerns).

☐☐☐ **Verbal Cues**   Use non-verbal and verbal cues, i.e. tone and pace of voice, and nod head where appropriate.

EXAMINER'S EVALUATION

0   1   2   3   4   5

☐☐☐☐☐☐ Overall assessment of explaining ectopic pregnancy

☐☐☐☐☐☐ Role player's score

Total mark out of 31

INSTRUCTIONS: You are a foundation year House Officer in a gynaecology outpatient clinic. Ms Atkin is a 29-year-old woman who has been referred to the clinic by her GP following a routine PV examination. The ultrasound scan demonstrated a 6.5 cm fluid-filled sac with regular borders on her right ovary. Explain these findings to the patient and tell her what will happen next.

HISTORY

0 1 2

☐☐☐ **Introduction**   Introduce yourself. Elicit her name, age and occupation. Establish rapport.

History   Take a brief history of her presenting complaint, including pain, irregular periods, nausea and vomiting.

☐☐☐ **Ideas**   Ask the patient if she has any ideas of what may be causing her symptoms.

☐☐☐ **Concerns**   Ask the patient if she has any worries or concerns about her symptoms.

Ovarian Cyst
Symptoms, Signs and Investigation Findings
Ovarian cysts are usually asymptomatic and are often discovered as an incidental finding on a pelvic ultrasound scan. If they are symptomatic they may present with irregular menses or vaginal spotting and produce symptoms secondary to a mass effect. They are found in nearly all premenopausal women, and in up to 15% of postmenopausal women. They can affect women at any age but are more common in women of childbearing age. Functional cysts are by far the most common type and include follicular cysts and corpus luteal cysts. Follicular cysts occur in the first two weeks of the cycle when the ovarian follicle fails to rupture and release an egg but instead continues to grow. When it does rupture it causes a sudden onset, sharp, severe, unilateral pain typically during mid-cycle (*mittelschmerz*). Luteal cysts represent failed degeneration of the corpus luteum and tend to produce symptoms when they become inflamed or haemorrhage spontaneously, often in the later half of the cycle. Others include theca lutein cysts (due to high HCG levels) and chocolate cysts (blood-filled cysts that are frequently painful). On ultrasound investigation, unilateral cystic lesions <10 cm in diameter with regular borders are most likely to be benign. Lesions that persist beyond 2 months and are >10 cm in diameter with irregular borders or thick septa should be investigated for possible malignancy.

☐☐☐ **Ultrasound**

Break the news empathetically, using pauses where appropriate. The information should be paced with good use of body language and silence.

'I have the results of your ultrasound scan. It shows there is a medium-sized fluid sac within your right ovary. This is known an ovarian cyst. Have you ever been told that you have an ovarian cyst and can you tell me what you understand by it?'

☐☐☐ **Ovarian Cyst**

Explain the diagnosis in simple terms the patient understands.

'Ovarian cysts are fluid-filled sacs located in the ovaries of women. They are quite common and most of them are quite harmless. During a woman's normal cycle, small cysts develop in the ovaries and usually disappear before the next cycle. Sometimes, for various reasons, your hormones may become unbalanced and, instead of disappearing, these cysts grow in size. Usually they are quite harmless and disappear within 6 weeks. On very rare occasions they can turn out to be cancerous.'

☐☐☐ **Observe**

Explain to the patient that a repeat US will be performed in 4 weeks time.

'In most cases we normally watch and wait to see what will happen with the cyst. We will repeat an ultrasound in 4 weeks time to see if the cyst has shrunk in size.'

☐☐☐ **Surgery**

Explain to the patient when surgery may be indicated.

'If you are suffering from symptoms due to the ovarian cyst such as severe pain, fever and vomiting, or if the cyst is exceptionally large, then we would advise that the cyst should be removed surgically.

'We will need to keep you in hospital and perform the surgery to drain the cyst. This will be done laparoscopically, which is otherwise known as keyhole surgery. You will be put to sleep and the surgeon will make two small incisions in your tummy. The cyst will be drained and a small sample removed and sent to the laboratory. In exceptional cases, open surgery may have to be carried out if keyhole surgery fails.'

☐☐☐ **Symptoms**

Advise the patient when to seek medical help.

'Although generally cysts do not cause any symptoms you should seek medical help if you begin to suffer from the following: pain with fever and vomiting, sudden severe abdominal pain, faintness or dizziness.'

□□□ **Recurrence**　Explain to the patient what treatments are available in case of recurrence.

'If you suffer from recurrent ovarian cysts, some treatments are available such as the combined oral contraceptive or the depot contraceptive injections that can reduce the rate of recurrence. You can discuss this further with your GP if the need arises.'

Summarise　Summarise back to the patient what you have explained so far.

CLOSING

□□□ **Understanding**　Confirm that the patient has understood what you have explained to her.

□□□ **Questions**　Respond appropriately to the patient's questions.

Leaflet　Offer to give her more information in the form of a handout. Advise that the leaflet contains much of the information you have mentioned.

COMMUNICATION SKILLS

□□□ **Rapport**　Attempt to establish rapport with the patient through the use of appropriate eye contact. Maintain appropriate body language and an open posture throughout.

□□□ **Listening**　Demonstrate an interest and concern in what the patient says. Show active listening and listen empathetically.

□□□ **Empathy**　Demonstrate an empathetic response (offer emotional support and validate concerns).

EXAMINER'S EVALUATION

0 1 2 3 4 5
□□□□□□ Overall assessment of explaining ovarian cysts
□□□□□□ Role player's score
Total mark out of 27

OBSTETRICS: **Nuchal Scanning**

INSTRUCTIONS: You are a foundation year House Officer in obstetrics. Mrs Chun Lee is a 41-year-old woman who is 8 weeks into her first pregnancy. She is due to have a nuchal scan and would like you to explain more about this. You will be assessed on your communication skills and on the information that you provide.

INTRODUCTION

0 1 2

☐☐☐ **Introduction** Introduce yourself. Elicit her name, age and occupation. Establish rapport.

☐☐☐ **Ideas** Ask the patient what she understands by the term nuchal scanning and what she thinks it will entail.

☐☐☐ **Concerns** Ask the patient if she has any worries or concerns about the nuchal scan (e.g. risk of Down's, miscarriage). Make sure to explore these appropriately.

MEDICAL ADVICE

☐☐☐ **Screening Test** Explain appropriately the purpose of the scan.

'The scan is an ultrasound screening test that is offered to all pregnant women to assess the risk of having a child with Down's syndrome. It helps identify those mothers who may need more invasive diagnostic testing. The nuchal ultrasound test is safe and carries no risk of harm to yourself or your baby (such as miscarrying).'

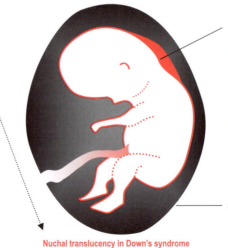

Nuchal Translucency

The area located posterior to the back of the skull and neck represents the nuchal translucency, which contains fluid. The widest part should be measured to evaluate the risk of developing Down's syndrome or a chromosomal abnormality. The diameter is normally less than 3mm. >3mm is considered abnormal and carries a 10% risk of an abnormality, while >6mm increases the risk to above 90%

CRL (Crown-Rump Length)

Nuchal translucency measurement should be obtained between 10 and 14 weeks or equivalent to a CRL between 45 and 84 mm

Amniotic fluid

Nuchal translucency in Down's syndrome

▢▢▢ Procedure

Appropriately explain when the scan will be performed and what will be investigated.

'The scan will be performed between 11 and 14 weeks of your pregnancy. An ultrasound probe will be placed on your tummy along with some jelly. The scan will focus particularly on the thickness of the fat pad behind your baby's neck as well as other soft markers in the heart or head.'

▢▢▢ Risk

Explain how a risk ratio is arrived at.

'Along with the ultrasound findings, your general risk of having a Down's baby is based upon your age and the results of the triple blood test. An overall risk will be calculated that represents the chance that your baby may have Down's syndrome. This figure will categorise you as being either at high risk (>1 in 250) or at low risk (<1 in 250).'

Low Risk

Explain that being at low risk does not mean the baby does not have Down's syndrome.

'The nuchal scan as well as the triple blood test is the most effective non-invasive way of identifying Down's syndrome. However, it is important to appreciate that being categorised as 'low risk' does not mean that your child definitely does not have Down's, but means that it is highly unlikely. You will be given a figure that represents the chance that your child will be affected. For example, a risk of 1 in 500 means that out of 500 births, one of these will be a Down's syndrome baby while the other 499 births will not.'

High Risk

Explain the procedure in the event of a positive result.

'If you are categorised as being at high risk (having greater than 1 in 250 chance that the child has Down's) then there are two options available to you. You can either choose to continue with the pregnancy without further investigation, or you may wish to pursue more invasive tests that check the baby's genes for Down's. It is important to remember that being told that you are at a higher risk does not mean that the baby definitely has Down's syndrome. This figure merely represents the probability that your child will be born with Down's. For example, a risk of 1 in 25 means that out of 25 births, one birth will be that of a Down's syndrome baby.

Risk of Down's Syndrome (DS) in a Baby
Association of Down's syndrome with maternal age
Until recently, maternal age was the only factor used to identify mothers who are at high risk of developing a Down's syndrome baby. As demonstrated by the graph below, the risk of developing Down's syndrome increases exponentially with maternal age. Women aged over 35 are routinely offered invasive diagnostic tests. Recent studies have

revealed that increasing paternal age also increases the risk of Down's, especially in older mothers.

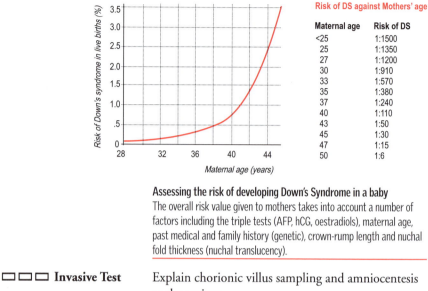

Risk of DS against Mothers' age

Maternal age	Risk of DS
<25	1:1500
25	1:1350
27	1:1200
30	1:910
33	1:570
35	1:380
37	1:240
40	1:110
43	1:50
45	1:30
47	1:15
50	1:6

Assessing the risk of developing Down's Syndrome in a baby
The overall risk value given to mothers takes into account a number of factors including the triple tests (AFP, hCG, oestradiols), maternal age, past medical and family history (genetic), crown-rump length and nuchal fold thickness (nuchal translucency).

☐☐☐ Invasive Test

Explain chorionic villus sampling and amniocentesis to the patient.

'We can take a sample from the placenta by passing a fine needle through the wall of your tummy. This is known as chorionic villus sampling and is carried out at 11 to 14 weeks of pregnancy. The other option, known as amniocentesis, is carried out at around 16 weeks and allows us to obtain the baby's cells from the surrounding fluid. Both of these tests carry a 1 in 100 chance of causing your pregnancy to miscarry.'

Pathology and Symptoms of Down's Syndrome
Mnemonic: 'DOWN'
Decreased alpha-fetoprotein and unconjugated estriol (maternal)
One extra 21 chromosome
Women of advanced age
Non-disjunction during maternal meiosis

☐☐☐ Follow-up

Make appropriate arrangements to discuss results.

'The results are normally ready within 2 weeks of your test. The results are sent back to your doctor, who will make arrangements to discuss this with you. Please feel free to bring your partner or a family member with you for support.'

☐☐☐ Pros and Cons

Discuss the pros and cons of nuchal testing.

'Having the nuchal scan is very useful as it can reassure you as to whether your baby is likely to be healthy. It will give you the option to consider terminating the pregnancy if you so wish. If you decide to carry on with the pregnancy, it can give you time to prepare for the arrival of a baby with special needs. However, having a nuchal scan is not conclusive as you may be categorised as being at high risk and yet go on to deliver a healthy baby. Hence, the procedure may cause undue anxiety and stress. If you have already decided that you want to keep a baby with Down's, then this procedure may result in unnecessary investigations.'

Summarise   Summarise back to the patient what you have explained so far.

CLOSING
☐☐☐ **Understanding**   Confirm that the patient has understood what you have explained to her.

☐☐☐ **Questions**   Respond appropriately to the patient's questions.

Leaflet   Offer to give her more information in the form of a handout. Advise that the leaflet contains much of the information you have mentioned.

COMMUNICATION SKILLS
☐☐☐ **Rapport**   Attempt to establish rapport with the patient through the use of appropriate eye contact. Maintain appropriate body language and an open posture throughout.

☐☐☐ **Fluency**   Speak fluently and do not use jargon.

☐☐☐ **Listening**   Demonstrate interest and concern in what the patient says. Show active listening and listen empathetically.

☐☐☐ **Empathy**   Respond empathetically (offer emotional support and validate concerns).

EXAMINER'S EVALUATION

0 1 2 3 4 5

☐☐☐☐☐☐ Overall assessment of explaining nuchal translucency
☐☐☐☐☐☐ Role player's score
Total mark out of 29

INSTRUCTIONS: You are a foundation year House Officer in a general practice. Mrs Gillord is due to give birth to her first child in a few weeks time. She has come to the practice as she is not sure whether to breast or bottle feed her child. Explore her concerns and give her appropriate advice. You will be assessed on your communication skills and on the information that you provide.

INTRODUCTION

0 1 2

☐☐☐ **Introduction** — Introduce yourself. Elicit the patient's name, age and occupation. Establish rapport.

☐☐☐ **Ideas** — Elicit the patient's ideas about breast-feeding.

☐☐☐ **Concerns** — Establish any concerns or fears she has about breast-feeding her child.

Expectations — Elicit how the patient would like to benefit from her consultation today.

ADVICE

☐☐☐ **Advantages** — Explain the advantages of breast-feeding over bottle feeding for the child.

'We generally advise all our mothers to breast-feed their newborn children. This is because breast-feeding has a number of advantages over bottle feeding. Breast-feeding provides all the nutrients and energy that a baby needs in the first six months of life. It also includes antibodies to help protect the baby from infections and helps to maintain the growth and development of the baby. Recent evidence has shown that it helps prevent illnesses such as asthma, eczema and diabetes.'

Explain that breast-feeding has many advantages for the mother as well.

'Breast-feeding will have many benefits for you as a mother as well. It helps develop a strong bond between you and the baby. It helps the womb to return to its normal size quicker. This process uses up calories and so will allow you to return to your normal weight sooner. Breast milk is always ready and available when your child needs it and will not cost you anything. Also, recent evidence has shown that breast-feeding will help you in the long term. In particular, it helps to reduce your risk of developing breast and ovarian cancer.'

Mnemonic: 'ABCDEFGH'

Benefits to Infant	Benefits to Mother
Allergic conditions reduced	**E**conomical (free)
Best nutritional food for infant	**F**itness (body shape returns quicker)
Close relationship with mother	**G**uards against breast, ovary and uterus cancer
Development of IQ	**H**aemorrhage (postpartum) reduced

☐☐☐ **Disadvantages**   Explain the possibility of the transfer of infection and drugs to the baby while breast-feeding.

'Unfortunately along with nutrients, other substances can be transferred from mother to child in the breast milk. These include viruses such as HIV and Hepatitis B may also be transmitted. Therefore if you are suffering from one of these illnesses you may be advised not to breastfeed.'

'It is also important to realise that whatever you eat or drink may be passed to your baby through your breast milk. Such things include alcohol, caffeine and nicotine, which may harm your baby. Also, if you are on any medication or if you are going to start any new medication, let your doctor or pharmacist know that you are breast-feeding.'

Drugs Contraindicated in Breast-feeding
Mnemonic: 'BREAST'

Bromocriptine, **B**enzodiazepines	**A**miodarone, **A**mphetamines
Radioactive isotopes	**S**timulant laxatives, **S**ex hormones
Ergotamine, **E**thosuximide	**T**etracycline

☐☐☐ **Breast to Bottle**   Explain to the patient that breast-feeding should always be attempted before bottle feeding. This is because it is usually more difficult to switch from the bottle to the breast than it is from the breast to the bottle. Also remind the mother that it is often more difficult to restart breast milk once it is stopped.

☐☐☐ **Method**   Explain to the mother the technique required for breast-feeding. Encourage her to breast-feed soon after birth.

'During the latter part of pregnancy your breast will be primed to produce breast milk. Once your baby is born this is a great time to start breast-feeding. This is because the first milk that you produce after giving birth will be extremely nutritious and beneficial to the baby.

'In order to breast-feed your child, you need to keep your baby's head and body in a straight line. Hold the baby close to you and keep the baby's nose opposite your nipple. Encourage the baby to latch on to your breast and hold the baby in a comfortable position. The more the baby sucks the more milk is produced.

'I would like to reassure you that although this may sound tricky, most mothers find that breast-feeding comes naturally and as time goes by you will feel more confident. Remember that you can always approach your heath visitor or your midwife for help and assistance.'

Breast-feeding Technique

Newborns commonly require on average eight feeds a day with each feed approximately 20 minutes in length. Hold the baby such that her whole body is facing your body. Ensure that her nose and chin is pressed against your breast while supporting her head, neck and back. Allow the baby's mouth to latch onto your nipple and areola. If you wish to break the attachment, avoid pulling the baby away from your breast. Instead insert your little finger into the corner of their mouth and gently detach the baby from your breast

☐☐☐ **Expressing**

Explain that breast milk can be given in expressed form.

Definition

'Breast milk does not have to be given only from the breast. You can also express it, which means squeezing the milk out of your breast with a pump.'

Reasons

'Expressing milk is useful for a number of reasons. Firstly, it can be used to give your child breast milk if it is it is having difficulty in suckling or when it is unwell and doesn't have enough energy.

'If your breasts feel uncomfortably full, you can express breast milk and store it to give to your baby later. If you wish to go back to work or are away from your baby you can express milk so that your baby can still be fed breast milk.'

Method

'It is a good idea to ask your midwife or health visitor for advice. To express breast milk by hand, cup your breast and feel back from the end of your nipple to where the texture of the breast changes. From this area you need to use your thumb and index finger to gently squeeze toward your nipple. Milk should begin to flow at this point. This technique should become easier with time. Change to the other breast when milk stops flowing or slows down to a drip. If you are using a pump please refer to the instruction manual.'

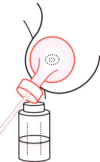

Using a Breast Pump

Breast pumps can come in two varieties, hand and electric models. Ensure that the pump is sterilised before and after use. Breast milk can be refrigerated for a maximum of 3 months. Refer to the instruction manual regarding use of hand and electric model

Storage

'Expressed milk can be stored in a fridge at a temperature of 2–4°C for 24 hours. It can also be stored in the ice compartment of a fridge for 1 week and for up to 3 months in a freezer. Always use a sterilised container for storage.'

□□□ **Enough Milk**

Explain that there are certain signs that indicate the baby has had enough milk.

'You will know the baby has had enough milk as it will stop feeding by itself and appear satisfied after the feed. A well-fed baby should be gaining weight after 2 weeks and should wet around six nappies a day.'

Other Fluids

Explain that other fluids should not be given during breast-feeding as this will reduce the amount of milk the mother will produce.

□□□ **Dummies**

Explain that dummies should be avoided during the early months of breast-feeding as the baby may lose the ability to suckle the breast correctly.

□□□ **Sore Nipples**

Explain that sore nipples can occur as a result of incorrect positioning during breast-feeding and that advice should be sought from the GP or health visitor.

□□□ **Mastitis**

Explain and give advice regarding mastitis.

'Mastitis is when the breast becomes hot and tender and can be caused by infection. During this time you may also feel as though you have the 'flu. It is OK to carry on breast-feeding but you should get your midwife or health visitor to check your feeding position. If there is no improvement you should go to your GP as you may need a course of antibiotics.'

Duration

Explain that there is no set limit to the time for breast-feeding. However, the mother should aim to breast-feed for between 6 to 12 months. Solids should be encouraged after 4 months.

Breast Size	Virtually all sizes and shapes of breasts can produce milk. After breast-feeding, some women notice that their breasts have become a little smaller or bigger. For other women there is no change
From One Breast	If there is only one functioning breast it is still possible to breast-feed effectively. If both breasts are being used, one breast should be drained completely before the other one is offered
Refusal to Feed	A baby's refusal to feed can sometimes be remedied by the mother simply resting and eating well before trying to feed the child again
Sickness	If the mother becomes sick with a minor illness such as a cold or cough, it is usually fine for her to continue breast-feeding
Alcohol	Mothers should be advised to avoid alcohol altogether while breast-feeding
Pregnancy	Although breast-feeding significantly reduces the chances of pregnancy, mothers should be advised to used additional methods of contraception

CLOSING

☐☐☐ **Understanding** Confirm that the patient has understood what you have explained to her.

☐☐☐ **Questions** Respond appropriately to her questions.

Leaflet Offer to give her more information in the form of a handout. Advise that the leaflet contains much of the information you have mentioned.

COMMUNICATION SKILLS

☐☐☐ **Rapport** Attempt to establish rapport with the patient through the use of appropriate eye contact.

☐☐☐ **Fluency** Speak fluently and do not use jargon.

☐☐☐ **Summarise** Check with the patient and deliver an appropriate summary.

EXAMINER'S EVALUATION

0 1 2 3 4 5
☐☐☐☐☐☐ Overall assessment of breast-feeding advice
☐☐☐☐☐☐ Role player's score
Total mark out of 31

Gynaecology

INSTRUCTIONS: You are a foundation year House Officer in an outpatient gynaecology clinic. Mrs Paborski, a 59-year-old woman, presents to you for the first time complaining of heavy vaginal bleeding. Take a full gynaecological history from the patient.

INTRODUCTION

0 1 2

□□□ **Introduction**   Introduce yourself appropriately and establish rapport.

□□□ **Name & Age**   Elicit the patient's name and age.

□□□ **Occupation**   Enquire about the patient's occupation.

HISTORY

□□□ **Concerns**   Elicit all the patient's presenting concerns. Use open questions and explore the patient's beliefs about her health. For each concern or complaint, elicit the patient's ideas, concerns and expectations.

□□□ **History**   For each complaint ascertain the time of onset, presenting features and associated symptoms. Explore each symptom systematically using appropriate mnemonics, e.g. SOCRATES (pain), ONE RESP (shortness of breath).

GYNAECOLOGICAL HISTORY

□□□ **Periods**   Establish the patient's age of menarche (first menstrual period). Enquire about the date of her last menstrual period (LMP), its duration and regularity. Ask if she has noticed any heavy bleeding (menorrhagia) and how much. Does she use tampons, pads or sanitary towels? Were they soaked and how many did she use? Did she soil her underwear? Were there any clots?

Causes of Vaginal Bleeding in a Non-Pregnant Woman

General	Thyroid disease, hepatic disorders, leukaemia and myeloproliferative disorders, thrombocytopenia, coagulopathies
Local	Vaginitis, fibroids, polyps, adenomyosis, endometriosis, infection (chlamydia, gonorrhoea), tumours (ovarian, endometrial and cervical), foreign body, trauma

Other	Dysfunctional uterine bleeding (DUB): no anatomical or systemic cause is found, foreign body (tissue paper), trauma (abuse)

⬜⬜⬜ **Irregular bleed**

Enquire about bleeding between periods (inter-menstrual) and following sexual intercourse (post-coital).

Causes of Inter-menstrual (IMB) & Post-coital bleeding (PCB)

IMB	**Vaginal bleeding occurring in the menstrual cycle other than normal menstruation**
Physiological	1–2% women spot around ovulation
Obstetric	Pregnancy, ectopic pregnancy, gestational trophoblastic disease
Uterine	Endometrial polyps, endometrial carcinoma, adenomyosis, fibroids
Vaginal	Vaginitis, vaginal malignancy
Cervical	Cervical cancer (commonly post-coital), cervical polyps, ectropion, cervicitis (blood-tinged discharge)
Iatrogenic	Contraceptive pills, tamoxifen, anticoagulants, SSRIs, corticosteroids
PCB	**Vaginal bleeding that occurs immediately after sexual intercourse**
Causes	Cervicitis, cervical and endometrial polyps, vaginal cancer, cervical cancer, infection (Chlamydia, gonorrhoea, trichomaniasis, yeast), trauma

⬜⬜⬜ **Menopause**

Establish if the patient is menopausal. If so, ask for how long she has been menopausal and if she has had any post-menopausal bleeding.

Causes of Post-Menopausal Bleeding (PMB)

PMB	**Vaginal bleeding 6 months after menopause. Any PMB should be treated as malignant until proved otherwise**
Causes	Atrophic vaginitis (90%), infections (chlamydia, gonorrhoea, trichomoniasis), polyps (cervical or endometrial), endometrial carcinoma, cervical carcinoma, ovarian carcinoma, vaginal carcinoma, uterine sarcoma
Other	Hormone replacement therapy (HRT), clotting disorder, trauma

⬜⬜⬜ **Pain**

Note any associated pain during her periods (dysmenorrhoea), particularly the timing in the cycle, its location, duration, radiation and severity. Note any other associated symptoms.

53

ASSOCIATED HISTORY

☐☐☐ **Sexual History**   Establish if the patient is sexually active. Is she suffering from any dyspareunia (if so, is the pain superficial or deep)? Is she with a regular sexual partner?

Discharge   Enquire if she is experiencing any vaginal discharge. Note its colour (clear, white, purulent, bloodstained), odour and amount. Is there associated pruritus? Is the partner experiencing any symptoms?

Gynae. History   Enquire about the date and result of her previous smear test. Did she have any previous abnormal results, if so, what was done (colposcopy)? Establish if the patient is using contraception (barrier methods, the pill, intramuscular contraception, the coil) and enquire about her current method.

OTHER ASSOCIATED HISTORY

☐☐☐ **Obstetric Hx.**   Has she ever been pregnant? If so, how many times and what were their gestations. Has she had any terminations of pregnancy, stillbirths or miscarriages?

Medical History   Has she had any previous surgery or any serious illnesses (e.g. breast, cervical or ovarian cancer)?

☐☐☐ **Family History**   Is there any history of any serious medical illness in the family such as breast or ovarian cancer? Enquire about the ages of the family member at the onset of such illnesses.

☐☐☐ **Drug History**   Is she taking any regular medications (tamoxifen, OCP, HRT) prescribed or over the counter? Does she have any allergies?

Risk Factors for Endometrial Carcinoma
Mnemonic: 'ENDOMET'
Elderly, **N**ulliparity, **D**iabetes, **O**besity, **M**enstrual irregularity, o**E**strogen therapy, hyper**T**ension

---

Social History   Does she drink alcohol or smoke?

Systemic Rvw   Does she have any constitutional symptoms, such as weight loss, loss of appetite, increased fatigue, sweating and hot flushes? Does she suffer from any urinary symptoms, such as abdominal pain or dysuria?

Questions to Ask about Urinary Symptoms

Pain	Have you experienced any pain passing water (dysuria) or pain in your loins?
Frequency	How frequently do you pass water (frequency >6/day)?
Nocturia	Do you ever go during the night (nocturia >2/night)?
Urgency	Do you have a strong desire to pass urine (urgency)? Have you ever had accidents (bedwetting – enuresis)?
Straining	Do you have episodes of incontinence with straining or coughing (stress)? Do you ever leak when you are just walking? Do you use pads to keep yourself dry? How many do you use in a day?
Haematuria	Have you noticed any blood in your urine?
Other	Associated fever? Do you have any sensation of a mass in your vagina or a dragging heavy sensation (prolapse)?

CLOSING

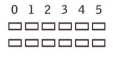 **Rapport**   Establish and maintain rapport and demonstrate listening skills.

Summarise   Check with patient and deliver an appropriate summary.

'This is Miss Paborski, a 59-year-old Polish woman with a three-months' history of vaginal bleeding. Her last LMP was 7 years ago. She states that the bleeding is progressively worsening, and has been occurring on a daily basis for the past 2 weeks. She has no abdominal pain but mentions that she has been unintentionally losing weight. She has been using HRT for the last 5 years but was stopped by her GP 2 months ago. In view of her gynaecological history, I suspect that this may be a case of endometrial cancer and I would like to perform a full pelvic examination, including a smear. I would also like to refer her for an urgent transvaginal ultrasound and hysteroscopy with biopsy, if indicated.'

EXAMINER'S EVALUATION

0 1 2 3 4 5

☐☐☐☐☐☐ Overall assessment of gynaecological history-taking
☐☐☐☐☐☐ Role player's score
Total mark out of 28

DIFFERENTIAL DIAGNOSIS

Menopause

In the UK the average age of menopause is between 51 and 52 years of age. It is usually preceded by the climacteric, which is a transitional phase in which there is an irregular response of the ovaries to pituitary stimuli manifesting as erratic ovulation and menstruation. Menopause before 40 years of age is considered premature. In the early stages of the menopause, a woman may experience a number of symptoms such as hot flushes, insomnia, poor concentration, fatigue, vaginal dryness and a reduced libido.

Amenorrhoea

Amenorrhoea is defined as the absence of a menstrual period in a woman of reproductive age. It is derived from the Greek word *amenorroia*, which means 'a lack of monthly flow'. It becomes clinically significant when there is a failure of menstruation lasting longer than 6 months (or six cycles) in a woman of reproductive age (16–40 years) who is not pregnant. It is subdivided into primary and secondary amenorrhoea depending on the time of onset. Primary amenorrhoea is the complete absence of menses in a 14-year-old with a lack of secondary sexual characteristics or in a 16-year-old with a normal development of sexual characteristics. Secondary amenorrhoea is the cessation of menstruation in a patient who has had periods previously for at least 6 months. Amenorrhoea can be normal in prepubertal girls, pregnancy, lactation, post-menopause and contraception.

Causes of Amenorrhoea	
Primary	**Absence of menses by 14 years with lack of 2° sexual characteristics or by 16 years with normal 2° sexual characteristics**
Familial	Constitutional delay (FH)
Structural	Imperforate hymen, haematocolpos
Genetic	Turner's syndrome, Prader-Willi syndrome
Congenital	Testicular feminisation
Organic	Hypo/hyperthyroidism, adrenal tumours/hyperplasia, PCOS
Other	Anorexia nervosa, psychological, athleticism, drugs (oral contraceptives)
Secondary	**Cessation of menstruation with no periods for at least 6 months**
Hypothalamic	Hypogonadism (Kallmann's syndrome), anorexia nervosa
Pituitary	Hyperprolactinaemia (pituitary hyperplasia/adenoma), Sheehan's syndrome
Ovary	Premature menopause, PCOS, ovarian dysgenesis (Turner's)
Other	Thyroid (hypo/hyperthyroidism), adrenal (hyperplasia, Cushing's syndrome, advanced Addison's disease), pancreas (diabetes)

Menorrhagia

Menorrhagia is defined as the loss of more than 80 mL of blood per cycle. It is often used to describe blood loss that has lasted longer than 7 days. Menstrual periods on average are expected to last a maximum of 5 days with total blood flow of between 25 and 80 mL. Apart from heavy bleeding, patients may complain of symptoms of anaemia. Causes can be both local and systemic (thyroid disease and clotting disorders). However, in around 60% of cases no abnormality can be found and this is known as dysfunctional uterine bleeding. Patients often complain of having to make increased use of sanitary towels or tampons, and they may experience floods or pass clots. Bleeding associated with secondary dysmenorrhoea, which occurs several days before the onset of menstruation, may be indicative of fibroids, endometriosis, adenomyosis or ovarian tumours.

Causes of Menorrhagia	
Structural	Fibroids, endometriosis, adenomyosis, cervical and endometrial polyps, endometrial carcinoma
Infection	Pelvic inflammatory disease (PID), STIs
Drugs	Aspirin, warfarin, chemotherapy
Systemic	Hypothyroidism, clotting disorders (Von-Willebrand's disease)
Other	Intra-uterine contraceptive device (IUCD), sterilisation

Dysmenorrhoea

Dysmenorrhoea, or pain during menstruation, affects approximately 50% of menstruating women. The pain is usually a cramping lower abdominal pain that occurs several days before menstruation and usually subsides by the end of the period. The incidence of dysmenorrhoea is greatest in women in their late teens and early twenties. Primary dysmenorrhoea refers to painful periods occurring in healthy women in the absence of pathology. Secondary dysmenorrhoea is menstrual pain that is due to an underlying disease such as PID, endometriosis, adenomyosis, fibroids, adhesions and endometriosis.

Dyspareunia

The word dyspareunia is derived from the Greek word *dyspareunos*, meaning 'badly mated'. It is defined as pain caused by sexual intercourse. It is broadly divided into two categories, superficial, pain during penetration felt in the introitus, and deep pain felt with penile thrusting deep within the pelvis and against the cervix.

Causes of Superficial and Deep Dyspareunia	
Superficial	**Painful intercourse during penetration felt in the introitus**
Psychological	Fear, ignorance, vaginismus
Infection	Candidiasis, chlamydia, trichomonas, UTI
Vaginal atrophy	Post-menopause (oestrogen deficiency), infrequent intercourse
Organic	Vaginal cancer, rectal cancer, endometriosis
Deep	**Painful intercourse felt with penile thrusting deep in the pelvis**
Cause	PID, cervicitis, endometriosis, adenomyosis

GYNAECOLOGY: **Cervical Smear Test**

INSTRUCTIONS: You are a foundation year House Officer in general practice. Ms Tanner, a 28-year-old lady, has come in for her routine smear test. Carry out the test and necessary examination, explaining to the examiner what you are doing as you proceed.

NOTE: In the OSCE setting you may be provided with a dummy instead of a real patient. Ensure that you treat it with the same courtesy and respect as you would a real patient.

INTRODUCTION

0 1 2

☐☐☐ **Introduction** Introduce yourself. Elicit the patient's name, age and occupation. Establish rapport.

The UK's National Cervical Cancer Screening Programme
The UK cervical cancer-screening programme was introduced in 1988 to prevent cervical cancer. Women are screened between the ages of 25 and 65 years with a 3-year interval for women aged over 25 and a 5-year interval for women aged over 50. Women aged over 65 are tested only if they have not been screened since the age of 50 or have had a recent abnormal test. Samples are taken from the squamo-columnar junction and are investigated for cervical intraepithelial neoplasms (CIN). Cellular abnormalities (dyskaryosis) are graded as mild, moderate or severe. CIN are pre-malignant cells that can develop into cervical cancer.

☐☐☐ **Explanation** Explain to the patient the nature of the examination before seeking consent.

'I will be performing a smear test today. This involves taking a sample from the neck of the womb, which will be checked to make sure there are no abnormalities. In order for me to take the cells, I will have to use a device known as a speculum to keep the walls of the vagina open. I will then place a wooden spatula in the opening to collect the cells from the neck of the womb, which will then be sent to the lab for investigation. The examination may feel a little uncomfortable but should not be painful.'

☐☐☐ **Chaperone** Inform the patient that you will obtain a chaperone.

Expose Adequately expose the patient before examining her.

'If I may ask you to remove the clothing below your waist, lie back on the couch and cover yourself with the sheet I'll provide you with. Call me when you feel comfortable and ready to proceed.'

EQUIPMENT

- Pair of gloves
- Speculum
- Lubricant
- Pencil and investigation form
- Wooden spatula
- Slide
- Alcohol fixative spray

SMEAR TEST

☐☐☐ **Position**

Ask the patient to bring her heels towards her bottom and allow the knees to flop apart.

☐☐☐ **Prepare**

Don a pair of sterile gloves. Adjust the light for maximum visibility and choose an appropriately sized speculum. A medium-sized speculum should be appropriate for most patients, but small and large sizes are also available.

☐☐☐ **Label**

Label the slide with a pencil with the patient's name, date of birth, hospital number and the date when the cervical smear was performed.

Labelling Slide

Label patient's name, date of birth, hospital number and date cervical smear was performed in legible writing

Inspection

Examine the vulva for any redness, irritation, discharge, cysts, warts or any abnormal distribution of hair.

☐☐☐ **Speculum**

Apply lubricant jelly just below the tip of the blades to avoid covering the cervix with the gel. Part the lips of the labia with your non-dominant hand. Hold the speculum so that the tip of the blade is held vertically and insert it gently into the vagina. Rotate through 90° as you progress so the handle is found anteriorly. Warn the patient before opening the blades. Opening the blades will stretch the wall of the vagina, bringing the cervix into view. Lock the blades into position by tightening the screw once the cervix is visualised.

☐☐☐ **Sample Cells**

Introduce the spatula so that the tip rests on the external os and then rotate 360° clockwise and anticlockwise. Remove the spatula and spread the sample firmly onto the slide and then spray with fixative spray.

59

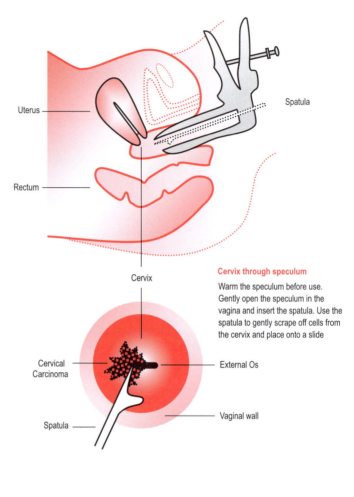

Uterus

Rectum

Spatula

Cervix

Cervical Carcinoma

Spatula

External Os

Vaginal wall

Cervix through speculum

Warm the speculum before use. Gently open the speculum in the vagina and insert the spatula. Use the spatula to gently scrape off cells from the cervix and place onto a slide

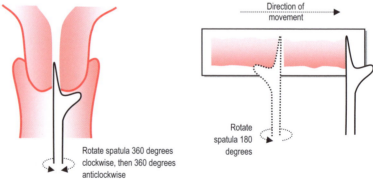

Rotate spatula 360 degrees clockwise, then 360 degrees anticlockwise

Direction of movement

Rotate spatula 180 degrees

☐☐☐ **Remove**	Carefully unlock the blades by loosening the screw and dislodge the speculum from the cervix. Permit the blades to close under pressure from the surrounding walls as you withdraw it from the vagina. Ensure the blades rotate through 90° as the speculum is removed in the reverse manner to how it was initially introduced.
☐☐☐ **Dispose**	Dispose of the speculum and spatula appropriately.

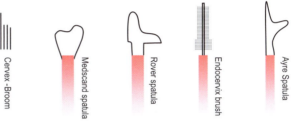

Different Types of Spatulas

Dress	Allow the patient the opportunity to dress herself in privacy.
☐☐☐ **Form**	Complete the investigation form with relevant patient's details (name, date of birth, hospital number), date of request, doctor's name and clinical details.
☐☐☐ **Results**	Tell the patient when the results will be available.

'The results will be sent through the post in 6–8 weeks with a copy sent to your GP. If the results are negative then the cells are healthy and we will see you again for routine check in 3 years' time. If the cervical smear is not negative it may need to be interpreted and explained by your GP. On occasion an inadequate sample may have been taken, which means that you may have to repeat the test.'

Management of Abnormal Cervical Smears

Result	Management
Negative	Inform patient and repeat after 3 years (>25 yr) or 5 years (>50 yr)
Inadequate	Repeat the test within 3 months. If three consecutive inadequate samples are collected, refer for colposcopy
Borderline	Borderline endocervical cells' change – refer for colposcopy

	Borderline squamous cells' change – repeat test within 6 months. Most smears will return to normal. If there are three consecutive borderline squamous cell samples, refer the patient for a colposcopy
Mild Dyskaryosis	Repeat test within 6 months. Most will return to normal. If two tests report mild dyskaryosis, refer for colposcopy
Moderate Dyskaryosis	Refer for colposcopy
Severe Dyskaryosis	Refer urgently for colposcopy

Complications   Inform the patient that she may experience some spotting for a day or two after the examination but it should not be heavy or painful.

Using a Cervex-Brush and Liquid Based Cytology (LBC) Vial

The Cervex-Brush broom is a soft, pyramid-shaped brush that allows the simultaneous collection of ectocervical, endocervical and transformation zone cells in a single sample. It is significantly more efficient than the wooden spatula in obtaining adequate cervical smears and ensuring fewer repeat smears. Numerous studies have showed that liquid-based cytology is more sensitive than conventional cytology.

To collect a cell sample, introduce the broom into the canal approximately 2 cm in length, similar to the length of the brush. Allow the central bristles to lie within the endocervical canal while the outer bristles rest against the ectocervix. Rotate the brush clockwise through only five cycles before removing it from the canal. Next check the expiry date of the liquid-based cytology vial. Apply gentle pressure against the back of the brush head, allowing it to snap off from the main stem and rest inside the preservative vial. Further samples can be placed into the same vial and must be documented in the request form. Apply the cap to the vial and tighten. Document the patient's name, date of birth and date of sample on the vial.

EXAMINER'S EVALUATION

```
0  1  2  3  4  5
☐  ☐  ☐  ☐  ☐  ☐   Overall assessment on performing a smear test
```
Total mark out of 20

GYNAECOLOGY: **Bimanual Examination**

2.3

INSTRUCTIONS: You are a foundation year House Officer in general practice. Ms Okuwawa, a 35-year-old woman, has been experiencing painful heavy periods for a number of years. You have taken a history and wish to perform a bimanual examination. Perform the examination and explain to the examiner what you are doing as you proceed.

NOTE: In the OSCE setting you may be provided with a dummy instead of a real patient. Ensure that you treat it with the same courtesy and respect as you would with a real patient.

INTRODUCTION

0 1 2

☐☐☐ **Introduction** — Introduce yourself. Elicit the patient's name, age and occupation. Establish rapport.

☐☐☐ **Explain** — Ensure the patient understands the nature of the examination before seeking her consent.

'I will be performing an internal examination to ensure the womb and ovaries feel healthy. This will involve introducing two gloved fingers into the vagina whilst lightly pressing on your tummy. The examination may feel a little uncomfortable but it should not be painful.'

Bladder — Ensure the patient has emptied her bladder before proceeding. A full bladder may conceal the vagina.

☐☐☐ **Chaperone** — Inform the patient that you will ask for a chaperone.

☐☐☐ **Expose** — Ask the patient to lie flat on the couch, take off her undergarments and bring her heels up to her bottom and allow her knees to flop apart. Expose her abdomen from the bra line to the pubic hairline. Cover her pelvic region with a towel or drape until you start the internal examination. Ensure that the patient is comfortable and maintain privacy throughout.

☐☐☐ **Abdomen** — Examine the suprapubic region and right and left iliac fossae for tenderness or masses.

BIMANUAL EXAMINATION

Gloves — Don a pair of gloves and adjust the light for maximum visibility.

☐☐☐ **Vulva**

Inspect the vulva for redness, irritation, ulceration, swellings, cyst, warts, prolapse (positive cough impulse) or any abnormal distributions of hair.

☐☐☐ **Labia**

Palpate along the length of the labia majora feeling for any masses (cysts, carcinomas of the vulva) and palpate Bartholin's gland. Normally the gland is not palpable; however, if a non-tender mass is palpable consider a Bartholin's cyst or a Bartholin's abscess if it is red, hot and tender.

☐☐☐ **Lubricate**

Lubricate the fingers of your gloved right hand with K-Y jelly. Part the labia with your thumb and index finger of your left hand.

☐☐☐ **Internal Exam.**

Warn the patient before introducing your index and middle fingers gently into the vagina. Introduce your fingers with the palm facing medially. Gradually turn your hand through 90° so that your palm faces upwards.

Palpation

Palpate the vaginal wall, cervix, uterus and both adnexae in sequence.

Vaginal Wall

Palpate the walls of the vagina before assessing the cervix. Note any tenderness or masses.

☐☐☐ *Cervix*

Palpate the cervix with the fingertips of your right hand checking for tenderness (excitation). Comment on its size, surface, consistency and mobility.

☐☐☐ *Uterus*

Rest your left hand over the suprapubic area. Next, ballot the uterus between your two hands and attempt to catch it between the opposed fingers. Note the uterine size (enlarged – pregnancy, fibroids, endometrial carcinoma), consistency (firm, hard), mobility (immobile – endometriosis), position (retroverted, anteverted), masses (endometrial carcinoma) or tenderness.

☐☐☐ *Adnexae*

Finally, palpate the right adnexae by shifting your left hand over the right iliac fossa and internal fingers towards the right lateral fornix. Palpate the ovary and Fallopian tube (normally impalpable) by attempting to catch the adnexae between the fingers of both hands. Note enlarged ovaries (benign cysts, ovarian carcinoma), masses (ovarian carcinoma) or tenderness (salpingitis).

Repeat the examination on the left side employing the same technique.

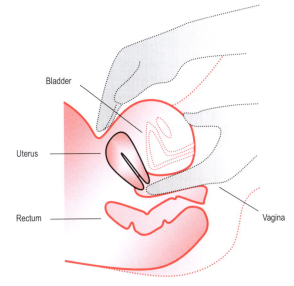

Bladder

Uterus

Rectum

Vagina

Bimanual Examination

Insert two lubricated gloved fingers into the vagina. Rotate your fingers clockwise through 90 degrees. Palpate the vaginal walls, cervix, uterus and adnexae in turn. Note the uterine size, consistency, mobility, position, masses or tenderness. Feel for the adnexae by palpating between the iliac fossa and fornix. Withdraw your fingers noting any blood or discharge

Withdrawal	Remove your fingers in same manner as they were inserted and inspect the glove for any signs of blood or discharge.
▢▢▢ **Dispose**	Throw away any remaining waste. Remove gloves and wash your hands.
Dress	Hand the patient some tissues to wipe herself while providing her an opportunity to dress herself in privacy.

EXAMINER'S EVALUATION

0 1 2 3 4 5
▢▢▢▢▢▢ Overall assessment at performing a bimanual examination
Total mark out of 23

DIFFERENTIAL DIAGNOSIS
Fibroids

Fibroids (also known as leiomyomata) are benign tumours of the smooth muscle of the uterus (myometrium). They are the most common form of neoplasm in females, affecting 40% of all women over 40 years of age and are more common in Afro–Caribbean women. They can be single or multiple and are often round, solid, well circumscribed, nodules that vary in size from a few millimetres to large tumours that can occupy most

65

of the abdomen. They often originate in the wall of the uterus (intramural) and may grow to bulge out of the uterus (subserosal, pedunculated) or inwards towards the cavity (submucosal, intracavitary polyps). Fibroids are oestrogen-dependent and hence increase in size during pregnancy and while the individual is on the combined pill. They reduce in size during the menopause. Patients are often asymptomatic. However, they can complain of heavy and prolonged periods (menorrhagia), dysmenorrhoea and inter-menstrual bleeding (submucosal fibroid). Submucosal fibroids can cause fertility problems including miscarriage and premature labour, whilst large fibroids can cause frequency of urinating or urinary retention due to the pressure applied on the bladder. On examination, a solid mass may be palpated that can be localised within the uterus. Multiple small fibroids may be felt as an irregular enlargement of the uterus.

Ovarian Carcinoma

Ovarian cancer is one of the most common causes of cancer-related deaths in women, commonly affecting western women in their seventh decade of life. In its early phase it exhibits very few symptoms and is only symptomatic once it has progressed and metastasised outside the pelvis. Ovarian cancers are categorised based upon their histology with epithelial carcinomas representing 90% of tumours. Risk factors are associated with the number of ovulations and as a result, early menarche, late menopause and nulliparous women have an increased risk whilst, those with multiple pregnancies, lactation, and a history of oral contraceptive use have a reduced risk. Patients who have a family history of ovarian or breast cancer have an increased risk. Ovarian carcinomas can also be familial via the BRCA1 and BRCA2 gene mutation. Symptoms include abdominal pain and distension, abnormal vaginal bleeding and changes in bowel habit. On examination, an ovarian or pelvic mass may be palpated with ascites. There may be evidence of a pleural effusion, bowel obstruction or breast symptoms due to metastasis.

Cervical Carcinoma

Cervical carcinoma is a malignant cancer of the cervix. It is the second most common female malignancy in the UK. However, its incidence has been falling since the introduction of the cervical screening programme. Overall, 70% of malignancies are squamous carcinomas, 15% are adenocarcinomas and 15% have a mixed pattern. Risk factors include HPV, sex at a young age, multiple sexual partners, promiscuous male partners, smoking and chlamydia infection. Early stages are often asymptomatic. Symptoms of established disease include post-coital bleeding and an offensive vaginal discharge. However, inter-menstrual and post-menopausal bleeding may also be seen. Late features include an altered bowel habit, painless rectal bleeding, haematuria and chronic urinary frequency. These are suggestive of rectum, urethra and bladder involvement, respectively.

Pelvic Organ Prolapse

Pelvic organ prolapse occurs when the pelvic ligaments and the muscular floor of the pelvis become lax and weaken causing the pelvic organs to drop. It is an umbrella term which encompasses a number of different conditions such as cystocele, urethrocele, enterocele, rectocele, uterine or vaginal vault prolapse. Symptoms often depend on the type of prolapse and can include incontinence, frequency of urination, urgency and incomplete bladder emptying (cystocele, cystourethrocele), constipation (rectocele, enterocele), impaired sexual function or heaviness or dragging sensation in the pelvic area, which patients often describe as 'my insides are falling out' (uterine prolapse). On examination, a bulge or fullness is noted in the posterior (enterocele, rectocele) or anterior (cystocele, urethrocele) vaginal wall.

Types of Pelvic Organ Prolapses

Cystocele	Bulging of the bladder into the upper two-thirds of the anterior vaginal wall
Urethrocele	Bulging of the urethra into the lower one-third of the anterior vaginal wall. Often occurs together with a prolapse of the bladder (cystourethrocele)
Enterocele	Herniation of the pouch of Douglas into the upper posterior vaginal wall. Often occurs with a rectocele or uterine prolapse
Rectocele	Prolapse of the rectum into the lower posterior vaginal wall, unlike a rectal prolapse (in which the rectum prolapses out of the anus)
Uterine	Uterus drops down into the vagina. Graded according to level of descent:
1st degree	Uterus drops slightly. Cervix remains in the vagina
2nd degree	Uterus drops further. Cervix protrudes through the introitus
3rd degree	Uterus lies entirely outside the introitus (procidentia)
Vaginal Vault	The top of the vagina (the vault) sags or bulges down into the vaginal canal. Often secondary to a hysterectomy

2.4

INSTRUCTIONS: You are a foundation year House Officer in obstetrics. Mrs Gandhi has grade 3 placenta praevia and has been admitted for elective Caesarean section at 36 weeks. You have been assigned the task of inserting a pre-op urinary catheter. Explain to the patient what you will do and insert the catheter with the equipment provided. Explain to the examiner what you are doing as you proceed.

INTRODUCTION

0 1 2

☐☐☐ **Introduction**   Introduce yourself. Elicit the patient's name, age and occupation. Establish rapport.

☐☐☐ **Explain**   Ensure that the patient understands the nature of the examination before seeking consent.

'As you will be having a Caesarean section we will need to monitor the amount of urine that you will be producing during the procedure. I will therefore have to insert a urinary catheter. This is a simple procedure that involves inserting a small flexible plastic tube through your water pipe and into your bladder. It should not be painful, but may feel a little uncomfortable. Do you have any questions or concerns?'

Consent   Obtain consent before beginning the procedure.

☐☐☐ **Chaperone**   Inform the patient that you will ask for a chaperone.

Equipment   Collect and set up the equipment and place it on the bottom shelf of trolley.

EQUIPMENT

- Catheterisation pack
- Catheter bag
- Sterile gloves
- Lignocaine gel (Instilagel prefilled)
- Three plastic prongs

- Foley catheter 12 or 14
- Antiseptic solution (chlorhexidine)
- Adhesive tape
- 10 mL syringe (+1 green needle)
- 10 mL sterile water

PROCEDURE

★ Trolley

☐☐☐ **Preparation**   Put on an apron, clean the trolley using bactericidal spray and wash hands.

☐☐☐ **Expose**   Ask the patient to lie flat on the couch and take off her undergarments, and bring her heels up to her bottom. Maintain the patient's dignity by covering her with a sheet. Ensure that the patient is comfortable and maintain privacy throughout.

☐☐☐ **Sterile Field** Peel the outer plastic covering of the catheterisation pack and slide the pack onto the trolley. Unwrap the paper covering, touching only the outside of the paper and form a sterile area. Stick the yellow disposable bag onto the side of the trolley. Place the above equipment in a sterile manner into the area. Check the expiry date of the chlorhexidine solution and then pour it into a small pot with swabs (found in catheter pack). Open a 10 mL vial of sterile water and then place it outside the sterile field.

☐☐☐ **Gloves** Don a pair of sterile gloves.

Preparation Squeeze a small amount of lignocaine gel into the cardboard receptacle. Take the 10 mL syringe and attach the green needle to draw up the sterile water. Dip the needle into the vial (outside the sterile field) without touching it (or ask assistance). After drawing up 10 mL, dispose of the needle in the sharps bin and replace the syringe in the sterile field. Finally remove the tip of the end of the catheter sheath.

★ **Patient**

☐☐☐ **Drape & Gauze** Make a hole in the drape and place it appropriately over the patient to maintain a sterile field.

☐☐☐ **Clean Labia** Holding a wet chlorhexidine-soaked swab with a plastic prong, wipe the right labia minor only. Dispose of the swab and prong. Taking a newly soaked swab and prong, cleanse the left labia minor once only, then dispose of this swab and prong. Finally, separate the labia with your left hand using a piece of gauze, take a new wet swab and prong and clean the urethral meatus with your right hand. Dispose of the swab as before.

If there has been any contact between the gloves and the non-sterile area while cleaning, it is important to put on a second pair of sterile gloves before inserting the catheter.

★ Catheter

☐☐☐ **Preparation** — Place the catheter (still in its plastic covering), into the cardboard receptacle and put it between the patient's legs.

Lignocaine — Massage the end of the catheter out by a few centimetres. Dip the tip of the catheter into the LA jelly previously deposited in the receptacle.

☐☐☐ **Insert Catheter** — Hold the labia open with one hand and introduce the catheter tip, via its sleeve, into the urethral orifice by approximately 5–6 cm. Keep the end of the catheter over the receptacle to catch any sudden flow of urine. Once urine starts to flow, advance the catheter a further 1–2 cm to ensure the balloon is in the bladder.

☐☐☐ **Inflate Balloon** — Inflate the catheter balloon with 1 mL of sterile water. Ask the patient to say if she feels any pain. Continue filling slowly with the remaining 9 mL asking patient if she is in any pain and observe the patient's face for grimacing as you inflate the balloon. Gently tug on the catheter to make sure that the balloon becomes lodged in the neck of the bladder.

☐☐☐ **Catheter Bag** — Attach the drainage bag to the end of the catheter and tape the catheter to the thigh.

☐☐☐ **Dispose** — Dispose of waste appropriately.

☐☐☐ **Document** — Document in the notes the size of catheter used and the residual volume of urine initially collected.

EXAMINER'S EVALUATION

0 1 2 3 4 5

☐☐☐☐☐☐ Overall assessment of inserting female catheter
Total mark out of 23

GYNAECOLOGY: **Pessaries and Suppositories**

INSTRUCTIONS: You are a foundation year House Officer in general practice. Mrs Begum is a 41-year-old woman suffering from chronic constipation and vaginal thrush. She has been prescribed Glycerine suppositories and Canesten pessaries as treatment. Explain to the patient how to use her medication and deal with her concerns appropriately.

2.5

INTRODUCTION

0 1 2

□ □ □ **Introduction**   Introduce yourself. Elicit the patient's name, age and occupation. Establish rapport.

□ □ □ **Ideas**   Elicit the patient's understanding of pessaries and suppositories.

'I understand that you have been prescribed Glycerine suppositories for your constipation and Canesten pessaries for your thrush symptoms. Have you ever used these medications before and can you tell me what you understand by them?'

□ □ □ **Concerns**   Elicit the patient's concerns and explore each one of them appropriately.

MEDICAL ADVICE

□ □ □ **Drug Prep.**   Explain why a pessary and suppository have been prescribed and the benefits of such preparations.

'Medications can be taken through a number of different ways other than by mouth. Special drug preparations that take the form of a pellet can be inserted into the back passage. This is known as a suppository. Alternatively, a similarly shaped tablet can be inserted into the vagina. This is known as a pessary. An advantage of these medications is that they can be absorbed locally at the site where the medicine is most needed. Consequently this reduces any side effects occurring elsewhere in the body.'

★ Suppositories

□ □ □ **Method**   Explain to the patient how to use the suppository, maintaining a sensitive approach throughout.

'Your suppository looks a bullet-shaped drug. It will need to be inserted into your back passage. The best time to insert it is after emptying your bowels and at night before you sleep. Before inserting it check that the medicine has not expired, wash your hand and then put on a pair of gloves. Position yourself on your side with one leg straight and the other bent at the knee. Gently insert the capsule about 2–3 cm into your back passage using a finger, making sure it does not slip out immediately. The suppository will then dissolve and be absorbed through the walls of your bowels.'

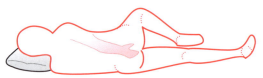

Suppositories

Moisten the suppository before use with water or lubricating jelly. Lie to one side and flex the leg to 90 degrees. Gently insert the suppository into the rectum so it is deep enough not to be expelled

□□□ **Advice**

Give the patent appropriate advice about opening her bowels after taking a suppository.

'You should avoid opening your bowels for at least an hour after inserting it. If you do open your bowels during that time, you may need to insert another suppository for the medicine to have an effect.'

★ Pessaries

□□□ **Method**

Explain to the patient how to use the pessary, maintaining a sensitive approach throughout.

'The pessary is similar to a suppository but instead is inserted in the vagina. Position yourself on the floor with your heels close to your bottom and with your knees relaxed and falling apart. Insert the capsule as far as it will comfortably go. Remain still for a short period afterwards so that it does not fall out of place. The pessary will then dissolve and be absorbed through the walls of your vagina.'

□□□ **Advice**

Give the patient appropriate advice about compliance, periods and contraception after taking a pessary.

'This treatment should not be performed during your menstrual period due to the risk that the pessary is washed out by the menstrual flow. If you are on your period, wait until your period is finished before taking the pessary. You must also be aware that using the pessary can cause damage to condoms and other barrier methods such as diaphragms. Therefore alternative methods of contraception should be considered.'

CLOSING

☐☐☐ **Understanding**   Confirm that the patient has understood what you have explained to them.

☐☐☐ **Questions**   Respond appropriately to the patient's questions.

☐☐☐ **Leaflet**   Offer to give her more information in the form of a handout. Advise her that the leaflet contains much of the information you have mentioned.

COMMUNICATION SKILLS

☐☐☐ **Rapport**   Attempt to establish rapport with the patient through the use of appropriate eye contact. Maintain appropriate body language and an open posture throughout.

☐☐☐ **Fluency**   Speak fluently and do not use jargon.

☐☐☐ **Summarise**   Check with patient and deliver an appropriate summary.

EXAMINER'S EVALUATION

0 1 2 3 4 5

☐☐☐☐☐☐ Overall assessment of pessaries and suppositories
☐☐☐☐☐☐ Role player's score
Total mark out of 28

Sexual Health

SEXUAL HEALTH: **Sexual History**

INSTRUCTIONS: You are a foundation year House Officer in a GUM clinic. Ms Franklin has presented with a vaginal discharge. Take a full sexual history from the patient. Elicit her concerns and answer any questions she may have. You will be marked on your ability to elicit a sexual history.

INTRODUCTION

0 1 2

☐☐☐ **Introduction** Introduce yourself. Elicit the patient's name and age. Establish rapport.

'I would like to ask you some personal questions about your sex life. It is OK if you prefer not to answer some of them. I just want to reassure you that any information you do give me will be treated in the strictest confidence.'

☐☐☐ **Occupation** Enquire about the patient's present occupation.

HISTORY

☐☐☐ **Concerns** Elicit all the patient's presenting concerns. Use open questions and explore the patient's beliefs about their health. For each concern or complaint, elicit the patient's ideas, concerns and expectations.

☐☐☐ **History** For each complaint ascertain the time of onset, presenting features and associated symptoms. Explore each symptom systematically.

☐☐☐ **Discharge** Have you noticed any discharge? Where have you noticed it (in the vagina, urethra, under foreskin, anal)? How long have you had it for? What colour is it? Does it smell (fishy)? Is it itchy?

Different Colours of Discharge

Clear/white	Physiological (increased in pregnancy, puberty, OCP)
White/yellow	Atrophic vaginitis (dyspareunia, soreness, light bleeding), chlamydia (discharge rare, dysuria)
White/grey	Bacterial vaginosis (fishy odour, no itchiness, dysuria, pH >4.5)
Cottage cheese	Candidiasis (redness, itchiness, dysuria, pH <4.5)
Green/grey	Trichomonas (frothy, odour, dyspareunia, itch, inflamed cervix, pH >4.5)
Green/yellow	Gonorrhoea (odour, dysuria)
Red/brown	Cervical/endometrial carcinoma (foul-smelling, weight loss)

☐☐☐ **Urinary Sympt.**   Do you get any burning or pain when passing urine (dysuria)? Are you passing urine more often (frequency)? Are you waking up at night to pass urine (nocturia)? Do you feel that when you want to go to the toilet you must go there and then (urgency)?

☐☐☐ **Pain**   Do you have any abdominal pain (male – penile, testicular)? When did it first start? Is it sharp or dull in nature?

☐☐☐ **Symptoms**   Have you noticed any fevers itchiness, rashes, pain during intercourse (dyspareunia) or joint pains?

SEXUAL HISTORY

☐☐☐ **Active**   Are you currently sexually active or have you been active in the last 3 months?

☐☐☐ **Contacts**   Do you have a regular or casual partner? Male or female? When was the last time you had sex? Currently how many partners do you have? Have they experienced similar symptoms?

☐☐☐ **Type**   Have you practised vaginal sex? Did you use protection? What type did you use (condoms, oral contraceptive pill, diaphragm)? Did you practice oral or anal sex? Did you give it or receive it? Did you use protection?

☐☐☐ **Location**   Have you had sex abroad? Where is your partner from? Do you know if your partner has had sex abroad?

☐☐☐ **STDs and HIV**   Have you or your partner ever had a sexually transmitted disease, such as chlamydia, gonorrhoea or syphilis? Was it successfully treated? Have you or your partner ever had an HIV test?

ASSOCIATED HISTORY

☐☐☐ **Menstrual Hx.**   When was your last period (LMP)? How long do your cycles last? Are your cycles regular? Do you have any pain or bleeding?

Obstetric Hx.   Do you have any children? How many? What type of delivery did they have? Have you had any miscarriages or terminations?

☐☐☐ **Gynae. History**   Have you had a smear test? Was it normal?

Medical History	Do you suffer from any medical illness? Have you ever been admitted to hospital?
☐☐☐ **Drug History**	Do you take any medications? Are you on any oral contraceptive pills?
Social History	Do you smoke? Do you drink alcohol? Do you take recreational drugs?

CLOSING

☐☐☐ **Follow-up**	Say that you would like to perform an examination and take a high vaginal swab (HVS) for culturing. Suggest that you wish check for chlamydia, gonorrhoea and syphilis.
☐☐☐ **Contact Tracing**	Explain to the patient the importance of testing their partners and provide a contact slip.
☐☐☐ **Safe Sex**	Educate the patient about the dangers of unprotected intercourse.

COMMUNICATION SKILLS

☐☐☐ **Rapport**	Establish and maintain rapport with the patient and demonstrate listening skills.
☐☐☐ **Response**	React positively to and acknowledge the patient's emotions.
☐☐☐ **Fluency**	Speak fluently and do not use jargon.
☐☐☐ **Summarise**	Check with the patient and deliver an appropriate summary.

'This is Ms Frankin, who is complaining of a 2-week history of a vulval itch, redness and discharge. She describes the discharge as thick and odourless and is cheese-like in consistency. She does not have any associated symptoms or pain. She is currently engaged in a long-term stable relationship that has lasted for over three years and uses the pill regularly. She has never been treated for STDs nor does her partner describe any symptoms of them. She was prescribed a course of antibiotics 1 month ago by her GP for a chest infection. She is deeply concerned that this is an STD and is worried that her partner is being unfaithful. In view of her history I suspect that this is candidiasis, however, I would like to perform an endocervical swab and HVS to rule out other differentials.'

0 1 2 3 4 5
☐ ☐ ☐ ☐ ☐ ☐ Overall assessment of taking a sexual history
☐ ☐ ☐ ☐ ☐ ☐ Role player's score
Total mark out of 38

DIFFERENTIAL DIAGNOSIS

Candidiasis (Thrush)

Candidiasis is a yeast-like fungal infection of which *Candida albicans* is the most common cause. It is not a sexually transmitted disease. It is the commonest cause of vaginitis, and is found in 20% of all women but it is often asymptomatic. Risk factors include pregnancy, diabetes and recent antibiotic use. Symptoms are often abrupt and include a thick, white cottage cheese-like discharge, with severe pruritus, vulval redness and irritation. The discharge adheres to the vaginal wall and leaves a reddened area on removal. The infection affecting the inner and outer parts of the vulva can spread to include the groin, pubic, inguinal areas and thigh. There may be superficial dyspareunia and dysuria. Symptoms can often be confused with bacterial vaginosis. In men, symptoms include red, irritable, patchy sores on the foreskin or near the head of the penis. These sores can be itchy and painful often burning in nature. Diagnosis is made by taking a swab. On testing the pH is less than 4.5. Alternatively a wet preparation under 10% potassium hydroxide (KOH) will show mycelia and spores.

Bacterial Vaginosis

Bacterial vaginosis is caused by the overgrowth of certain bacteria including *Gardnerella vaginalis*. It is not a sexually transmitted disease but it is the most common vaginal infection in women of childbearing age and can be found in 12% of women. It has been associated with pelvic inflammatory disease, pre-term labour and increased susceptibility to STDs and HIV. It is also more common with women who have had an IUD in situ. Symptoms include a greyish white discharge with a distinct unpleasant fishy odour that occurs especially after intercourse, with an absence of itchiness. However up to 50% of sufferers remain asymptomatic. Diagnosis is made by a swab, with the vaginal pH greater than 4.5, a positive 'whiff' test (the 10% KOH added produces a fishy odour) and the presence of clue cells under microscopy.

Features of Bacterial Vaginosis
Mnemonic: 'Take a whiff and get a clue for fishy bacteria'
Bacterial vaginosis discharge has fishy odour when 10% KOH is added to wet preparation. Clue cells can be seen under microscopy for organism identification

---

Chlamydia

Chlamydia is a common sexually transmitted infection caused by the bacterium *Chlamydia trachomatis*. Around 10% of women below the age of 25 are infected by it, while 75% remain asymptomatic. It can be spread through sexual contact and from the mother to the child at childbirth. If patients are symptomatic they usually present within 1 to 3 weeks after exposure. Chlamydia may initially infect the cervix and the urethra causing lower abdominal pain and a yellow mucopurulent odourless discharge with features of urethritis (dysuria and frequency). If left untreated, the infection may cause chronic pelvic pain, dyspareunia and inter-menstrual bleeding. It may spread to the uterus and Fallopian tubes causing pelvic inflammatory disease (a major cause of infertility), ectopic pregnancies and miscarriages. Men with a chlamydial infection may experience urethral discharge, penile irritation, urethritis and are at risk of epididymitis. Genital chlamydial infection can also cause Reiter's syndrome (arthritis, conjunctivitis, urethritis). Diagnosis is often made by an endocervical swab using immunofluorescent staining or via a urine sample (PCR and ligase chain reaction testing).

Gonorrhoea

Gonorrhoea, otherwise known as the 'clap', is a sexually transmitted disease that is caused by *Neisseria gonorrhoeae*. Overall 80% of women remain asymptomatic. However, when symptoms do appear they usually do so between 2 to 10 days after sexual contact with an infected partner. It presents with urethritis (dysuria and frequency), a greenish yellow foul-smelling discharge, Bartholinitis and cervicitis. Men are more symptomatic and complain of dysuria and yellowish-white discharge from the penis. Homosexual men can develop gonorrhoea in the rectum. Symptoms include pruritus and a painful discharge of bloody pus from the anus. Diagnosis is confirmed by an endocervical swab which on gram staining will reveal gram-negative intracellular diplococci (GNID).

Genital Warts

Genital warts (*Condylomata acuminata*) are a sexually transmitted condition caused by the human papilloma virus (HPV). They can range from flesh-coloured, flat lesions to large cauliflower-shaped structures. They can usually be seen in and around the vagina or cervix, or around the anus, and can be singular or clustered. In men they occur with equal prevalence and appear as warts that affect the tip or, less commonly, the shaft of the penis, scrotum or anus. They can also affect the cervix where they are associated with cervical carcinoma. They do not appear until 2–4 weeks after infection and can be itchy but are usually not painful. Diagnosis is through clinical examination or a swab.

Genital Herpes

Genital herpes is a sexually transmitted disease caused by the herpes simplex viruses type 2 (HSV-2) and occasionally by type 1 (HSV-1). Most individuals are asymptomatic;

however, symptoms can include tiny painful, erythematous vesicles accompanied by ulcers on the labia, vagina, cervix and thighs. Other symptoms include localised oedema, tender inguinal lymph nodes, dysuria, fever and malaise. The primary infection tends to be the most painful, occurring within 2 weeks after initial exposure and lasting up to 2–4 weeks. Secondary infections are less severe and are shorter in duration with the incidence of reactivation decreasing over a period of years. Diagnosis is through clinical examination or viral swab. Serology can be used to show a fourfold rise in an antibody titre.

Trichomoniasis

Trichomoniasis is caused by the single-celled pear-shaped flagellate motile protozoan parasite called *Trichomonas vaginalis*. About 70% of patients are asymptomatic. Symptoms occur within 7 to 28 days after exposure. It presents with profuse amounts of a frothy, greenish yellow, mucopurulent discharge with an offensive fishy odour and dysuria. Other symptoms include superficial dyspareunia, itchiness of the vulva and an inflamed vaginal wall and cervix. It is distinguished from bacterial vaginosis by punctuate 'strawberry' spots found on the cervix. Complications include pre-term labour, low birth weight and increased risk of HIV transmission. Diagnosis is made by directly observing motile trichomonads through a microscope (wet film microscopy) and using a swab (pH >5).

Features of Trichomoniasis
Mnemonic: Five Fs of Trichomoniasis

Flagella shaped protozoan Frothy discharge
Fishy odour (occasionally) Fornication (a STD)
Flagyl (treated with metronidazole)

Syphilis

Syphilis is a sexually transmitted disease caused by the bacterium *Treponema pallidum*. After 21 days from initial exposure, a small, solitary, firm, round painless vulval sore or ulcer, called a chancre, appears denoting the primary stage. The chancre denotes the site of inoculation and usually heals after 4 weeks without treatment. Secondary syphilis may develop a few weeks later with a rough brownish-red papulosquamous rash, which is generalised, symmetrical and non-pruritic in nature affecting the palms of the hand and the soles of the feet. There may be accompanying warty genital or oral growths known as condylomata lata. Other associated symptoms include flu-like symptoms such as fever, swollen lymph glands, sore throat, muscle aches and 'snail-track' ulcers. As secondary syphilis resolves, the infection can progress to the latent phase. This may cause dementia, aortic regurgitation, tabes dorsalis and paralysis. A blood test for syphilis serology (VDRL) reveals an infection but diagnosis is confirmed by examining the exudate from the ulcer, via a swab, through a microscope under dark-ground illumination.

SEXUAL HEALTH: **HIV Assessment and Pre-counselling**

3.2

INSTRUCTIONS: You are a foundation year House Officer in a sexual health clinic. Mr McFadden has attended today, anxious and concerned about a sexual encounter he had on the weekend. Take an appropriate history and deal with his request sensitively.

HISTORY

1 2 3

☐ ☐ ☐ **Introduction** — Introduce yourself. Elicit the patient's name and age. Establish rapport with him.

☐ ☐ ☐ **Occupation** — Enquire about patient's present occupation.

☐ ☐ ☐ **Concerns** — Ask the patient if they have any specific concern that they wish to discuss today (HIV).

'I would like to ask you some personal questions about your recent sexual encounter. It is OK if you prefer not to answer some of our questions. I would like to reassure you that any information you do tell me will be treated with the strictest of confidence.'

'I know this may be difficult to talk about, however, the more information you give to me the more I can help you with your problem.'

FOCUSED SEXUAL HISTORY

☐ ☐ ☐ **Encounter** — When and where (abroad) did it occur?

☐ ☐ ☐ **Partner** — Male or female, regular or casual partner?

☐ ☐ ☐ **Method** — Oral, anal, vaginal? Were they giving or receiving?

☐ ☐ ☐ **Contraception** — Do they normally use condoms, were they using one on this occasion?

☐ ☐ ☐ **Risk** — Do they use any injectable recreational drugs, have they ever paid for sex?

HIV COUNSELLING

☐ ☐ ☐ **Understanding** — Elicit patient's understanding of HIV and testing.

'Have you ever had an HIV test before? Can you please tell me what you understand by HIV?'

☐ ☐ ☐ **HIV and AIDS** — Explain in clear and simple terms the difference between HIV and AIDS.

'HIV is a virus that invades the body and weakens its defences against other infections. It can be passed in different ways, the most common being through unprotected sexual intercourse (between male and female or male and male); or by sharing infected needles. AIDS is a condition, which is caused by HIV and is characterised by specific infections that infect the body as a result of the weakened immune system. The time period between HIV and developing AIDS varies from person to person and can often be many years.'

☐☐☐ **HIV Test**   Explain how the HIV test works.

'We will take some blood from your arm and send this to the laboratory for analysis. When a person has HIV, the body produces antibodies that we can test for. If these antibodies are present it means HIV has been detected; if not, it means you do not have HIV.'

☐☐☐ **Window Period**   Give appropriate advice regarding a possible negative test.

'It is important to appreciate that it can take up to 3 months after being infected with HIV for these antibodies to be produced. In essence we are assessing your HIV status 3 months ago. If you were recently infected because of unprotected sex, then the antibodies may not be present yet and you may get a negative result. This is known as the 'window period' and we may need to repeat the test in a few months to be sure of your status.'

TEST RESULTS

☐☐☐ **Results**   Explain how he will be informed of results.

'As I mentioned previously, everything that we have discussed remains confidential. The same applies for your blood results. We will not ring you or write to you with your results. Rather we will send you an appointment to attend the clinic. Some clinics have the facility to text a negative result to your mobile phone. Would this be of benefit to you?'

☐☐☐ **Implications**   Explain the possible advantages and disadvantages of having the test.

'Before taking the HIV test you may wish to consider what implications the results may have on you. One of the advantages of doing the test is knowing whether you have HIV or not. If positive, we can commence treatment immediately. Although treatment is not curative, it can delay progression to AIDS. Also by knowing your status you can take precautions from spreading the virus to your partner. However, knowing your status may have a negative impact on your relationship with your partner and you may also have to inform your insurance company.'

☐☐☐ **Support Group** Enquire about support network and whether he would like more counselling.

'If the results are positive is there anyone from your friends or family you think you can talk to? We have specially trained professionals who can counsel you if the test is positive. I can put them in touch with you if you think that may help?'

Advantages and Disadvantages of Taking the HIV test
Advantages
1 A positive HIV test result will permit you to start medical treatment as soon as possible to slow the progression of disease
2 Knowing your HIV status will allow you to take steps to prevent transmitting the infection to others

Disadvantages
1 Knowledge that you have acquired the infection
2 An adverse effect on your relationship with your partner since you are at risk of transmission
3 A restriction on your travelling to certain countries
4 A threat to your current employment and future employment prospects especially if you are expected to perform exposure-prone procedures
5 A threat to your ability to obtain new life insurance cover and mortgages that require such cover

CLOSING
☐☐☐ **Understanding** Confirm that the patient understands what has been discussed. Encourage them to ask questions and deal with their concerns accordingly.

☐☐☐ **Follow-up** Mention the need for an outpatient follow-up to review symptoms.

'I'd like to see you in a couple of months' time so that we can discuss the test results with you and see how you're getting on. In the meantime, it is important that you avoid intercourse with your partner or anyone else or at least use barrier condom protection until we are certain you do not have an infection to pass on. If your result does come back as negative it is important that you avoid high risk activities such as sharing needles and having unprotected sex.'

Leaflet Close the interview and offer HIV information leaflet.

COMMUNICATION SKILLS

☐☐☐ **Rapport**   Establish and maintain rapport and demonstrate listening skills.

☐☐☐ **Response**   React positively to and acknowledge patient's emotions.

☐☐☐ **Fluency**   Speak fluently and do not use jargon.

☐☐☐ **Summarise**   Check with patient and deliver an appropriate summary.

EXAMINER'S EVALUATION

0 1 2 3 4 5

☐☐☐☐☐☐ Overall assessment of HIV risk counselling
☐☐☐☐☐☐ Role player's score

Total mark out of 33

INSTRUCTIONS: You are a medical student on an attachment in a family planning clinic. You have been asked to see a patient who wants advice on how to put on a condom correctly. Elicit any concerns and give the appropriate instructions using the plastic training model provided. You will be marked on your communication skills, practical skills and the information given.

3.3

INTRODUCTION

0 1 2

☐☐☐ **Introduction**   Introduce yourself. Elicit the patient's name, age and occupation. Establish rapport with him.

'I understand that you have attended the family planning clinic today to find out more about contraception? Before I discuss this topic, I would like to ask you some questions.'

☐☐☐ **Ideas**   What do you already know about using a condom?

☐☐☐ **Concerns**   Do you have any issues or concerns you would like to raise regarding using condoms?

EXPLANATION

☐☐☐ **Mechanism**   Explain in simple terms what the condom is and how it works.

'The condom is a barrier method of contraception. This means that it works by preventing the sperm from reaching the egg. It fits over the erect penis and is made out of thin latex rubber.'

☐☐☐ **Benefits**   Explain the benefits of using a condom.

'Wearing condoms greatly reduces chances of pregnancy. They also provide considerable protection against sexually transmitted infections (STIs), including HIV, but this protection is not 100%.'

☐☐☐ **Efficacy**   Explain to the patient the efficacy and failure rate.

'When used correctly, a condom is about 98% effective. This means only 2 in every 100 women would get pregnant in the course of a year. This is more effective than other forms of contraception, such as withdrawal or using spermicide on its own.'

☐☐☐ **Partner**   Explain that condom use should be discussed with partner and put on before any genital contact.

'It is important that you discuss with your partner your wish to use condoms. It is important that you put the condom on before there is any genital contact between you and your partner.'

Quality	Stress the importance of using British kite-marked condoms which have undergone thorough quality checks.
□□□ **Expiry Date**	Advise the patient to check the expiry date on the condoms and not to use them if they have expired.
Damage	Advise the patient to check the condom for damage and not to inadvertently tear it with nails or rings when removing it from its packet.

Explaining use of a Condom

Advise the patient to expel the air from the teat and then demonstrate how to successfully roll on a condom on a model. Check for the kite and expiry date before using it. Be careful when opening packet not to inadvertently damage the condom

□□□ **Method**	Advise the patient to expel the air from the teat and then demonstrate how to successfully roll on a condom on a model.

'It is important to squeeze the air out of the 'teat' at the end, otherwise the semen will not be able to collect or enter it if it is full of air. Now roll the condom onto the erect penis, as shown on this model. Do not try putting it on before the penis is erect. Roll it down to the base of the penis, and hold the base down as you penetrate.'

□□□ **Lubricants**	Recommend the patient to avoid oil-based lubricants, such as K-Y jelly or vaseline, which can weaken the condom and predispose it to tears.
□□□ **Withdrawal**	State the importance of holding condom onto base of penis during withdrawal and when removing it to ensure that it has not spilt.

'As soon as you've climaxed, hold the condom firmly onto the base of your penis with your fingers, and withdraw from the vagina, taking care that no fluid is spilt. This is very important. You should check that the condom has not been damaged because this would mean that there is a possibility that semen has escaped and entered the vagina.'

Dispose	Advise the patient to remove the condom, wrap it in paper or tissue, and dispose of it in bin. Warn the patient it is not advisable to reuse a condom. If he

wishes to have sexual intercourse again he should
wash his penis and use a new condom.

☐☐☐ **Fails** Inform the patient of the availability of emergency
contraception if the condom is unsuccessful.

'If the condom tears or you discover that it tore during intercourse, or
it slipped or anything else happened, your partner should consult the
GP or the family planning clinic as soon as possible, where emergency
contraception can be provided.'

CLOSING

☐☐☐ **Understanding** Check and confirm for patient's understanding.

☐☐☐ **Questions** Respond appropriately to patient's questions.

Leaflet Offer to give them more information in the form of a
handout. Advise that the leaflet contains much of the
information you have mentioned.

COMMUNICATION SKILLS

☐☐☐ **Rapport** Establish and maintain rapport and demonstrate
listening skills.

☐☐☐ **Fluency** Speak fluently and do not use jargon.

☐☐☐ **Summarise** Check with patient and deliver an appropriate
summary.

EXAMINER'S EVALUATION

0 1 2 3 4 5
☐☐☐☐☐☐ Overall assessment of explaining the use of a condom
☐☐☐☐☐☐ Role player's score
Total mark out of 29

INSTRUCTIONS:
You are a medical student on an attachment in a family planning clinic. You have been asked to see a patient who wants advice on how to put on a diaphragm and cap correctly. Elicit any concerns and give appropriate instructions. You will be marked on your communication skills and the information given.

3.4

INTRODUCTION

0 1 2

☐☐☐ **Introduction**

Introduce yourself. Elicit the patient's name, age and occupation. Establish rapport with her.

'I understand that you have attended the family planning clinic today to find out more about contraception? Before I discuss this topic, I would like to ask you some questions.'

☐☐☐ **Ideas**

What do you already know about using a diaphragm or cap?

☐☐☐ **Concerns**

Do you have any issues or concerns you would like to raise regarding this type of contraception?

EXPLANATION

☐☐☐ **Mechanism**

Explain in simple terms what the diaphragm and cap are and how they work.

'Diaphragms and caps are barrier methods of contraception. This means that they work by preventing the sperm from reaching the egg. They also work with spermicides, which are chemicals that destroy sperm. The diaphragm and cap fit inside your vagina and cover the neck of the womb. The diaphragms are larger and dome shaped with flexible rims, while cervical caps are similar but are smaller in size.'

☐☐☐ **Benefits**

Explain the benefits of using a diaphragm and cap.

'Wearing a diaphragm or cap greatly reduces your chances of pregnancy. They also provide some protection against STIs, but this protection is far from 100%.'

Advantages and Disadvantages of the Diaphragm or Cap

Advantages	Can be put on at any time before sex
	The woman is in control of the method and can use it as required
	It provides some protection against cervical cancer and STIs (should be used in conjunction with condoms)

	Effective with no serious health risks if used with care
Disadvantages	May take time to put on correctly with loss of spontaneity
	Requires handling of own genitalia
	Insertion may disrupt sex with some loss of sensation (uncommon)
	Spermicides can be untidy and cause irritation
	Urine infections can be associated with diaphragms
Contraindicated	Uterovaginal prolapse, poor vaginal tone, recurrent UTIs, rubber allergy, toxic shock syndrome, acute vaginitis, aversion to touching genitalia

☐☐☐ **Efficacy**

Explain to the patient the efficacy and failure rate.

'When used correctly, a cap or diaphragm is about 92–96% effective. This means between 4 to 8 people in every 100 women using this method would get pregnant in the course of a year. However, if it is not used according to the instructions, it is likely that more women will get pregnant.'

☐☐☐ **Partner**

Explain that the cap or diaphragm should be put on before any genital contact.

☐☐☐ **Damage**

Advise the patient to check the diaphragm or cap for damage and not to inadvertently tear it with her nails or rings when removing it from its packet.

☐☐☐ **Insertion**

Advise the patient how to insert the diaphragm and cap into the vagina.

Diaphragm

'Wash your hands. Apply two strips of contraceptive (spermicide) cream, 1 inch in length to both sides of the diaphragm. Add a small amount to the rim as well. Find a suitable position that is comfortable for you when inserting it. You can stand with one leg propped up or squat with your knees apart. Alternatively you can lie on your back with your knees kept up. Hold the diaphragm by putting your index finger in the dome and squeezing the rim with your thumb and fingers. Slide the folded diaphragm into the vagina pushing it downwards and backwards. Use your index finger to push the rim and fit it into place. Check that it covers your cervix by feeling the neck of the womb underneath the dome. Ensure that the diaphragm is secure in place at the front and back of the cervix.'

Cervical Cap

'Wash your hands. Fill one-third of the cap with contraceptive cream but do not apply it to the rim as the cap stays in place by suction. Squeeze the cap between your thumb and two fingers. Insert into the vagina and place the cap tightly over the neck of the womb. Once it is in place add more spermicide cream.'

☐☐☐ **Removal**   Explain how to remove the cap and diaphragm.

'If the cap or diaphragm is not securely in place or you wish to take it out, hook your finger under the rim and gently pull it downwards and out. Do not remove it for at least 6 hours after intercourse. However, do not leave it in for more than 30 hours at a time.'

Lubricants   Recommend that the patient avoids oil-based lubricants, such as K-Y jelly or vaseline, which can weaken the seal of the cap or diaphragm.

☐☐☐ **Reusable**   Explain to the patient that the diaphragm or cap can be reused. Ensure that it is regularly washed in warm soapy water and rinsed thoroughly. Check it regularly for tears or holes.

Bath   Advise the patient to insert the device after a bath since the spermicide may be washed away if it is inserted before bathing.

☐☐☐ **Check-up**   Advise the patient to visit her GP or nurse every 6 to 12 months to ensure that the device fits correctly.

☐☐☐ **Failure**   Inform the patient of the availability of emergency contraception if the diaphragm or cap is unsuccessful.

CLOSING

☐☐☐ **Understanding**   Check and confirm that the patient has understood the instructions.

☐☐☐ **Questions**   Respond appropriately to the patient's questions.

Leaflet   Offer to give her more information in the form of a handout. Advise that the leaflet contains much of the information you have mentioned.

COMMUNICATION SKILLS

☐☐☐ **Rapport**   Establish and maintain rapport and demonstrate listening skills.

☐☐☐ **Fluency**   Speak fluently and do not use jargon.

☐☐☐ **Summarise**   Check with the patient and deliver an appropriate summary.

0 1 2 3 4 5

☐ ☐ ☐ ☐ ☐ ☐ Assessment of explaining the use of diaphragm
☐ ☐ ☐ ☐ ☐ ☐ Role player's score

Total mark out of 30

3.5

INSTRUCTIONS: You are a foundation year House Officer in a general practice. Ms Johnson has asked to be started on the oral contraceptive pill. Elicit any concerns she has and give appropriate instructions. You will be marked on your communication skills and the information given.

INTRODUCTION

0 1 2

☐☐☐ **Introduction** — Introduce yourself. Elicit the patient's name, age and occupation. Establish rapport with her.

☐☐☐ **Ideas** — Why do you want to start using the oral contraceptive pill? What do you understand about the oral contraceptive pill?

☐☐☐ **Concerns** — Do you have any specific concerns regarding the oral contraceptive pill?

ASSOCIATED HISTORY

☐☐☐ **Sexual History** — Are you currently sexually active? Are you using any forms of contraception? What type have you been using and for how long? Have you been using it occasionally or all the time? Have there been any problems with the current type or method?

☐☐☐ **STIs** — Have you or your partner ever had a sexually transmitted infection, such as chlamydia, gonorrhoea or syphilis? Was it successfully treated?

☐☐☐ **Menstrual Hx.** — When was your last period (LMP)? How long do your cycles last? Are your cycles regular? Do you have any pain or bleeding?

☐☐☐ **Obstetrics Hx.** — Do you have any children? Are you currently breast-feeding? Is there any chance that you could be pregnant?

SUITABILITY AND CONTRAINDICATIONS

☐☐☐ **Explain** — 'I need to ask you a few questions to find out if the pill is suitable for you or whether you need some other form of contraception.'

Absolute	Breast-feeding (<6 wk postpartum), PE, DVT, IHD, CVA, migraine with aura, breast cancer, chronic liver disease or liver tumours, smoker (>15/day + >35-years old)
Relative	Smoker (<15/day + >35-years old), HTN, obesity, risk factors for arterial disease, DM with vascular disease, cervical cancer
Drugs Reducing Efficacy	Rifampicin, carbamazepine, phenytoin, phenobarbitone, antibiotics

MEDICAL ADVICE

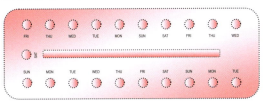

Oral Contraceptive Pill (OCP)

OCP should be taken continuously for 21 days without interruption. Then allow for a 7-day break. Not all patients are suitable for the pill

□□□ **Mechanism**

Explain in simple terms how the contraceptive pill works.

'The oral contraceptive pill contains two hormones, oestrogen and progesterone, which are similar to the two the body naturally produces. It works by changing the body's hormone balance so that you do not release an egg each month from your ovary. It also makes it difficult for sperm to enter the womb to fertilise an egg and thins the uterus lining making it difficult for a fertilised egg to attach to.'

□□□ **Method**

Explain to the patient how to take the combined oral contraceptive pill.

'Begin the pill on the first day of your next period. Then take the pill at the same time once a day for the next 21 days. Take a break for 7 days, during which time you may have a withdrawal bleed. However, during this break you will continue to be protected as long as you restart the next pack on time.'

□□□ **Efficacy**

Explain to the patient the efficacy and failure rate.

'If taken properly the pill is 99% successful in preventing pregnancy. However you need to take the pill regularly and at the same time each day.'

□□□ **Mishap**

Inform the patient what will happen if she misses a single pill.

'If you miss a pill, the advice we give is to carry on taking your regular pills and take the missed pill as soon as possible. You will not need to use protective barrier methods or an emergency contraceptive pill.'

'If you vomit within 3 hours of taking a pill, take another pill as soon as possible. If you are able to keep this pill down then you will continue to be protected from pregnancy.'

Latest Guidelines for 'Missed Pill Rule' – 2005

Mishap	Women are advised to 'just keep going' and take the missed pill as soon as possible and return to their normal routine
Missed a Pill	If she has missed only one pill, she should take the missed pill as soon as possible and continue taking the remaining pills at the regular time. This may mean that she takes two pills on the same day and even takes them at the same time (depending when she remembers missing a pill). She will not require barrier methods nor emergency contraception
> One Pill	If she misses more than one pill, she should take the last missed pill and continue taking the remaining pills as per usual. However, abstinence or condoms should be considered for 7 days if:
'Two for 20':	2 (or more) of 20 mcg ethinylestradiol pills are missed
'Three for 30':	3 (or more) of 30 mcg ethinylestradiol pills are missed
Week 1	She should consider emergency contraception if she has missed pills (2 for 20 mcg, 3 for 30 mcg) in the first week and had unprotected sex
Week 3	She should not have a pill-free interval if the missed pills (2 for 20 mcg, 3 for 30 mcg) occurred in the third week. She should then start a new pack immediately once the current pack is completed. This will mean she does not need to use emergency contraception

☐☐☐ **Advantages**

Explain to the patient the benefits of taking the pill.

'The pill is a very effective form of contraception. It often makes periods lighter, less painful and more regular. It reduces the risks of developing certain cancers such as ovarian and endometrial cancer.'

☐☐☐ **Disadvantages**

Explain to the patient the disadvantages of taking the pill.

'Most women who take the pill do not develop any side effects. However, common side effects can include nausea, headache, weight gain and mood alterations. It is also known to be associated with an increased risk of developing blood clots in the legs (DVT) and lung (PE). There is also a slightly increased risk of developing breast and cervical cancer.'

STIs

'It is also important to be aware that the pill does not protect against sexually transmitted infections and so will require barrier protection with condoms in addition if at risk.'

Side Effects of Oral Contraceptives
Mnemonic: 'CONTRACEPTIVES'

Cholestatic jaundice	**E**levated blood sugar (DM)
Oedema (corneal)	**P**orphyria, **P**igmentation, **P**ancreatitis
Nasal congestion	**T**hyroid dysfunction
Thromboembolism (DVT, PE)	**I**ntracranial hypertension
Raised BP	**V**omiting (progesterone only)
Acne, **A**lopecia, **A**naemia	**E**rythema nodosum, **E**xtrapyramidal effects
CVA, TIA	**S**ensitivity to light

Interaction

Explain to the patient the common drug interactions that reduce the efficacy of the pill (antibiotics, anti-TB drugs, antiepileptic medication).

'There are a number of drugs that can reduce the effectiveness of the pill. It is important to inform your GP or your pharmacist that you are taking the pill when you take other medications such as common antibiotics, anti-epileptic medication and treatment for tuberculosis. You may need to use additional forms of contraception (condom) for at least 2 weeks.'

Alternatives

Suggest other forms of contraception if the patient is not suited to using the oral contraceptive pill. Explain to the patient the reasons for the incompatibility.

CLOSING

Understanding

Check and confirm that the patient understands the instructions.

Questions

Respond appropriately to the patient's questions.

Leaflet

Offer to give her more information in the form of a handout. Advise that the leaflet contains much of the information you have mentioned.

COMMUNICATION SKILLS

Rapport

Establish and maintain rapport and demonstrate listening skills.

☐☐☐ **Fluency**   Speak fluently and do not use jargon.

☐☐☐ **Summarise**   Check with the patient and deliver an appropriate summary.

EXAMINER'S EVALUATION

0   1   2   3   4   5

☐☐☐☐☐☐   Assessment of explaining the combined pill

☐☐☐☐☐☐   Role player's score

Total mark out of 34

INSTRUCTIONS: A 15-year-old girl visits you in the A&E department. She appears frightened and scared. She states that her previous form of contraception has failed and wants emergency contraception. Deal with her request appropriately.

3.6

NOTE: It is unlawful for doctors to provide contraceptive advice and treatment to a child under the age of 16 without parental consent unless he or she is 'Fraser competent'. The child can give consent to treatment only if she understands its nature, purpose and hazards and if the proposed treatment is in the child's best interest. Also, reasonable efforts have to be made to persuade the child to consult her parents.

HISTORY

0 1 2

☐☐☐ **Introduction** — Introduce yourself. Elicit the patient's name, age and occupation. Establish rapport with her.

☐☐☐ **Ideas** — Why do you want to use the emergency contraceptive pill?

☐☐☐ **Concerns** — Do you have any specific issues or concerns you would like to raise regarding the emergency contraceptive pill?

ASSOCIATED HISTORY

☐☐☐ **Sexual History** — Take a detailed sexual history including the time and type of intercourse and the reason for failure.

Time — When was the last time you had sexual intercourse? Several hours or days ago?

Type — Did you practise penetrative sex? Did you use protection? What type did you use (condoms, oral contraceptive pill, the diaphragm)?

Mishap — Was there a failure with the contraception (condom split, hole in diaphragm, forget to take pill)? Has this ever occurred in the past?

☐☐☐ **Menstrual Hx.** — When was your last period (LMP)? How long do your cycles normally last? Are your cycles regular?

Obstetrics Hx. — Do you think you are pregnant? Have you been pregnant in the past?

| **Medical History** | Do you suffer from any medical illnesses? Have you ever been admitted to hospital? |
| **Drug History** | Do you take any medications? Are you on any oral contraceptive pills? |

SUITABILITY AND CONTRAINDICATIONS

☐☐☐ **Explain**   Ascertain whether the patient has any contraindications for taking this form of contraception. Use the table below to guide you.

Contraindications of Emergency Contraceptive Pill (ECP)
Pregnancy, vaginal bleeding, arterial disease, liver adenoma, porphyria

---

MEDICAL ADVICE

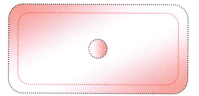

Emergency Contraception

The emergency contraceptive pill should be taken within 72 hours of unprotected sexual intercourse. It comes as a single 1.5 mg levonorgestrel (Levonelle 1500) tablet (previously two 0.75 mg tablets)

☐☐☐ **Mechanism**   Explain in simple terms how the emergency contraception works.

'The emergency contraceptive pill contains a high dose of a progestogen hormone that is similar to what the body naturally produces. It works by changing the body's hormone balance and therefore prevents or postpones an egg from being released (ovulation) and makes it more difficult for the fertilised egg to settle in the womb.'

☐☐☐ **Method**   Explain to the patient how to take the emergency contraceptive pill.

'Take the pill as soon as possible after unprotected sex. It should be taken within 72 hours of intercourse.'

☐☐☐ **Efficacy**   Explain to the patient the efficacy and failure rate.

'We advise all patients that the emergency contraceptive pill should be used only in an emergency as it is not as effective as other forms of contraception. It prevents around 95% of pregnancies from developing if it is taken within 24 hours of unprotected sex; and the sooner it is taken the more effective it is.'

Efficacy of Emergency Contraception (Levonorgestrel)	
Time after intercourse	% of pregnancies prevented
<24 hours	95
24–48 hours	85
48–72 hours	58

☐ ☐ ☐ **Side Effects** — Explain to the patient the side effects of taking the emergency contraceptive pill.

'Side effects include feeling nauseous, vomiting, breast tenderness, headaches, dizziness and tiredness. Often side effects are mild and tend to disappear after a few hours. If you are sick and vomit within 3 hours of taking the pill then you will require a replacement dose.'

Period — Explain to the patient possible alteration of her monthly cycle.

'By taking this pill your next period may be a few days earlier or later than expected. However, do visit your GP or a doctor if your next period is more than 7 days later than expected, as you may require a pregnancy test.'

Abdo Pain — Explain to the patient the warning symptoms of ectopic pregnancy.

'Visit your doctor directly if you notice any lower abdominal pains or vaginal bleeding over the next 2–6 weeks (ectopic pregnancy).'

☐ ☐ ☐ **Alternatives** — Suggest other forms of emergency contraception including the intra-uterine device.

'The IUD or intra-uterine device works by stopping an egg from being fertilised or implanted in the womb. It can be fitted up to 5 days after unprotected sex and is more effective (prevents 98% of pregnancies) than the emergency contraceptive pill. However, it is considered more invasive than the pill.'

☐ ☐ ☐ **Contraception** — Explain that the emergency contraceptive pill should not replace her usual form of contraception; rather it should solely be used for emergencies.

☐ ☐ ☐ **Education** — Stress the importance of practising safe sex with contraception.

☐ ☐ ☐ **Pregnancy Test** — Offer the patient a pregnancy test prior to prescribing the emergency contraceptive pill.

CLOSING

☐ ☐ ☐ **Understanding** — Confirm that the patient has understood what you have explained to her.

□□□ **Questions**   Respond appropriately to the patient's questions.

   Leaflet   Offer to give her more information in the form of a handout. Advise that the leaflet contains much of the information you have mentioned.

COMMUNICATION SKILLS

□□□ **Rapport**   Establish and maintain rapport and demonstrate listening skills.

□□□ **Fluency**   Speak fluently and do not use jargon.

□□□ **Summarise**   Check with patient and deliver an appropriate summary.

EXAMINER'S EVALUATION

0 1 2 3 4 5

□□□□□□ Assessment of explaining emergency pill

□□□□□□ Role player's score

     Total mark out of 33

INSTRUCTIONS: You are a foundation year House Officer in a general practice. Mrs Shakespeare is a 30-year-old teacher who is interested in taking Depo-Provera and would like to know more about it. Deal with her request appropriately.

3.7

HISTORY

0 1 2

□ □ □ **Introduction**   Introduce yourself. Elicit the patient's name, age and occupation. Establish rapport with her.

□ □ □ **Ideas**   Why do you want to use Depo-Provera?

□ □ □ **Concerns**   Do you have any specific issues or concerns you would like to raise regarding this form of contraception?

Depo-Provera (Injectable Contraception)
Depo-Provera is a progestogen-containing contraceptive injection. The active ingredient is 150 mg of depot medroxyprogesterone acetate (DMPA). It is given every 3 months (12–13 weeks) intramuscularly. It works by inhibiting follicular development and preventing ovulation. Under 'perfect attendance' the first year failure rate is 0.3%. However, its average efficacy is 97%. Because of its prolonged action it should never be given without counselling the patient

SUITABILITY AND CONTRAINDICATIONS

□ □ □ **Explain**   Ascertain whether the patient has any contraindications for taking this form of contraception. Use the information below to guide you.

Contraindications of Depo-Provera
Absolute   Pregnancy (delay 6 weeks postpartum before commencing), DVT, PE, CVA, serious liver disease (hepatitis, cirrhosis, tumours), breast cancer, undiagnosed vaginal bleeding, known hypersensitivity to Depo-Provera

MEDICAL ADVICE

□ □ □ **Mechanism**   Explain in simple terms how Depo-Provera works.

'Depo-Provera is a form of contraception that is delivered as an injection. It contains progesterone (medroxyprogesterone acetate), which is a chemical that is naturally found in your body. It works in three different ways. Firstly, it puts your ovaries to sleep, preventing the release of an egg. Secondly, it thins the lining of your womb, preventing the egg from attaching securely. Finally, it makes the mucus in the neck of your womb thicker, preventing sperm from reaching your womb.'

☐☐☐ **Efficacy**

Explain to the patient the efficacy and failure rate.

'It is very effective and has a failure rate of less than 1%, which means that in every 100 sexually active women using it only 1 on average will become pregnant over the course of a year.'

☐☐☐ **Method**

Explain to the patient how the Depo-Provera is administered.

'The injection is given into the buttock every 12 weeks. If it is given in the first 5 days of your menstrual cycle it provides immediate protection. On any other day you will require extra protection for 7 days using barrier methods, such as the condom.'

Depo-Provera Injections

150mg of DMPA IM injections taken every 12 weeks. Effective immediately if taken during the first 5 days of the menstrual cycle. Requires 7 days to take effect if given after the period cycle. Does not protect against STIs

☐☐☐ **Advantages**

Explain to the patient the benefits of using intramuscular contraception.

'Depo-Provera provides long-lasting protection against pregnancy without the side effects of the combined pill. It is also highly effective and does not interfere with sex. It is safe while breast-feeding and offers some protection against cancer of the womb.'

☐☐☐ **Disadvantages**

Explain to the patient the disadvantages of using intramuscular contraception.

'It is important to note that 9 out of 10 women who take Depo-Provera will stop having periods after a year of use, whilst others may

| | | experience irregular periods. Once the injections have stopped, there is usually a delay of up to 18 months before fertility returns fully.' |

Side Effects		'Side effects include headaches, weight gain, breast tenderness and mood swings.'
STIs		'The Depo-Provera does not protect against STIs so you will require barrier protection with condoms in addition if you are at risk.'

CLOSING

☐☐☐ **Alternatives**   Suggest other forms of contraception if the patient is not suited to use Depo-Provera or the treatment is contraindicated. Explain to the patient the reasons for such incompatibility.

☐☐☐ **Understanding**   Confirm that the patient has understood what you have explained to her.

☐☐☐ **Questions**   Respond appropriately to the patient's questions.

Leaflet   Offer to give her more information in the form of a handout. Advise that the leaflet contains much of the information you have mentioned.

COMMUNICATION SKILLS

☐☐☐ **Rapport**   Establish and maintain rapport and demonstrate listening skills.

☐☐☐ **Fluency**   Speak fluently and do not use jargon.

☐☐☐ **Summarise**   Check with the patient and deliver an appropriate summary.

EXAMINER'S EVALUATION

0 1 2 3 4 5

☐☐☐☐☐☐   Assessment of explaining the Depo-Provera method
☐☐☐☐☐☐   Role player's score
Total mark out of 28

SEXUAL HEALTH: **Contraceptive Implant**

INSTRUCTIONS: You are a foundation year House Officer in general practice. Mrs Butt is a 30-year-old housewife who is interested in using the Implanon device and would like to know more about it. Deal with her request appropriately.

HISTORY

0 1 2

☐☐☐ **Introduction**   Introduce yourself. Elicit the patient's name, age and occupation. Establish rapport.

☐☐☐ **Ideas**   Why do you want to use the Implanon device?

☐☐☐ **Concerns**   Do you have any specific issues or concerns you would like to raise regarding this form of contraception?

Implanon (Contraceptive Implant)
Implanon is a single-rod contraceptive subdermal implant that is inserted into the medial aspect of the non-dominant upper arm. It releases approximately 40 mcg of etonorgestrel a day over a 3-year period. It works primarily by preventing ovulation but also increases cervical mucus viscosity inhibiting sperm penetration. The typical failure rate is 0.05% and it must be inserted by a trained health professional. Its effects are rapidly reversible with normal fertility returning within days of its removal

SUITABILITY AND CONTRAINDICATIONS

☐☐☐ **Explain**   Ascertain whether the patient has any contraindications for taking this form of contraception. Use the table below to guide you.

Contraindications of Implanon

Absolute	Pregnancy (delay 6 weeks postpartum before commencing), DVT, PE, CVA, serious liver disease (hepatitis, cirrhosis, tumours), breast cancer, breast-feeding (<6 wks postpartum), undiagnosed vaginal bleeding, known hypersensitivity to Implanon

MEDICAL ADVICE

☐☐☐ **Mechanism**   Explain in simple terms how the Implanon device works.

'Implanon is a small flexible tube that is 40 mm long and 2 mm wide (the size of a matchstick) which is placed under the skin of the upper arm. It contains a chemical that is similar to the naturally occurring female sex hormone, progesterone. Progesterone is released slowly into the blood stream at a steady rate. It works by changing the body's hormone balance and therefore prevents an egg from being released (ovulation) and makes it difficult for the fertilised egg to settle in the womb by making the lining of the womb thinner. It also makes the mucus in the neck of the womb thicker, preventing the sperm from entering the womb.'

☐☐☐ **Efficacy**

Explain to the patient the efficacy and failure rate.

'It is very effective and has a failure rate of less than 1%, which means that in 100 sexually active women using it only 1 will become pregnant over the course of a year.'

☐☐☐ **Inserted**

Explain to the patient how the Implanon is placed.

'Implanon is put in the inner side of the upper arm. A local anaesthetic is injected to numb the skin. Then an incision is made where the implant will be placed using an applicator. The procedure can take less than a minute. Some patients may have pain and bruising for a few days.'

☐☐☐ **Protection**

Give appropriate advice regarding the insertion of the Implanon device in relation to the patient's cycle.

'If inserted in the first 5 days of your menstrual cycle it provides immediate protection. However, on any other day of your cycle, you will require extra protection for 7 days by using barrier methods, such as condoms.'

☐☐☐ **Remove**

Explain to the patient when and how the Implanon device should be removed.

'Implanon provides contraception for 3 years and requires replacing after this. In order to remove the Implanon device a small cut is made under local anaesthetic and then it is removed with small forceps.'

☐☐☐ **Advantages**

Explain to the patient the benefits of the Implanon device.

'One of the advantages of the Implanon device is that it lasts for 3 years and you do not need to worry about contraception during this time. It is extremely reliable, does not interfere with sex and is safe while you are breast-feeding. It is also rapidly reversible in that within a very short time after its removal, your blood hormone levels return back to normal.'

☐☐☐ **Disadvantages**

Explain to the patient the disadvantages of the Implanon device.

'Some of the disadvantages include unpredictable changes to your periods. Most women experience irregular bleeding in the first year. However, after 1 year most settle back to a regular pattern. Some women experience infrequent and light periods and occasionally no periods at all (amenorrhoea).'

Side Effects	'Side effects include headaches, weight gain, breast tenderness and mood swings.'
STIs	'Implanon does not protect against STI so you will require barrier protection with condoms in addition if you are at risk of STDs.'
☐☐☐ **Alternatives**	Suggest another form of contraception if the patient is not suited to Implanon or there are contraindications for using it. Explain to the patient the reasons for her incompatibility.

CLOSING

☐☐☐ **Understanding**	Confirm that the patient has understood what you have explained to her.
☐☐☐ **Questions**	Respond appropriately to the patient's questions.
Leaflet	Offer to give her more information in the form of a handout. Advise that the leaflet contains much of the information you have mentioned.

COMMUNICATION SKILLS

☐☐☐ **Rapport**	Establish and maintain rapport and demonstrate listening skills.
☐☐☐ **Fluency**	Speak fluently and do not use jargon.
☐☐☐ **Summarise**	Check with the patient and deliver an appropriate summary.

EXAMINER'S EVALUATION

0 1 2 3 4 5

☐☐☐☐☐☐ Assessment of explaining the Implanon device

☐☐☐☐☐☐ Role player's score

Total mark out of 30

SEXUAL HEALTH: **Intra-uterine Device (IUD)**

You are a foundation year House Officer in General Practice. Mrs Anderson is a 35-year-old housewife who is interested in using the intra-uterine device and would like to know more about it. Deal with her request appropriately.

INTRODUCTION

0 1 2

☐☐☐ **Introduction** — Introduce yourself. Elicit the patient's name, age and occupation. Establish rapport.

☐☐☐ **Ideas** — What do you already know about the intra-uterine device?

☐☐☐ **Concerns** — Do you have any specific issues or concerns you would like to raise regarding this form of contraception?

ASSOCIATED HISTORY

☐☐☐ **Menstrual Hx.** — When was your last period (LMP)? How long do your cycles last? Are your cycles regular? Do you have any pain or bleeding?

☐☐☐ **STIs** — Have you or your partner ever had a sexually transmitted infection, such as chlamydia, gonorrhoea or syphilis? Was it successfully treated?

Obstetric Hx. — Do you have any children? Are you currently breast-feeding? Is there any chance that you could be pregnant?

SUITABILITY AND CONTRAINDICATIONS

☐☐☐ **Explain** — Ascertain whether the patient has any contraindications for using this form of contraception. Use the table below to guide you.

Contraindications of IUD	
Absolute	Pregnancy, fibroids, severe anaemia, STI, unexplained vaginal bleeding, uterine malignancy, PID, copper allergy, Wilson's disease

MEDICAL ADVICE

☐☐☐ **Mechanism** — Explain in simple terms how the intra-uterine device works.

'The intra-uterine device is a small T-shaped apparatus, often containing copper, that is inserted into the womb. It is approximately the size of a matchstick with threads that should hang out a little from your vagina. These help you to identify whether the device is in place. It works by making it difficult for the fertilised egg to settle in the womb and grow.'

☐☐☐ Efficacy

Explain to the patient the efficacy and failure rate.

'It is a highly effective form of contraception and tends to have a failure rate between 0.2–2%. This means that in 100 sexually active women using it less than 2 will become pregnant over the course of a year.'

☐☐☐ Method

Explain to the patient how the IUD will be placed.

'The intra-uterine device can be inserted only by a trained health professional. This usually takes place during your period. While you are lying on a couch a speculum is inserted into the vagina, similar to having a smear taken. The device is then inserted through the neck of your womb. The procedure is quite straightforward but you may suffer from some slight discomfort.'

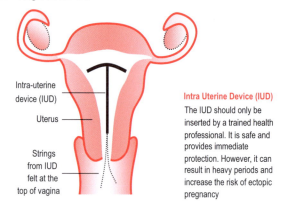

Intra-uterine device (IUD)

Uterus

Strings from IUD felt at the top of vagina

Intra Uterine Device (IUD)
The IUD should only be inserted by a trained health professional. It is safe and provides immediate protection. However, it can result in heavy periods and increase the risk of ectopic pregnancy

☐☐☐ Advantages

Explain to the patient the benefits of using the intra-uterine device.

'One of the advantages of the IUD is that it is very safe. It provides immediate protection and doesn't interfere with intercourse. It also has a long lifespan of up to 8 years and can be removed at any time.'

☐☐☐ Disadvantages

Explain to the patient the disadvantages of using the intra-uterine device.

'Some of the disadvantages include experiencing painful, heavy periods and an increased risk of developing infection or inflammation of the pelvis (PID). There is a very small possibility (1 in 1000) of the device puncturing the womb. There is also a slight chance that the device could fail and that a pregnancy takes place outside of your womb (ectopic pregnancy). In this unlikely event, you should seek urgent medical advice.'

STIs 'An IUD does not protect against STIs so you will require barrier protection with condoms in addition if you are at risk of STDs.'

Side Effects of Intra-Uterine Devices (IUDs)
Mnemonic: 'PAIN'

Period that is late	**I**ncrease in body temperature
Abdominal cramps	**N**oticeable vaginal discharge

☐☐☐ **Check Threads** Stress the importance of checking the threads of the IUD.

Alternatives Suggest other forms of contraception if the patient is not suited to an IUD or there are contraindications for using it. Explain to the patient the reasons for the incompatibility.

Contraindications for Intra Uterine Devices
Mnemonic: 'Please Don't Ever Put-up Contraceptives'
Pregnancy, **D**UB, **E**ctopic pregnancy, **P**ID, **C**arcinoma (cervical)

CLOSING

☐☐☐ **Understanding** Confirm that the patient has understood what you have explained to her.

☐☐☐ **Questions** Respond appropriately to her questions.

Leaflet Offer to give her more information in the form of a handout. Advise that the leaflet contains much of the information you have mentioned.

COMMUNICATION SKILLS

☐☐☐ **Rapport** Establish and maintain rapport with her and demonstrate listening skills.

☐☐☐ **Fluency** Speak fluently and do not use jargon.

☐☐☐ **Summarise** Check with patient and deliver an appropriate summary.

EXAMINER'S EVALUATION

0 1 2 3 4 5
☐☐☐☐☐☐ Assessment of explaining the IUD
☐☐☐☐☐☐ Role player's score
Total mark out of 30

Paediatrics

INSTRUCTIONS: You are a foundation year House Officer in paediatric outpatients. Mrs Cooper has brought in her 7-year-old son for an appointment. Take an appropriate history. You will be marked on your interviewing skills and ability to elicit the history.

NOTE: When taking a paediatric history, it is important to adapt your history-taking around the child's age. Certain questions become more significant for a toddler than a teenager. Ensure you address questions to both the parent and the child when appropriate.

4.1

INTRODUCTION

0 1 2

☐☐☐ **Introduction**   Introduce yourself and establish rapport.

☐☐☐ **Name & Age**   Elicit the child's name (preferred as well as official) and confirm the relationship of the adult accompanying the child. Elicit the age of the child in years and months or days and weeks for babies.

HISTORY

☐☐☐ **Complaint**   Elicit all the patient's presenting complaints.

☐☐☐ **History**   When did it first start? What did you first notice? When was the child last well? Did it come on suddenly or gradually? Is it getting better or worse? Have you ever had it before? Has the child been exposed to unwell individuals (e.g. siblings)?

Cough   Has he had a cough? Is it worse during the day or the night? Is it made worse by exercise? What does it sound like (barking, a whoop, wet or dry)? Is there an associated wheeze? Any sputum or catarrh?

Fever   Have you been feeling hot? How high did the temperature go? Is it a swinging fever? Any shaking (rigors) or fits (seizures)? Have you taken any medication? Any headaches or intolerance to light (photophobia)? Any rashes (face/trunk/nappy area)? What does it look like? Does it change colour when pressed (blanching/non-blanching)?

Number of Days Rash Appears after Initial Infection
Mnemonic: 'Very Sick People Must Take Early Retirement'

Day 1	Varicella	Day 5	Typhus
Day 2	Scarlet fever	Day 6	Enteric fever (typhoid)
Day 3	Pox (small)	Day 7	Rubella
Day 4	Measles		

D and V

How many times has he passed stools (neonates – wet nappies)? Are the stools loose, watery or fully formed? Any blood, mucus or tummy pain? Is there any pain associated with feeding? Does he pass urine everyday? How many times has he vomited? Is the vomiting related to meals? Is there projectile vomiting (pyloric stenosis)? Is there any associated fever? Does he feel nauseous? What colour is the vomit? Is there any blood?

Seizures

Did he have a fever before the fit? How long did it last for? Did he bite his tongue? Did he wet himself or lose consciousness? Were his limbs jerking? Did he feel sleepy or drowsy afterwards?

Systemic Rvw

Does he have any pain anywhere? Has he been constipated? Is he playing normally? Has he passed urine? Has he been drowsy or irritable? Does he have any lumps anywhere? Any sweats?

☐☐☐ **Concerns**

Do you have any particular concerns or worries about the symptoms your child is experiencing? Do you know what may be causing them?

☐☐☐ **Impact on Life**

How have these symptoms affected his life? And his family?

Principles of Good Paediatric History Taking

1 **Listen attentively to the mother (or the parents):** The mother is correct until proven otherwise. Elicit her ideas and worries regarding her child's illness
2 **Take a thorough history:** Ascertain the chronological order of the symptoms and explore each one individually, taking note of the speed of onset, duration, character and frequency of pattern. Include a detailed past medical, family, social, developmental, immunisation and birth history
3 **Engage the child:** Listen to the child carefully. He may be able to give a surprisingly detailed account of their illness. Ensure their account of events is corroborated by their parents

4 **Tailor the history:** Take into account the child's age. Use appropriate vocabulary and props (toys and teddy bears). Do not be patronising or dismiss anything the child may say

ASSOCIATED HISTORY

□□□ **Medical History**   Ascertain a history of any serious medical illnesses (asthma, epilepsy, diabetes) or operations. Any skin problems (eczema)? Has he ever been jaundiced or suffered from seizures? Is there a history of repeated GP or A&E attendance? Any previous SCBU admissions?

□□□ **Birth History**   How was the childbirth? Were there any maternal illnesses during pregnancy (diabetes, blood pressure, IUGR, viral infections)? Any problems or complications (prolonged labour)? Normal or assisted delivery? Full term or early birth? Any illnesses or problems after birth (growth, heart, breathing, jaundice)?

□□□ **Maternal Hx.**   Any problems during pregnancy (oligohydramnios, pre-eclampsia, diabetes, medication, harmful substances, viral illness such as hepatitis B, varicella, HIV? Any problems after pregnancy (over/underweight)?

Feeding   Ask when solids were introduced, whether the child was breast-fed or bottle-fed and if there were any problems during weaning. If the patient is an infant, ask the parent if the infant is being breast-fed or bottle-fed, how often they are fed and how many bottles per day.

Development   Ask for the child's red book, if appropriate. Check the child's height, weight and head circumference and record the centiles. Ask the parents if they have any concerns regarding the child's growth, weight and development. If appropriate for the child's age, ask about developmental milestones achieved so far (see chapter 4.5 on child development).

Failure to Thrive in Children
Assessing for failure to thrive in young children
The term, 'failure to thrive' is used to describe infants or toddlers whose rate of weight gain or growth is suboptimal. It is important that regular and accurate measurements of height and weight are taken and recorded

over time. The values are then plotted on a centile chart, which can reveal signs of failure to thrive. A single observation out of context provides little information but a consistent fall across two major centile lines over time is suggestive of failure to thrive

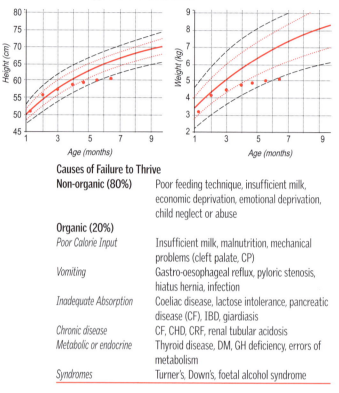

Causes of Failure to Thrive

Non-organic (80%)	Poor feeding technique, insufficient milk, economic deprivation, emotional deprivation, child neglect or abuse
Organic (20%)	
Poor Calorie Input	Insufficient milk, malnutrition, mechanical problems (cleft palate, CP)
Vomiting	Gastro-oesophageal reflux, pyloric stenosis, hiatus hernia, infection
Inadequate Absorption	Coeliac disease, lactose intolerance, pancreatic disease (CF), IBD, giardiasis
Chronic disease	CF, CHD, CRF, renal tubular acidosis
Metabolic or endocrine	Thyroid disease, DM, GH deficiency, errors of metabolism
Syndromes	Turner's, Down's, foetal alcohol syndrome

□□▫ **Well-being**

What is the child's mood or demeanour usually like? Have there been any changes recently? Is the child eating and drinking normally? Does the child have any sleeping problems?

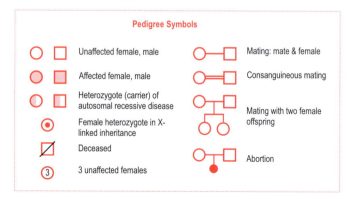

☐☐☐ **Immunisations** Confirm with the parents which immunisations the child has had to date. Ask the parents if they have brought with them a record of immunisations.

☐☐☐ **Family History** Are there any illnesses that run in the family (cystic fibrosis)? Are the parents related (consanguinity)? How are the other siblings? Draw a pedigree chart to assist you.

☐☐☐ **Drug History** Does the child take any regular medication? Does he have any allergies (to medications, food, pets)?

☐☐☐ **Social History** Take a detailed history of the home and school circumstances.

Home Who lives at home with the child? Are there any problems at home? What do the parents do for a living? Does anyone at home smoke?

School How are things going at school? Is the child in the appropriate year? Is he performing well? Any concerns of bullying?

COMMUNICATION SKILLS

☐☐☐ **Rapport** Establish and maintain rapport with the child and parent whilst demonstrating listening skills.

☐☐☐ **Summarise** Check with the patient (and parent) and deliver an appropriate summary.

'This is Johnny, a 7-year-old boy brought in by his mother, with a 3-day history of wheezing. The wheeze is worse at night and is associated with temperature and dry cough. There is no shortness of breath on exertion or whilst playing. He is eating and drinking well and passing a good volume of urine. The mother has not noticed any rash nor has the child been drowsy at any time. He suffered from eczema as a child, and his eldest sister suffers from asthma. He has been feeling tired and has not attended school for the last 2 days. Mum has not given any medication and is concerned that her son may be asthmatic. In view of the history, I suspect that Johnny is suffering with an upper respiratory tract infection (viral wheeze). However, I would like to exclude asthma as a possible cause.'

EXAMINER'S EVALUATION

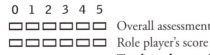

0 1 2 3 4 5
☐☐☐☐☐☐ Overall assessment of paediatric history
☐☐☐☐☐☐ Role player's score
Total mark out of 28

COMMON CHILDHOOD PRESENTATIONS
Headache

Headaches occur commonly in children and are rarely due to underlying organic disease. One of the most important conditions to consider in any sick child and particularly in a sick child with a headache is meningitis. In all ages, symptoms to look for include fever, nausea and vomiting, drowsiness and fitting. In infants, a heightened irritability, high pitched crying and a bulging fontanelle should alert you to meningitis, whilst in older children early symptoms include a headache with photophobia and neck stiffness. Where there is a strong suspicion of bacterial meningitis, early initiation of treatment with intravenous antibiotics is vital.

Tension headaches are common and usually present with a generalised ache or tightness around the head, typically of mild to moderate severity. They usually last for a few hours and can occur on a daily basis for a number of weeks. They have no associated aura or neurological features. They are often associated with poor sleep and problems at home or school.

Migraines are recurrent headaches which are usually severe or moderate and last for up to 72 hours. They are often unilateral and throbbing in nature and can be associated with nausea, vomiting, abdominal pain, photophobia and visual aura (in some cases aura can occur without headache). It is quite common for there to be a strong family history. Management involves avoiding known or common triggers (e.g. bright lights, certain foods), analgesia for acute episodes and preventative drugs as prophylaxis.

Further investigation following history and examination should be considered if there has been an increase in the severity and frequency of headaches, a history of behavioural change, neurological signs present on examination or if there are features in the history and examination suggestive of raised intracranial pressure.

Fits (Seizures)

Fits are fairly common in children. By the age of 11 years approximately 6% of children would have experienced one. Neonatal seizures can occur as a result of birth injury, infections, developmental problems or metabolic disorders. They are especially common in the first few weeks following birth.

Febrile convulsions are the most common form of seizures seen in pre-school children. They are caused by elevated body temperature (usually as a result of upper respiratory tract infections), can occur from a few months after birth and can affect children until about the age of 5 years. The seizures are usually generalised and clonic in nature and do not last for longer than 15 minutes. Management is mainly aimed at educating parents in the use of antipyretic drugs, cooling the child and seeking emergency help when appropriate.

Idiopathic epilepsy is the term used for recurrent seizures that are not associated with fever and have an unknown cause. It should always be considered following a seizure in a previously healthy child. Seizures can present as either generalised (including tonic-clonic, absence and myoclonic seizures) or partial (either simple partial or complex partial). Investigations include EEG testing (which is abnormal in more than half of cases) although it is often extremely difficult to make a definitive diagnosis. Management aims to prevent seizures through the use of prophylactic anticonvulsant therapy.

Respiratory Complaints

Upper respiratory tract infections occur more commonly than lung disease in children and are usually viral. A history should always enquire about general malaise and fever. Examination should always include the ears, nose and throat. Asthma is becoming increasingly common in children, and a history should focus on looking for diurnal variation in symptoms, dry cough, wheeze (although children with asthma may cough instead of wheeze), environmental irritants (dust, smoke), associated illness (eczema) and family history. Common causes of a persistent cough in children include asthma, postnasal drip, chronic rhinorrhoea and environmental irritants (e.g. cigarette smoke). In a child with a history of recurrent cough productive of sputum, cystic fibrosis should be considered.

Rash

Napkin dermatitis (nappy rash) is common and can occur as a result of irritation from wet nappies, prolonged contact with urine or faeces, infections (bacterial and candida) and other skin disorders (e.g. psoriasis). Treatment involves changing wet nappies promptly, careful perineal washing and drying and application of barrier creams.

Cradle cap is a crusty, thick, brownish rash occurring on the scalp of infants. It is non-itchy and can be treated with oils and shampoos. It can develop into seborrhoeic dermatitis, a generalised inflammatory skin reaction affecting other parts of the body. Areas commonly affected include the neck, axillae and groins (sebum-gland rich areas). Like cradle cap, seborrhoeic dermatitis is not irritant and is self limiting, resolving within a few weeks.

Impetigo is a highly contagious skin infection (spread via direct contact with lesions) which mainly occurs in young children and is usually caused by *Staphylococcus aureus* (*Streptococcus pyogenes* is also implicated in complicated cases). Following infection, a blister forms which ulcerates and produces pus which dries and produces golden brown crusts. The skin underneath is often itchy and this increases risk of spread to other areas or close contacts. Due to the highly contagious nature of this condition, children should be kept away from school until they are better and must also use separate towels. Treatment is initially by washing with water and a suitable antiseptic soap, with topical (and oral if indicated) antibiotics if necessary.

Atopic eczema is characterised by red, flaky and itchy skin following exposure to triggers such as certain foods, allergens and irritants. It is increasing in prevalence, currently affecting about 15–20% of school children. There is also a strong association with a family history of atopy, asthma and hay fever. The condition has a fluctuating course and resolves in about 50% of children by the age of two, with the remainder continuing to suffer from it. Treatment involves avoidance of all soaps and scented body washes, and using copious amount of emollients and ointments instead. Other agents that can be used when necessary include topical steroids, antihistamines and antibacterial creams. Oral antibiotics are reserved for systemic infections. Measures aimed at reducing symptoms and severity include cotton underclothes (rather than wool), mittens worn at night to prevent scratching and light bandaging of limbs at night.

Psoriasis is a condition affecting the skin (and joints) in which there is a development of red circumscribed patches topped with silvery plaques. The lesions are non-itchy and are usually found over extensor surfaces (e.g. elbows and knees) as well as the scalp. Psoriasis appears to have a strong genetic component, usually affects sufferers after the age of 10 and precipitant factors in children include stress. Coal tar preparations form the mainstay of treatment.

Gastrointestinal Complaints

Presenting symptoms include abdominal pain, vomiting, diarrhoea and constipation. Acute abdominal pain is highly non-specific in children. Non-organic origin is suggested by pain which is central, the presence of a family history, vomiting, a tense personality and the absence of abnormal signs, abnormal growth and normal blood tests. Appendicitis classically presents with a history of central abdominal pain which has moved to the right iliac fossa and is worsened on moving and coughing. Mesenteric adenitis also presents with right iliac fossa pain. Pyelonephritis presents with loin pain and a positive urine dipstick. Intussusception is bowel prolapse into an adjacent section and usually occurs at the terminal ileum or ileo-caecal junction. It is the most common cause of bowel obstruction in the first two years of life and presents with paroxysmal pain, vomiting, indrawing of the legs to the chest, followed by 'red currant jelly' stool (stool mixed with mucus and blood). Immediate treatment is by performing a barium enema which reduces the intussusception and also confirms diagnosis. However, if unsuccessful, surgery is indicated.

Chronic abdominal pain is a common problem affecting around 1 in 10 school children. In the majority of cases no organic cause is found. Appropriate investigation following history and examination would include urinalysis, routine blood tests and culture. In many cases the abdominal pain is coexistent with emotional problems and a family history of irritable bowel syndrome may also be present. Where an organic cause is suspected, further investigation may include abdominal ultrasound and upper gastrointestinal endoscopy.

Bedwetting (Enuresis)

Enuresis is generally regarded as inappropriate voiding of urine when the child is of an age where control is expected. A more specific definition is repeated urination into bed or clothes in a child aged 5 or more years, which has occurred for a duration of 3 or more months at a frequency of at least two times a week. It usually occurs at night (nocturnal enuresis). Nocturnal enuresis occurs more commonly in boys and in lower social classes and is associated with a positive family history. Causes include a general developmental delay and stressful events (especially around the time when micturitional control is being learnt). Underlying illness or side effects of medication need to be reliably excluded before a diagnosis is made. Most children with enuresis do not suffer from psychological disorders or other illnesses, and conditions associated with urinary symptoms (e.g. urinary tract infection, diabetes) rarely present with enuresis. Treatment strategies begin with encouragement (e.g. enuresis diary, with rewards for dry nights), followed by conditioning therapy (enuresis alarm systems which detect bed wetting, sound the alarm, and cause the child to waken and go to the toilet). Drugs are used to a limited extent in the treatment of nocturnal enuresis as the rate of relapse following withdrawal of medication is high. Drugs used include tricyclic antidepressants and antidiuretics. Daytime enuresis occurs more commonly in girls and is usually due to urge incontinence secondary to bladder instability. Management involves eradicating any associated urinary infection, encouraging the child to go to the toilet more frequently and timed voiding.

INSTRUCTIONS: You are a foundation year House Officer in paediatrics. Mrs Ridley has brought James, an 11-year-old boy, to see you. She is very concerned about the headaches and is demanding a CT scan. Take an appropriate history and offer advice. You will be marked on your interviewing skills, ability to elicit the history and on the advice that you give.

4.2

INTRODUCTION

0 1 2

☐☐☐ **Introduction** — Introduce yourself and establish rapport.

☐☐☐ **Name & Age** — Elicit child's name and age as well as relationship to the adult.

☐☐☐ **Ideas** — Elicit patient's (mother's) ideas about what may be causing the headaches.

☐☐☐ **Concerns** — Establish any concerns (CT scan to exclude brain tumour) or fears the mother may have regarding the symptom.

FOCUSED HISTORY

Headaches — Ask the patient (and mother) all relevant questions regarding the headaches including site, onset, character, radiation, etc. (**mnemonic – SOCRATES**).

☐☐☐ *Site* — Where exactly is the pain? Could you please point to it? Does it affect one side or both sides of your head?

☐☐☐ *Severity* — How bad are these headaches? Are they affecting your school work? Have you missed any days off school?

Onset — When did you first notice the pain? What were you doing at the time? Did it come on quickly or slowly?

☐☐☐ *Character* — Can you describe what the pain feels like? Does it feel like it is beating (pulsating), a needle prick (sharp) or aching (dull) pain? Does it feel like a tightening rope passing across your forehead (band-like)?

Signs and Symptoms of Migraines
Mnemonic: 'POUNDing'

Pulsating	**N**ausea
HOurs (between 1 and 72 hrs)	**D**isabling
Unilateral	

Radiation — Does the pain move anywhere?

Relieving	Does anything make the pain better (posture)? Does sleeping make it go away? Are the headaches better on weekends or days off school (stress/school related)?
▢▢▢ *Aggravating*	Does anything make the headache worse? Such as coughing, moving your head, foods (caffeine, cheese, chocolates), flashing lights, lack of sleep?

Triggers for Migraines

Triggers can be behavioural, environmental, dietary, chemical or hormonal

Behavioural	Stress (school, bullying), anxiety, too much or too little sleep, missing meals
Environmental	Smoking (passive/active), bright lights, flickering lights (computer screens), loud noises, perfumes, motion sickness
Dietary	Tyramine-containing products (aged cheese, red wine, smoked fish), nitrates and nitrites (preserved meat, bacon, hotdogs, pork) and monosodium glutamate (MSG – flavour enhancer). Others include chocolate, citrus fruits, dairy products, lack of water, alcohol, caffeine (coffee, tea, colas)
Hormonal	Oral contraceptives, menstruation
Chemical	Excessive use of analgesics (NSAIDs)

Timing	When do the headaches come on (morning, afternoon, after school)? Do they wake you up? How long do they last for?
Exertion	Is the pain worse on playing or doing sports?
▢▢▢ *Symptoms*	Have you noticed anything else such as feeling sick, vomiting or tummy pain? Have you had a fever or skin rash? Do get pain when you look at a strong light (photophobia) or hear loud sounds (phonophobia)? Have you had any blurred vision or flashing lights? Do you have any stiffness in your neck (meningeal irritation)? How is your concentration? Have you had any change in your behaviour (angry and irritable, sad and depressed)? Have you had any pins or needles over your face or body? Do you feel sleepy all the time (drowsiness)?

Early Signs of Meningitis

1 Pale dusky skin with cyanotic discolouration of lips
2 Temperature and cold peripheries
3 Severe leg pain

☐☐☐ **Head Injury**   Have you hit your head or had a fall recently?

☐☐☐ **Medical History**   Ascertain a history of any past serious medical illnesses (asthma, epilepsy, diabetes) or operations. Has he ever been jaundiced or suffered from seizures? Is there any history of repeated GP or A&E attendances? Does the patient wear glasses (or have difficulty reading the blackboard)? When was the last eye test?

☐☐☐ **Family History**   Does anyone in the family suffer with migraines? Are there any inherited family disorders?

Drug History   Current medications and what medicines have been attempted for the headache. Any drug allergies?

☐☐☐ **Social History**   Any stress at home or bullying at school? Is the child in the appropriate year? Is he performing well or have there been concerns with poor performance?

COMMUNICATION SKILLS

☐☐☐ **Rapport**   Establish and maintain rapport with the child and parent whilst demonstrating listening skills.

☐☐☐ **Response**   React positively to and acknowledge patient's and mother's emotions.

☐☐☐ **Fluency**   Speak fluently and do not use jargon.

☐☐☐ **Summarise**   Check with the patient and deliver an appropriate summary.

'Thank you very much for telling me about your son's problems and bringing him today. I understand you are very concerned about his headaches, in particular about the possibility of a brain tumour, and that you would like a computed tomography scan to exclude this. I would like to reassure you, having taken a full history from both you and your son, that I believe it is highly unlikely that James has a brain tumour. Brain tumours are extremely rare in children and in addition to this James's symptoms are highly suggestive of a common migraine. As a result a CT scan would not be indicated or assist the diagnosis.'

EXAMINER'S EVALUATION

0 1 2 3 4 5

☐☐☐☐☐☐ Assessment of taking the headache history

☐☐☐☐☐☐ Role player's score

Total mark out of 32

DIFFERENTIAL DIAGNOSIS
Childhood Migraine

The word 'migraine' is derived from the Greek words *hemi-* and *krania*, meaning 'half-sided headache'. It can affect up to 5% of children, with prevalence increasing throughout childhood. Classically, migraines present as severe pulsating headaches frequently located in the temples or frontal head regions. They are different from adult forms of migraine in that the headaches are more often bilateral and shorter in duration. They may be associated with visual (scotoma, fortification spectra, hemianopia) or gastrointestinal disturbances (nausea, vomiting and abdominal pain) as well as photophobia and phonophobia. The headaches may last between 1 and 72 hours and are aggravated by physical activity but relieved by sleep. Occasionally, there is a history of migraines amongst other first-degree or second-degree relatives. They are broadly categorised into four different groups: migraine without auras, migraine with auras, childhood periodic syndromes (abdominal migraines) and retinal migraines. An abdominal migraine is a variant that occurs in young children in which the child complains of nausea, vomiting, anorexia and abdominal pain. The abdominal pain is a paroxysmal midline pain lasting less than 72 hours. Aura and headaches are often minimal. Unfortunately, most children with abdominal migraine will develop migraine headaches later on in life.

Migraine Classification	
Without Aura	Common migraine (5 or more episodes, headache <72 hours, pulsating, moderate to severe, bilateral or unilateral, aggravated by movement, nausea and vomiting, photophobia and phonophobia)
With Aura	Migraines that are preceded (by 30 min) with visual sensations (flashes, lines, hemianopia, blurred vision, blindness, visual hallucinations) or motor (hemiplegia) symptoms. Overall 5% of children have auras without a headache
Periodic Syndrome	Childhood periodic syndromes include cyclical vomiting, abdominal migraine, benign paroxysmal vertigo of childhood
Retinal Migraine	Migraine headaches with repeated attacks of monocular visual symptoms, including scintillations, scotomata or blindness

Tension Headaches

Tension headaches are the second most common form of headaches in children and often occur in the older school-aged child. They differ from migraines in that they have greater chronicity and frequency but are less severe and associated features can be absent. They are brought on by emotional and psychological factors such as stress, anxiety and depression. The headaches are bilateral and non-pulsating in nature described as band-like aches. They last from 30 minutes to 7 days, are mild to moderate in severity but are not aggravated by movement. They occur in the absence of nausea or vomiting but can present with either photophobia or phonophobia, but not both.

Sinusitis

Sinusitis is the infection or inflammation of one or more of the paranasal sinuses (frontal, ethmoid, maxillary, sphenoid) resulting in the obstruction of the normal drainage mechanisms. It can be acute (<4 weeks), subacute (4–12 weeks) or chronic (>12 weeks) in nature. Symptoms include facial pain over the affected sinuses, headache, fever, facial swelling and tenderness, nasal congestion and purulent discharge. Children may also complain of a daytime cough and persistent nasal discharge. The condition often resolves within 10 days of onset.

Raised Intracranial Pressure

A child with suspected raised intracranial pressure constitutes a medical emergency. However, it is important to note that this is a very rare cause of headache in children but represents the greatest anxiety in parents. Raise intracranial pressure increases the risk of a cerebral herniation where the brain shifts from its normal compartments within the skull across dural structures distorting the cortex, brainstem and vascular supply, and results in potential irreversible injury or death. Clinical manifestations vary with age but commonly the patient describes a headache that is worse on lying down and is associated with blurred vision, nausea, morning vomiting, irritability and lethargy. The headache and vomiting are usually worse in the morning and often wake the child from sleep. There may be an associated change in personality or a change in school performance. On examination, the child is hypertensive, bradycardic and with irregular respiration (Cushing's triad). A sixth nerve palsy may be noted that is a false localising sign. Papilloedema is the most reliable sign for raised ICP but often appears late in presentation. Other features include a change in pupil reaction, seizures, increased confusion, a tense or bulging fontanelle and distended scalp veins (in infants). The most common causes include cerebral oedema (a tumour, abscess, haemorrhage or infarct), hydrocephalus, trauma, infection and space-occupying lesions.

PAEDIATRICS: **Neonatal Examination**

INSTRUCTIONS: You are a foundation year House Officer in paediatrics. Ms Turner delivered a new baby boy 12 hours before and now wishes to be discharged. Please carry out an appropriate examination of the neonate and determine whether the newborn may be discharged. Explain to the examiner what you are doing as you proceed.

NOTE: In the OSCE setting you will be provided with a manikin instead of a real neonate. It is important to handle the manikin and exam it with the same respect as if it were a child.

EXAMINATION

0 1 2

☐☐☐ **Introduction** Introduce yourself. Establish rapport with the mother.

Request Request the maternal obstetric notes. Check blood results, ultrasound scans and general comments.

☐☐☐ **History** Take a brief obstetric and birth history from the mother. Establish if there were any maternal illnesses during the pregnancy. Ascertain the type of delivery and whether any anaesthesia or instruments had been used.

Enquire about the condition of the child at birth and the Apgar scores at 1 and 5 minutes. Establish if there were any resuscitative measures used or problems during the birth. Briefly ask if the baby had passed urine (in first 12 hours) and meconium (passed within 48 hours of birth).

Signs	Score of 0	Score of 1	Score of 2
Appearance	Blue	Blue at extremities, pink trunk	Normal pink
Pulse	Absent	<100 bpm	>100 bpm
Grimace (reflex irritability)	None	Grimace/feeble cry	Sneeze/cough/ pulls away, cries
Activity	None, floppy	Some flexion	Active movement
Respiration	Absent	Weak or irregular	Loud cry

APGAR Score (out of 10)

The APGAR score is a useful tool that allows an instant assessment of a newborn to determine if he or she requires immediate medical care

| **Consent** | Explain the examination to the mother and seek consent to perform it. |
| ☐☐☐ **Wash Hands** | Wash your hands, and undress the baby completely, including removing the nappy. If you are unsure whether the baby will be calm by the end of the examination you may wish to consider auscultating the heart now before he or she becomes restless. |

INSPECTION

| **General** | Stand at the edge of the bed and observe the baby. Note the baby's appearance, colour, posture, tone, movements and breathing. |
| ☐☐☐ *Appearance* | Check for dysmorphic features, signs of birth trauma, rashes and baby's size. |

Appearance in the Neonatal Examination

Colour	Jaundice, peripheral cyanosis, pallor, rashes, petechiae (purple spots)
Dysmorphic changes	Dysmorphia, cleft lip, epicanthic folds, single palmar crease, large tongue (Down's syndrome), small jaw and tongue (Pierre-Robin syndrome)
Birth trauma	Caput succedaneum, subconjunctival haemorrhages, moulding, cephalhaematoma, forceps marks
Birth marks	Mongolian blue spots, stork bite, strawberry mark, erythema toxicum, miliaria, congenital melanocytic naevi, café au lait spots
Baby's size	Foetal malnutrition. Weigh the baby and check the weight for length ratio

Posture	Look for hemiparesis, 'pithed frog' position or opisthotonos (rigidity, arched back, head thrown backwards).
Tone	Look at the head, arms and legs for generalized hypertonicity (stiff) or hypotonicity (floppy – Down's syndrome).
☐☐☐ *Movements*	Watch limb movements for asymmetrical or abnormal movements (myoclonus, convulsions).
☐☐☐ *Breathing*	Observe the neonate's pattern of breathing, respiratory rate, and chest wall movements and note any added sounds.

Chest Shape	Pectus carinatum, pectus excavatum, over-inflation
Pattern of Breathing	Regular or irregular
Respiratory Rate	Normal (30–50 breaths per minute)
	Dyspnoea (laboured breathing)
	Tachypnoea (>60 breaths per minute)
Type of Breathing	Periodic apnoea (cessation of breathing for 15–20 seconds)
	Tracheal tug, sub/intercostal recession, nasal flaring, grunting, use of accessory muscles, asymmetrical movements
Additional Sounds	Cough, wheeze, stridor (harsh, high/low pitched, continuous)

PALPATION
✳ Head
▭▭▭ **Fontanelle**

Palpate the anterior and posterior fontanelles noting if they are depressed and soft (dehydrated) or tense (ICP – hydrocephalus). Start at the frontal bone and follow to the apex of the head. Ascertain if the cranial sutures are fused.

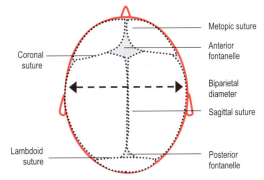

▭▭▭ **Measure**

Measure the head circumference and state that you would like to plot it on a growth centile chart.

Measuring the Head Circumference in a Baby

The head circumference gives an accurate approximation of the volume of the cranial content. It should be measured midway between the child's eyebrows and hairline at the front to the occipital prominence at the back with the tape passing over the ears. An inelastic plastic tape should be employed. The best of several measurements should be documented. The normal-term newborn head circumference is between 33 to 38 cm. Measurements are based on sex and age (weeks, months)

✳ Face

Ears   Note the presence of any ear tags. Draw an imaginary line from the corner of the eye to the ear and establish if the baby has low-set ears (Down's syndrome). Check the patency of the ears and nostrils.

☐☐☐ **Eyes**   Ask for an ophthalmoscope to look for the presence of a red reflex. The absence of a red reflex suggests congenital cataracts, while a white reflex suggests a retinoblastoma. Redness of the sclera could indicate a subconjunctival haemorrhage (birth trauma). Check for abnormal eye movements (squint) and Brushfield spots (Down's syndrome) in the iris.

☐☐☐ **Mouth**   Establish the presence of the rooting reflex by stroking with your finger the corner of the baby's mouth. The baby should turn towards the finger. Insert your finger into the baby's mouth and note if the baby starts to suckle (sucking reflex). Whilst it is in the mouth, raise your finger to palpate the soft palate for a cleft palate (ideally also using a torch for better vision).

✳ Hands

General   Note the presence of palmar creases (Down's syndrome). Count the fingers looking for accessory digits (polydactyly) or fused digits (syndactyly).

✳ Chest and Heart

☐☐☐ **Capillary Refill**   Check for the capillary refill time by placing your thumb on the baby's sternum and noting the time it requires to restore its natural colour. The normal duration is less than 3 seconds.

☐☐☐ **Pulse**   Palpate the femoral and brachial pulses sequentially then simultaneously. Note if they are weak, absent or delayed (brachio-femoral delay – coarctation of the aorta). Use the pads of your fingers, avoiding the thumb, when examining for the pulse. A normal heart rate should be 100–160 bpm.

☐☐☐ **Heart**   Palpate the praecordium and feel and look for the apex beat. Listen to the heart using the bell of the stethoscope. Listen over the four cardiac areas, similar to an adult, for the presence or absence of murmurs.

☐☐☐ **Lungs** Auscultate the lung fields using the diaphragm of the stethoscope. Listen for asymmetrical air entry, crepitations, rhonchi and bowel sounds.

✳ **Abdomen**

General Inspect the abdomen noting the presence of a scaphoid abdomen (diaphragmatic hernia) or a distended abdomen (bowel obstruction) with visible gastric or bowel movements.

☐☐☐ **Umbilicus** Carefully inspect the umbilical stump at the infant's end, counting three umbilical vessels (two arteries and one vein). Look for signs of infection, bleeding or discharge from the stump. The stump should spontaneously separate within a week.

☐☐☐ **Palpation** Palpate the abdomen, in particular the liver (hepatomegaly), spleen (splenomegaly), bladder (outlet obstruction) and masses. Ballot the kidneys to check their presence and size by resting your thumbs in the flank area and your fingers in the loin region.

✳ **Genitalia**

☐☐☐ **Boy** Gently palpate the testes, noting if they have descended, and the scrotum for the presence of a hydrocele. If the testes are not in the scrotum, palpate downwards from the inguinal region. Observe for hypospadias (absent urethral orifice, baby urinates via anus).

Girl Make an attempt at separating the vulva, noting for the presence of a vulval fusion, vaginal cysts, tags and discharge.

Hernias Palpate over the inguinal canals for presence of inguinal hernias.

✳ **Hips**

☐☐☐ **Special Tests** Perform Barlow's and Ortolani's test to assess for congenital dislocation of the hip.

Barlow's Test Perform the Barlow manoeuvre by stabilising the pelvis with the index and middle fingers over the greater trochanter and the thumb over the inner aspect of the infant's thigh. Adduct and flex the hip while applying a gentle downward force in line with the shaft of the femur. In a dislocatable hip, dislocation is felt as a palpable 'clunk' as the femoral head slips out of the acetabulum posteriorly (positive Barlow's sign). The Barlow's manoeuvre tests for an unstable hip that lies in the normal position but can be dislocated.

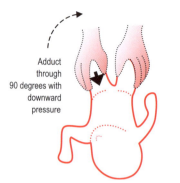

Adduct through 90 degrees with downward pressure

Barlow's Sign

Flex and adduct the baby's hips while applying downward pressure noting for a 'clunk'. Positive sign suggests hip can be dislocated

Ortolani's Test

Perform the Ortolani's manoeuvre by flexing the baby's hips and knees to 90° with the examiner's thumbs resting on the inner aspect of the infant's thigh, and the index fingers over the greater trochanter. Next gently abduct the hip through 90° feeling for and listening for a distinctive clunk which is palpable and audible as the femoral head is reduced back into the acetabulum. A positive Ortolani's sign indicates the hip is dislocated but reducible. However, a restriction of abduction may suggest an irreducible dislocation.

Significance of the Ortolani's Test
Mnemonic: Ortolani = OUT
Ortolani tests if the hip is **OUT** (dislocated). It is performed by abducting the hip **OUT**wards

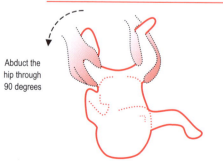

Abduct the hip through 90 degrees

Ortolani's Sign

Flex the baby's hips and knees to 90 degrees and gently abduct the hip through 90 degrees noting for a 'clunk'. Positive sign suggests hip is dislocated

✶ Feet

□□□ **General**   Inspect the feet looking for plantar skin creases and clubbed feet (talipes equinovalgus). Count the digits on each foot checking for accessory digits. Look for calcaneovalgus (abducted forefoot and dorsiflexed ankle). Check full range of movements including dorsiflexion and plantar flexion. Inability to dorsiflex and externally rotate the foot is suggestive of talipes. Turn baby over and now assess the back.

✶ Back

□□□ **Spine**   Palpate along the spine from the head to the bottom noting any defects (spina bifida occulta, meningomyelocele, meningocele), dermal sinuses or dimples. Look for lipomas, tufts of hair (spina bifida) and port wine stains.

□□□ **Anus**   Look at the anus and assess if it is patent (anal atresia).

✶ Posture and Reflexes

□□□ **Head Lag**   Pick up the baby from the supine position by the arms to test for the presence of any head lag.

□□□ **Moro Reflex**   Elicit the Moros reflex by securing the baby's back with the palm of your hand while holding the baby's head with the other hand. Next, release the head by dropping your hand causing it to extend momentarily before supporting it again. The baby will symmetrically abduct, flex and extend his upper limbs. This can be followed by an adduction phase and an audible cry. Asymmetrical movement suggests unilateral paralysis caused by brachial plexus (Erb's palsy, Erb–Duchenne paralysis) or clavicle injury (birth trauma). Bilateral paralysis suggests damage to the central nervous system (brain or spinal cord).

Allow the head to momentarily extend

Moro Reflex

Allow the baby's head to suddenly extend. The infant will bilaterally abduct their arms and flex their elbows. Note for a bilateral, unilateral or absent response

Other Reflexes   Elicit the grasp reflex by placing your finger in the baby's palm and observing for finger closure.

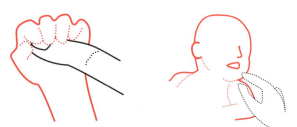

Age Limits for Primitive Reflexes

Plantar Grasp   Stroking the baby's palm or sole causes his fingers or toes to grasp. From birth to 4 months. Persistence may suggest a frontal lobe lesion

Moro Reflex   Also known as the startle reflex. It occurs as a response to unexpected loud noise or when the infant feels that he is falling. The child shows a startle response, abducts and then adducts his arms. From birth until 4 months

Rooting Reflex   Associated with the sucking reflex, both reflexes assist breast-feeding. The newborn baby turns his head towards anything that strokes his cheek or mouth. From birth until 4 months

Tonic Neck Reflex   The asymmetric tonic neck reflex (ATNR), or parachute reflex, occurs when the child's head is turned to one side, when the ipsilateral arm and leg extend. From birth to 6 months

Galant's Reflex   (Trunk incurvation) Hold the baby in ventral suspension and stroke his skin along one side of his back. The baby will swing his trunk and hips to the ipsilateral side being stroked. From birth to 4 months

☐☐☐ **Weigh**   Weigh the child on appropriate paediatric scales and state that you would like to plot it on a growth centile chart.

Weight and Height Measurements in a Baby

A baby's growth is best assessed by plotting the baby's height and weight on appropriate charts. Babies should be weighed naked (or with a clean dry nappy) on a self-calibrating or regularly calibrated scale. In an older child, weighing can be performed on a standing scale with minimum clothing. An infant's height should be measured on a calibrated length board. Similarly, babies should be measured naked or with a clean dry nappy. An assistant should hold the baby's head against the headpiece with the head facing upwards. The measurer then brings the footboard gently into contact with the baby's heels with a downward pressure required at the knees to extend both the legs to full length

	Request	Tell the family that you would like to perform a heel-prick test, (Guthrie test) which tests for phenylketonuria and hypothyroidism, on day 6 of his life.
☐☐☐	**Summarise**	Thank the baby's parent. Answer any questions and summarise findings.

Traffic Light System for Identifying Risk of Serious Illness*

Signs or symptoms in the 'red' column are considered as high risk. Symptoms solely in the 'amber' column are recognised as being at intermediate risk. Symptoms and signs only in the 'green' column are deemed low risk.

	Green – low risk	Amber – intermediate risk	Red – high risk
Colour	Normal colour of skin and tongue	Pallor reported	Pale/mottled/blue
Activity	Responds to social cues Content/smiles Stays awake Strong normal cry	Not responding normally to social cues Wakes only with prolonged stimulation Decreased activity No smile	No response to social cues Appears ill Does not wake Weak, continuous cry
Resp.		Nasal flaring, crackles RR >50 bpm, age 6–12 months RR >40 bpm, age >12 months O_2 saturation ≤95% in air	Grunting, RR >60 bpm Severe or mod. chest indrawing
Hydration	Normal skin and eyes Moist mucous membranes	Dry mucous membranes Poor feeding in infants CRT ≥3 seconds Reduced urine output	Reduced skin turgor
Other	No amber or red symptoms	Fever for ≥5 days Swelling of a limb or joint Non-weight bearing/not using an extremity A new lump >2 cm	Age 0–3 months, temp ≥38°C Age 3–6 months, temp ≥39°C Non-blanching rash, bulging fontanelle, neck stiffness, status epilepticus, focal neurological signs Focal seizures Bile-stained vomiting

CRT: Capillary refill time, RR: Respiratory rate.

Adapted from the NICE guidance on 'Feverish illness in children: Assessment and initial management in children younger than 5 years'

EXAMINER'S EVALUATION

0 1 2 3 4 5

☐☐☐☐☐☐ Assessment of the neonate examination

Total mark out of 38

DIFFERENTIAL DIAGNOSIS

Developmental Dysplasia of the Hip (DDH)

Developmental dysplasia of the hip includes a range of developmental hip disorders from mildly dysplastic to severely dysplastic, and dislocated hips. It describes a displacement of the femoral head from the acetabulum disturbing the normal development of the joint. It occurs in 1.5 per 1000 births and is eight times more frequent in girls than in boys. Of note, the left hip is twice as often dislocated as the right. This is believed to be due to the foetal position where the baby's left hip rests against the mother's sacrum, thereby restricting its movement. Risk factors include breech birth, first baby, restriction of movement (oligohydramnios) and Down's syndrome. Clinical features include limited abduction of the flexed hip, asymmetry of the inguinal or thigh skin folds, shortening of one leg, positive Ortolani's sign and Barlow's test, abnormal Trendelenburg's test and a waddling gait.

Caput Succedaneum

Caput succedaneum is the accumulation of subcutaneous fluid in the scalp. It is caused by mechanical trauma during childbirth as the presenting portion of the scalp is pushed through the cervix. It is more likely to occur during prolonged labour or vacuum extraction. As opposed to a cephalohematoma, the effusion overlies the periosteum with poorly defined margins, may cross the midline and over suture lines and consists of serum rather than blood. It is often associated with head moulding. The soft tissue swelling usually resolves over the first few days of life.

Cephalhaematoma

Cephalhaematoma is a subperiosteal collection of blood caused by the rupture of blood vessels between the skull and the periosteum. The bleeding is limited by the suture lines with the parietal region commonly affected. Causes include prolonged labour and instrumental delivery (ventouse, forceps). It presents as a well-demarcated fluctuant swelling that does not cross the suture lines. There is no overlying skin discolouration. It normally appears after 2–3 days of life and takes several weeks to resolve as the blood clot is slowly absorbed from the periphery towards the centre.

Inguinal and Umbilical Hernias

Umbilical hernias are congenital malformations that are common in infants of African descent and more frequent in boys. The incidence of umbilical hernias increases with low birth weight, Down's syndrome and Beckwith–Wiedemann syndrome. They are often asymptomatic and can get quite large in size, but fortunately strangulation is extremely rare. Up to 95% of umbilical hernias spontaneously close within 5 years. A surgical opinion should be sought if it persists for prolong periods. Inguinal hernias are protrusions of the abdominal cavity contents through the inguinal canal. They are more frequently found in boys (8:1) with the right side (70%) being more common than the left (25%). They are divided into two categories, direct and indirect hernias. Indirect hernias occur when the abdominal contents herniate through the deep inguinal ring. Direct hernias occur when the abdominal contents protrude and herniate through a weakening in the abdominal wall fascia and into the inguinal canal. They usually present as a painless intermittent lump in the inguinoscrotal region in boys and the inguinolabial region in girls, which increases in size when crying or straining. An inconsolable child with a tender, firm, discoloured lump should be treated with a high suspicion of incarceration.

Undescended Testes

Cryptorchidism is derived from the Greek words *krypto* and *orchis*, which literally mean 'hidden testicle'. It is the absence of one or both testes from the scrotum. However, although cryptorchidism is subtly different from 'undescended testes,' the terms are often used interchangeably. Undescended testes are associated with reduced fertility, an increased risk of testicular germ cell tumours and testicular torsions. They are commonly unilateral (66%) but can be bilateral and affect up to 2–3% of male neonates. Most of the time the testis remains palpable along the inguinal canal. However, in a minority of cases the testis is impalpable and resides in the abdomen or is absent. Cryptorchidism can be caused by a congenital absence (anorchia), maldescent or retractile testis (moving between the scrotum and canal). Most descend within the first year of life. Corrective surgery (orchidopexy) should be performed in infancy if the problem persists in order to minimise the risk of complications.

PAEDIATRICS: **Developmental Assessment**

INSTRUCTIONS: This scenario will test your observational skills and ability to make a diagnosis. For this you will need knowledge of developmental milestones and the presentation of certain childhood illnesses. Watch the video closely and complete the questionnaire provided.

DEVELOPMENTAL ASSESSMENT

4.4

0 1 2

☐☐☐ **Video**   Observe the video and watch the child playing in their environment.

☐☐☐ **Development**   Assess the four major categories including fine motor, gross motor, language and social categories (see table).

☐☐☐ **Milestones**   When assessing milestones, consider them in 3-month categories. Determine the child's age by observing for a milestone they can perform within a particular field before assessing for a milestone the child cannot carry out. The child's developmental age will fall within the two limits. It is important to note the developmental age may not be equal across the four developmental categories. This can be normal for a child.

Age	Fine motor	Gross motor	Language	Social
Birth	Follows face in midline	Symmetrical movements, head lag, flexed posture	Stills to voice Startled by loud noise	Smiles (6 weeks)
3 months	Fixes and follows through 90° (6 weeks), opens hand	Pushes up with arms, head control	Cries, laughs, vocalisation (4 months)	Laughs and squeals
6 months	Reaches, transfers objects, palmar grasp	Sits unsupported	Babbles	Solid food in mouth
9 months	Pincer grasp (9–10 months)	Sits well, pulls to stand	Says Daddy (non-specifically)	Stranger anxiety, plays peek-a-boo
12 months	Mature pincer grasp, releases object	Walks or shuffles	Says Mummy and Daddy (specific)	Waves bye-bye, drinks from cup
18 months	Scribbles, builds 3-cube tower	Adult walk, walks upstairs	5–10 words	Domestic mimicry
2 years	Circular scribbles and lines, builds 6-cube tower	Kicks ball, runs	2-word sentences	Uses spoon and fork, undresses, symbolic and parallel play
3 years	Draws a circle, builds bridge of 3 cubes	Jumps, throws ball, pedal tricycle	Says first and last name, knows colours	Dresses, has friend, interactive play

Age	Fine motor	Gross motor	Language	Social
4 years	Draws a cross or man, builds steps of bricks	Stands on one leg, hops	Counts to 10+	Does buttons, undress
5 years	Draws a triangle	Bicycle, catches ball, skips	Good speech	Ties shoe laces (or good attempt)

□ □ □ **Age Limits**

Observe for red flag features that suggest delayed development.

Age Limits for Developmental Milestones

Age	Development sign	Age	Development sign
8 weeks	Smiling, asymmetrical Moro	**12 months**	Stands upright
3 months	Fixes and follows	**12 months**	Pincer grip
4 months	Head control (no head lag)	**18 months**	Walks unsupported
6 months	Reaching out for objects	**18 months**	Feeds self with spoon
7 months	Polysyllabic babble	**30 months**	Speaks in phrases
8 months	Transfers	**2.5 years**	Symbolic play
9 months	Sits unsupported	**3.5 years**	Interactive play

Motor problems often present early in life (first year) as the child makes an effort to learn how to walk. Language concerns manifest in the second year of life during the period when the child attempts to speak a few words. Behavioural and social issues occur in the third year of life when the child should become more autonomous and interactive.

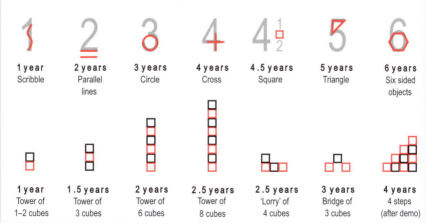

Developmental Milestones

1 year Scribble	**2 years** Parallel lines	**3 years** Circle	**4 years** Cross	**4.5 years** Square	**5 years** Triangle	**6 years** Six sided objects
1 year Tower of 1–2 cubes	**1.5 years** Tower of 3 cubes	**2 years** Tower of 6 cubes	**2.5 years** Tower of 8 cubes	**2.5 years** 'Lorry' of 4 cubes	**3 years** Bridge of 3 cubes	**4 years** 4 steps (after demo)

Milestones in Development of Children

Mnemonic:	1 year	Speaks single words
	2 years	Two word sentences, understands two step commands
	3 years	Three word combinations, repeats three digits, rides tricycle
	4 years	Draws four-sided square, counts four objects

EXAMINER'S EVALUATION

0 1 2 3 4 5

☐ ☐ ☐ ☐ ☐ ☐   Assessment of child development

Total mark out of 13

DIFFERENTIAL DIAGNOSIS

Down's Syndrome (Trisomy 21)

Down's syndrome was first described by John Langdon Haydon Down in 1866. It is one of the most common genetic disorders to cause learning disability in children and affects approximately 1 in 800 births. It is characterised by the presence of an extra copy of genetic material from the 21st chromosome. Up to 95% of children with Down's syndrome obtain the extra chromosome 21 from non-dysjunction at the time of gamete formation. The remaining 5% are the result of either translocation, involving part of the 21st chromosome attaching to another (chromosome 14), or by mosaicism. The incidence of Down's syndrome is strongly associated with maternal age, with the probability of conceiving a 'Down's baby' rapidly increasing after the age of 40 (risk at the age of 30 is 1:900, while at the age of 44 it is 1:37). It is often suspected in children because of a characteristic dysmorphic facial appearance including a round face, epicanthic folds, protruding tongue, Brushfield spots (speckled iris), single palmar creases (simian crease), incurved little finger (clinodactyly), a flat occiput and small stature. Patients also suffer from congenital abnormalities including cardiac defects (AVSD, VSD, ASD, PDA, tetralogy of Fallot), duodenal atresia, moderate to severe learning disability, atlantoaxial instability and increased risk of chest infections and leukaemias.

Symptoms of Down's Syndrome

Mnemonic: 'CHILD HAS PROBLEM'

Congenital heart disease (AVSD, VSD, ASD, PDA, T of F), **C**ataracts

Hypotonia, **H**ypothyroidism

Increased gap between 1st and 2nd toe, **I**ncurved little finger (clinodactyly)

Leukaemia risk (increased twofold), **L**ung problems (recurrent chest infections)

Duodenal atresia, **D**ysmorphic facial appearance

Hirschsprung's disease

Alantoaxial instability, **A**lzheimer's disease

Squint, Short neck
Protruding tongue, Palmar crease
Round face, Rolling eye (nystagmus)
Occiput flat, Oblique eye fissure
Brushfield spots, Brachycephaly
Low nasal bridge, Language problem
Epicanthic fold, Ear folded
Mental retardation, Myoclonus

Attention Deficit Hyperactivity Disorder (ADHD)

Attention deficit hyperactivity disorder (ADHD), also known as hyperkinetic disorder, is a syndrome diagnosed in approximately 0.1% of British children. It affects boys four times more than girls and is associated with behavioural problems. Features include hyperactivity, poor concentration or inattention, impulsive behaviour, restlessness and becoming easily distracted. Diagnosis is made when symptoms persist for more than 6 months, occur in more than one environment (school, home, shopping) and affect or impair the child's normal function. Affected children are prone to having often unprovoked temper tantrums and behaving recklessly. The disorder is associated with learning difficulties and is treated under specialist supervision using appropriate drugs (amphetamine or methylphenidate based) and behavioural therapy.

Autism Spectrum Disorder

Autism is a disorder beginning in early childhood (first 3 years of life) which is associated with impairment of social interaction, communication and abnormal behaviour. Autistic children appear to lack what is widely regarded as normal intuition about the people around them. They exhibit a reduced response to social stimuli (e.g. by not responding to their own name), show reduced social understanding and associated emotional responses (e.g. make poor eye contact and poor use of facial expression). They may also appear to be socially detached individuals although they do form attachments with their main carers. Impairment of communication normally presents as a delayed onset of cooing or babbling. Later, an inability to articulate useful speech is shown in association with restricted use of non-verbal communication. Autistic children may express an echolalia phenomenon whereby they repeat sounds and words that other people say. They may also ignore grammatical rules in their speech and exhibit pronoun reversals. Abnormal behaviour includes stereotypical movements (hand clapping, hand waving, body swaying), daily ritualistic behaviour and self-injurious behaviour. Autistic children may also exhibit poor imitation of others and a lack of imagination (e.g. during play).

Features of Autism
Mnemonic: 'AUTISTICS'
Again and again (repetitive behaviour)   Three years at onset
Unusual abilities (Asperger's syndrome)   Inherited component

Talking (language) delay	Communication poor (echolalia)
IQ subnormal	Self-injurious behaviour
Social development poor (less eye contact)	

Cerebral Palsy

Cerebral palsy (CP) describes a variety of persistent and non-progressive motor syndromes affecting movement and posture due to disturbances occurring in the foetal or neonatal period up to the age of 3 years. Sensation, cognition and behaviour may also be affected. Although clinical features can depend on the type of cerebral palsy presented, general classical features can include abnormal posture (for example, a slouched posture while sitting), an unsteady gait (including scissoring gait and toe walking), facial gestures (due to involuntary movements) and movements which appear to be clumsy.

INSTRUCTIONS: You are a foundation year House Officer in paediatrics. Examine this child's cardiovascular system. Explain to the examiner what you are doing as you proceed and present a differential diagnosis.

NOTE: When conducting a paediatric examination, it is important to be opportunistic. Be prepared to tailor your examination to the child and be flexible in your approach.

4.5

EXAMINATION

0 1 2

☐☐☐ **Introduction**   Introduce yourself. Establish rapport with the child.

Explain   Explain the purpose of the examination and obtain consent from the parent (and child where appropriate) to expose and examine the child.

☐☐☐ **Position**   Sit the child at a 45° angle and expose the patient appropriately. Maintain the child's dignity throughout.

INSPECTION

☐☐☐ **General**   Stand at the edge of the bed and observe the patient. Confirm the child's age and comment on their height and appearance in context of their age. Say that you will check their height and weight on growth charts standardised for age and sex.

General Observations in the Cardiovascular Examination	
General Health	Nutritional status, failure to thrive
Breathing at Rest	Comfortable, dyspnoeic, cough. Check respiratory rate
Colour	Pale, cyanosed (bluish discolouration)
Presence of Scars	Midline sternotomy (TGV, valve replacement) Left thoracotomy (Blalock–Taussig shunt, PDA ligation, COA repair, pulmonary artery banding) Right thoracotomy (Blalock–Taussig shunt, PDA ligation)
Dysmorphic Features	Check for features of Down's, Turner's and Marfan's syndrome
Turner's Syndrome	Webbed neck, short stature, cubitus valgus (COA, AS)
Down's Syndrome	(AVSD, ASD, VSD, tetralogy of Fallot)

Marfan's Syndrome	Tall for age, wide arm span and high arched palate (COA, AR, MR, MVP)
Others	Williams syndrome (AS), Noonan's syndrome (PS)

Abbreviations: TGV – transposition of great vessels, VSD – ventricular septal defect, COA coarctation of aorta, ASD – atrial septal defect, AVSD – atrioventricular septal defect, AR/MR – Atrial/mitral regurgitation, MVP – mitral valve prolapse, PDA – patent ductus arteriosus

▭▭▭ **Hands**

Feel the hands for any temperature change. Look in the hands for:

Hand Signs in the Cardiovascular Examination
Appearance	Arachnodactyly (Marfan's syndrome)
Temperature	Warm and well perfused/poor perfusion (capillary refill normal if <3 secs)
Peripheral Cyanosis	Blue nail beds
Clubbing	Endocarditis, cyanotic congenital heart disease
Endocarditis (SBE)	Osler nodes and Janeway lesions, splinter haemorrhages

▭▭▭ **Pulse**

In young children the brachial or femoral pulses are easier to palpate and more useful than the radial pulse. Check for the presence of a brachial pulse on either side. Assess the rate, rhythm, volume and character of the right brachial pulse.

Causes of Absent Brachial Pulse
Absent left side	Left Blalock–Taussig shunt, repair of coarctation of aorta
Absent right side	Right Blalock–Taussig shunt
Absent bilaterally	Cardiac catheterisation

▭▭▭ *Rate*

Count for 10 seconds and multiply the rate by six. Note if it is normal, bradycardic (athletic, heart block, drugs – β-blocker) or tachycardic (anxiety) depending on the normal range for the child's age.

Normal Heart Rates for Healthy Children
Age	Normal range (Beats per minute)
Infant (birth–1 years)	120–160
Toddler (1–3 years)	90–150
Preschool (3–6 years)	80–140
Young children (6–12 years)	70–120
Adolescent (12–18 years)	60–100

☐☐☐ *Rhythm* Establish the quality of the rhythm. Auscultate at the apex for the apical rate (true heart rate).

Normal Heart Rates for Healthy Children

Regular	Normal healthy children
Regularly irregular	Pulsus bigeminus, extrasystoles
Irregularly irregular	Multiple extrasystoles (common), AF (ASD, surgery, rheumatic MS)

Volume Establish the pulse volume.

High and Low Pulse Volumes

Low volume	Low cardiac outputs (hypovolaemia), heart failure, aortic stenosis, pericardial effusion
Large volume	Carbon dioxide retention, anaemia, AR, thyrotoxicosis

☐☐☐ *Character* Assess the character of the pulse.

Assessing the Character of the Pulse

Normal Pulse
Best appreciated in the carotid artery

Slow Rising Pulse
'Plateau'
Aortic Stenosis

Collapsing Pulse*
'Water hammer pulse'
PDA, AR

Bisferien Pulse
'Double peaks'
AS with AR

* To feel the collapsing pulse, raise the patient's arm while feeling the pulse with your fingers

– Aortic stenosis is often associated with other lesions such as a mitral stenosis and coarctation

☐☐☐ **Delay** Compare the pulses in both arms assessing for delay (aortic arch aneurysm, e.g. connective tissue diseases) and assess for radio-femoral delay (coarctation of the aorta). Absent femoral pulses indicate coarctation of the aorta.

☐☐☐ **Arms** Indicate that you would like to measure the patient's blood pressure.

☐☐☐ **Face** Look at the sclera for signs of anaemia and jaundice. Inspect the mouth for central cyanosis and a high arched palate (Marfan's syndrome).

Carotid Pulse Warn older children before feeling the carotids. Palpate the pulse gently with your thumb to assess its character. Never compress or palpate both carotids simultaneously.

JVP The jugular venous pressure (JVP) is not an essential element of the paediatric cardiovascular system since it can only be measured in older children. An elevated JVP is indicative of right heart failure, fluid overload or pericardial tamponade.

PALPATION

☐☐☐ **Apex Beat** Locate the apex beat by palpating the most inferior and lateral position at which the cardiac impulses can be detected. Use the manubriosternal angle (2nd intercostal space) as well as the mid-clavicular line, anterior and mid-axillary lines as landmarks when describing its location. Above the age of 8 years it is normally located in the 5th intercostal space mid-clavicular line, below 8 years it is in the 4th intercostal space. Note the character of the apex beat and whether it is displaced laterally (left ventricular hypertrophy, pectus excavatum). If it is impalpable consider dextrocardia or pericardial effusion.

Assessing the Character of the Apex Beat	
Tapping	Mitral stenosis
Thrusting	Aortic stenosis
Heaving	Mitral regurgitation, aortic regurgitation
Diffuse	Left ventricular failure, dilated cardiomyopathy

☐☐☐ **Heave & Thrills** Feel for the presence of thrills (palpable murmurs – AS, VSD, PS) by using the flat of the hand to palpate over the praecordium. Use the hypothenar aspect of the hand palpating to the left of the sternum feeling for a parasternal heave (right ventricular hypertrophy).

AUSCULTATION

☐☐☐ **Listen** Auscultate over the four areas of the heart with a stethoscope listening for heart sounds, additional sounds (extra heart sounds, clicks or snaps) and murmurs. Time the murmurs with the right brachial pulse using your thumb to establish if it is a systolic or diastolic murmur.

Auscultation Areas of the Heart
Mnemonic: 'All Patients Take Meds'
Aortic area, Pulmonary area, Tricuspid area, Mitral area

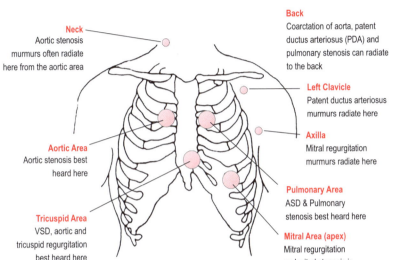

Neck
Aortic stenosis murmurs often radiate here from the aortic area

Back
Coarctation of aorta, patent ductus arteriosus (PDA) and pulmonary stenosis can radiate to the back

Left Clavicle
Patent ductus arteriosus murmurs radiate here

Aortic Area
Aortic stenosis best heard here

Axilla
Mitral regurgitation murmurs radiate here

Tricuspid Area
VSD, aortic and tricuspid regurgitation best heard here

Pulmonary Area
ASD & Pulmonary stenosis best heard here

Mitral Area (apex)
Mitral regurgitation and mitral stenosis is best heard here

Characteristics of Heart Sounds

Loud 1st heart sound	ASD, mechanical prosthetic valve, mitral stenosis
Loud 2nd heart sound	Includes pulmonary flow (PDA, ASD, large VSD), pulmonary hypertension
Soft 2nd heart sound	Tetralogy of Fallot, pulmonary stenosis
Split 2nd heart sound	Normal variation, atrial septal defect (fixed split)
3rd heart sound	Normal variation, left or right ventricular failure
4th heart sound	Left or right ventricular failure, pulmonary hypertension

☐☐☐ *Mitral*

Located around the left 5th intercostal space, mid-clavicular line. Listen for mitral stenosis here using the bell to hear the low-pitched murmur. Ask the patient to hold their breath in expiration, leaning over to the left-hand side. Next listen for

	mitral regurgitation by using the diaphragm of the stethoscope at the apex. Check for radiation of the murmur to the axilla.
Pulmonary	Located around the 2nd intercostal space, left sternal edge. Listen for pulmonary stenosis here using the diaphragm.
☐☐☐ *Aortic*	Located around the 2nd intercostal space, right sternal edge. Listen for aortic stenosis in this area. Check for radiation of the murmur to the carotids.
Tricuspid	Located around the 5th intercostal space, left sternal edge. Listen for aortic regurgitation by sitting the child forward and asking them to take a deep breath in and out holding it in full expiration no longer than 3 seconds.
Back	Remember to listen over the back between the shoulder blades for PS, PDA or COA.
☐☐☐ **Murmurs**	Listen for cardiac murmurs noting the timing, intensity, site, character, pitch, radiation and the effect of respiration and position.
Timing	Establish if the murmur is systolic, diastolic or continuous in nature.

Systolic, Diastolic and Continuous Murmurs

Systolic	Ejection (AS, PS, ASD), pansystolic (VSD, COA, MR, TR)
Diastolic	Early diastolic (AR, PR), mid-diastolic (MS, TS)
Continuous	Venous hum (innocent murmur), COA, PDA (machinery sound)

Intensity	Murmurs are graded in intensity, between one and six.

Grading the Intensity of a Murmur

Grade 1-3 (Thrill absent)	1	Faint and hard to hear with stethoscope
	2	Louder and heard easily with stethoscope
	3	Moderately loud and heard easily with stethoscope
Grade 4-6 (Thrill present)	4	Loud with stethoscope on chest with thrill just palpable
	5	Very loud and easily palpable thrill
	6	Very, very loud and audible without stethoscope

146

Site	Determine the location on the praecordium where the murmur is best heard. Note if it is best heard in the mitral, pulmonary, aortic or tricuspid area.
Character	Note if the murmur is rumbling (MS), blowing (MR) or harsh (AS) in character. Assess if it is a crescendo–decrescendo, decrescendo, crescendo or plateau type of murmur.
Pitch	Assess the pitch of the murmur. High-pitched murmurs are best heard with the diaphragm (AS) while low-pitched murmurs are best heard with the bell (MS).
Radiation	Check if the murmur radiates to the carotids (AS), axilla (MR), left sternal edge (AR) or to the back (PDA, PS and coarctation of aorta).
Respiration	(Mnemonic for the effect of respiration on murmurs: **RILE** – **R**ight-sided murmurs are heard with greatest intensity in **I**nspiration while **L**eft-sided murmurs are heard with greatest intensity in **E**xpiration.)
Position	Note if the murmur is best heard in the supine position (most murmurs), leaning forward with breath held in exhalation (AR) or in the left lateral position (MR).

Signs and Symptoms of Innocent Murmurs
The Mnemonic of multiple Ss
The **S**ymptom-less patient that has a **S**ystolic murmur in a **S**mall area (**S**ite), which is **S**hort in duration, **S**oft in sound with a possible **S**plit **S**econd heart sound. There are no **S**igns present with normal **S**pecial tests (ECG, X-ray, echo)

☐☐☐ **Lung Bases**

Keep the patient leaning forwards and auscultate the lung bases listening for crepitations and pleural effusion (heart failure).

☐☐☐ **Oedema**

Examine for sacral oedema by applying firm pressure for at least 15 seconds against the lower back and for pedal oedema by pressing down over the distal shaft of the tibia. Observe pitting oedema by looking for an indentation of your finger after applying pressure. Ensure that you ask the child if they feel any pain when being pressed.

| **Liver** | Lie the child flat and palpate and percuss for hepatomegaly (heart failure). |

Characteristic Features of Heart Failure

Symptoms	Breathlessness on feeding or exertion, sweating, poor feeding and weight gain, recurrent chest infections
Signs	Tachypnoea, tachycardia, galloping rhythm, heart murmur, sweating, cool peripheries, failure to thrive, cardiomegaly, hepatomegaly
Investigations	X-ray (cardiomegaly), ECG, echo (congenital heart disease)

ADDITIONAL POINTS

☐☐☐ **Pulses** — Palpate the peripheral pulses (femoral, popliteal, post tibial, dorsalis pedis).

Request — Ask to measure the blood pressure, take an ECG tracing and a chest X-ray of the patient. Mention that you would like to have a look at the patient's oxygen saturations and temperature chart.

☐☐☐ **Summarise** — Check with the patient and deliver an appropriate summary.

EXAMINER'S EVALUATION

0 1 2 3 4 5

☐☐☐☐☐☐ Assessment of cardiovascular system

☐☐☐☐☐☐ Role player's score

Total mark out of 36

DIFFERENTIAL DIAGNOSIS

Dextrocardia

The term 'dextrocardia' originates from the Latin word *dexter*, meaning 'on the right side'. This is a rare congenital condition in which the heart is situated on the right side of the thorax, as opposed to its usual left-sided position. If the patient's heart, in addition to their visceral organs are mirrored onto the opposite side, this is known as *situs inversus*. Patients with isolated dextrocardia have a high incidence of congenital heart defects compared to individuals with *situs inversus*. Kartagener syndrome can affect up to 20% of patients with *situs inversus*. This is an autosomal recessive condition that causes ciliary dyskinesia. It is characterised by a triad of abnormalities including sinusitis, bronchiectasis and dextrocardia. Other symptoms include respiratory infections, hearing loss, nasal polyps and infertility. On examination, an absent apex beat and heart sounds may warrant a brief check of the right side for this condition.

Ventricular Septal Defect (VSD)

Ventricular septal defects are the most common congenital heart anomalies and represent 30% of all newborn congenital heart defects. This is a defect in the ventricular septum resulting in an abnormal communication between the two ventricles that permits the mixture of oxygenated and deoxygenated blood. Most will close spontaneously during the first year of life with only a small percentage requiring surgery. They are frequently associated with chromosome abnormalities including Edward's, Pateau's and Down's syndrome. If the murmur is accompanied by cyanosis, Fallot's tetralogy should be considered. On examination, a harsh pansystolic murmur that radiates throughout the praecordium can be heard at the lower left sternal edge. The volume of the murmur is inversely proportional to the size of the defect, with large defects producing quiet murmurs. Other associated features include a displaced apex beat, an increased cardiac impulse, the presence of heaves and palpable thrills. Large defects may present with right to left shunts with central cyanosis, clubbing of the fingers and a loud second heart sound.

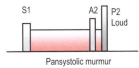

Pansystolic murmur

Atrial Septal Defect (ASD)

Atrial septal defect is an abnormal communication between the left and right atria caused by a defect in the interatrial septum. Consequently a shunt may form, resulting in the abnormal fusion of deoxygenated and oxygenated blood. It is categorised as ostium primum (atrioventricular septal defect) and ostium secundum (foramen ovale and the surrounding atrial septum). The ejection systolic murmur is best heard in the pulmonary area, due to the left to right shunt, with an associated rumbling or short mid-diastolic murmur heard in the tricuspid area due to increased flow across the valve. The murmurs are created by the flow across the valves rather than from the defect itself. There is also a fixed widely-split second heart sound and a displaced apex beat.

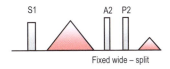

Fixed wide – split

Pulmonary Stenosis (PS)

Pulmonary stenosis is a condition that causes right ventricular outflow obstruction. It may occur in isolation or be associated with more complicated congenital heart

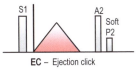

EC – Ejection click

disorders such ASD, VSD, PDA or with Fallot's tetralogy. It is also associated with other inherited conditions including Noonan, Ehlers–Danlos and William's syndromes. On examination, a parasternal heave and systolic thrills may be noted. An ejection systolic murmur with an ejection click is heard in the pulmonary area and radiates to the back. Only where there is a significant obstruction is P2 delayed and soft.

Aortic Stenosis (AS)

Aortic stenosis represents 5% of all congenital heart defects. It is classified as valvular, subvalvular or supravalvular. It is often associated with mitral stenosis and coarctation of the aorta. Most children with moderate AS are asymptomatic. Symptoms of exercise intolerance, chest pain, fatigability or syncope may be present with more severe forms of AS and are relative to the degree of obstruction. On auscultation, there is an ejection systolic murmur with ejection click best heard in the aortic area that can radiate to the neck. There is a carotid thrill, and a slow-rising pulse with soft second heart sound.

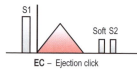

EC – Ejection click

Patent Ductus Arteriosus (PDA)

Patent ductus arteriosus is a congenital heart defect where a child's ductus arteriosus fails to close after birth. The ductus arteriosus is a shunt that connects the pulmonary artery to the descending aorta and permits blood to bypass the inactive lungs in utero. As the newborn takes his first breath, there is a reduction of pulmonary resistance as the lungs open, resulting in more blood flowing to the lungs and to the left side of the heart. This increases the aortic pressure and thus reverses the pressure gradient across the ductus arteriosus as blood no longer flows from the pulmonary artery to the aorta. At the same time, the release of bradykinin causes the constriction of the smooth muscle around the ductus arteriosus. These factors combine to cause the duct to close within 15 hours of birth but true closure can take up to 3 weeks. If the ductus arteriosus fails to close, the duct remains patent and will create a left to right shunt between the pulmonary artery and aorta. On examination, there is a continuous machine-like murmur that engulfs the second heart sound and is best heard in the pulmonary area. This may radiate to just beneath the left clavicle. Peripheral pulses are bounding (collapsing pulse) due to the wide pulse pressure.

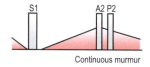

Continuous murmur

Coarctation of Aorta (COA)

Coarctation of the aorta derives its name from the Latin word *coarctatio*, meaning 'tightening or pressing together'. It is a condition that results in the localised narrowing of the aorta, particularly of the isthmus, located just distal to the origin of the left subclavian artery. Due to the location of the obstruction, there are unequal blood pressures between the upper and lower limbs with higher readings noted in the arms accompanied with a radial (brachial)-femoral delay or absent femoral pulses. The child may complain of dizziness, shortness of breath, headaches and leg claudication on exercise. On auscultation, an ejection systolic murmur can be heard between the shoulder blades. Conditions associated with coarctation include Turner's syndrome, Marfan's, neurofibromatosis, bicuspid aortic valves and berry aneurysms. Surgery is recommended, leaving the patient with a left thoracotomy scar and an absent left-sided brachial pulse.

Fallot's Tetralogy

Fallot's tetralogy was named after the French physician Etienne Louis Arthur Fallot. It is the commonest congenital heart defect that causes cyanosis in a newborn. It is classically characterised by four abnormalities including a VSD, pulmonary stenosis (causing tight ventricular outflow obstruction), an overriding aorta with biventricular connections (which may override the VSD) and right ventricular hypertrophy (**mnemonic**: 'Problems Of Small Hearts,' Pulmonary stenosis, Overriding aorta, Septal defect [ventricular], Hypertrophy of right ventricle). Amongst other anatomical anomalies, it may also be associated with an atrial septal defect, in which case the syndrome is called a pentalogy of Fallot. Due to the large VSD and right ventricular outflow obstruction, deoxygenated blood is allowed to mix with oxygenated blood on exiting the aorta, resulting in cyanosis from birth. Other symptoms include growth retardation, breathlessness, inconsolable crying, pallor and squatting to rest during exercise in older children (right to left shunt). On examination there is right ventricular predominance, a palpable thrill and a loud ejection systolic murmur best heard in the pulmonary area, which is associated with an aortic ejection click, single second heart sound and clubbing of the fingers.

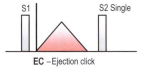

EC –Ejection click

PAEDIATRICS: **Respiratory Examination**

INSTRUCTIONS: You are a foundation year House Officer in paediatrics. Examine this child's respiratory system. Explain to the examiner what you are doing as you proceed and present a differential diagnosis.

NOTE: When conducting a paediatric examination, it is important to be opportunistic. Be prepared to tailor your examination to the child and be flexible in your approach.

4.6

EXAMINATION

0 1 2

☐☐☐ **Introduction**   Introduce yourself. Establish rapport with the child.

Explain   Explain the purpose of examination and obtain consent from the parent (and child where appropriate) to expose and examine the child.

☐☐☐ **Position**   Sit the child at a 45° angle and expose the patient appropriately. Maintain the child's dignity throughout.

INSPECTION

☐☐☐ **General**   Stand at the edge of the bed and observe the patient. Look for oxygen masks, nebulisers, peak flow meters and sputum pots surrounding the patient.

General Observations in the Respiratory Examination

Development	Height and weight for age (offer to check this against a growth chart)
Breathing at rest	Dyspnoea, pursed lips, nasal flaring, grunting, tracheal tug
Added sounds	Coughing, wheezing, stridor, barking cough (croup)
Chest shape	Barrel chest (air trapping), pectus excavatum (sunken sternum), pectus carinatum (pigeon chest – chronic airway obstruction), Harrison's sulcus (diaphragm insertion – asthma)
Chest movements	Asymmetrical expansion, accessory muscles, sub/intercostal recession
Skin, scars, misc.	Eczema (atopic), engorged superficial veins (SVC obs), thoracotomy scar, operative scars, gastrostomy, portacath, chest drain

---

☐☐☐ *Rate*   Count the respiratory rate for 10 seconds and multiply it by six. Note if it is normal, tachypnoeic or dyspneic in nature.

Normal Respiratory Rates for Healthy Children

Age	Normal range (Breaths per minute)
Infant (birth–1 year)	30–60
Toddler (1–3 years)	20–30
Preschool (3–6 years)	22–34
Young children (6–12 years)	18–30
Adolescent (>12 years)	12–16

□□□ **Hands**

Feel the hands for any temperature change. Look at the hands for:

Hand Signs in the Respiratory Examination

Temperature	Warm and well perfused/poor perfusion
Tremor	Resting tremor (beta agonist – salbutamol)
Peripheral cyanosis	Blue nail beds
Clubbing	Bronchiectasis, cystic fibrosis

Pulse

Feel the radial pulse (in small children the brachial) and assess the rate and rhythm. Assess for the presence of a bounding pulse (CO_2 retention).

□□□ **Arms**

Indicate that you would like to measure the patient's blood pressure.

□□□ **Face & Neck**

Look at the conjunctiva for signs of anaemia. Inspect the mouth for central cyanosis. Examine the jugular venous pressure (only in older children) between the two heads of the sternocleidomastoid muscle.

PALPATION

□□□ **Lymph Nodes**

Observe for any enlarged lymph nodes. Sit the patient forward and palpate the lymph nodes in the cervical region and supraclavicular fossa.

Trachea

Palpate the tracheal position by placing the index and middle finger on either side of the trachea. Be gentle and warn the child that it may feel uncomfortable. Determine if it is central or deviated to one side.

□□□ **Apex Beat**

Palpate the apex beat by feeling the furthest pulsating point of the heart. It is normally located in the 4th or 5th (depending on age) intercostal space mid-clavicular line. Determine if the apex beat is displaced (effusion, tension pneumothorax, collapse).

□□□ **Expansion**

Assess chest expansion by placing your hands on the patient's chest with the thumbs just touching in the midline and fingers spread along the ribcage. Ask

153

the patient to breathe normally and then to take
deep breaths in. Measure the distance between your
thumbs. Note if chest expansion is bilaterally or
unilaterally reduced.

PERCUSSION
□ □ □ **Chest**

Place the middle finger of one hand on the patient's
chest wall and percuss the centre of the middle
phalanx with the middle finger of the other. Percuss
the upper, middle and lower zones including the
apex, lateral areas and axilla comparing the percussion
note on both sides.

Character of Percussion Note

Stony dull	Pleural effusion
Dull	Consolidation, lung collapse, fibrosis
Resonant	Normal lung
Hyper-resonant	Pneumothorax, air trapping (asthma)

AUSCULTATION
□ □ □ **Chest**

With the child relaxed, request them to breathe
deeply through their mouth demonstrating how to
do so if necessary. Use the bell of your stethoscope
to listen to the apices of the lung and then the
diaphragm to listen over the different lung areas
mentioned above for breath sounds (bronchial
breathing, vesicular breathing, present or absent) or
added sounds (wheezes, crackles).

Breath Sounds (BS) on Auscultation

Vesicular breathing	Inspiration followed by expiration without interruption (normal)
Bronchial breathing	Audible gap between inspiratory and expiratory (consolidation, fibrosis)
Reduced BS	ARDS, asthma, pleural effusion, pneumothorax, collapse
Increased BS	Consolidation
Prolonged expiration	Asthma, emphysema
Added sounds	Check for the presence of wheezes, crackles or a pleural rub
Wheezes (rhonchi)	Asthma, pulmonary oedema, HF
Crackles (crepitations)	ARDS, bronchiectasis, consolidation, pulmonary oedema, early HF
Pleural Rub	Pneumonia, pneumothorax

154

▭▭▭ **Vocal Res.** If the child is mature enough to follow commands, assess vocal resonance by asking the patient to say '*ninety-nine*' while listening over the lung areas.

Sit the patient forward and repeat the chest expansion, percussion and auscultation on the back.

Differentials for Stridor
Mnemonic: 'ABCDEFGH'

Fever	**A**bscess, **B**acterial tracheitis, **C**roup, **D**iphtheria, **E**piglottitis
Without fever	**F**oreign body, **G**as (toxic gas), **H**ypersensitivity

ADDITIONAL POINTS

▭▭▭ **Oedema** Examine for sacral oedema by applying firm pressure for at least 15 seconds over the sacrum and, for ankle oedema, by pressing down over the distal shaft of the tibia. Observe pitting oedema by looking and feeling for an indentation of your finger after applying pressure. Ensure that you ask the patient if they feel any pain while you are pressing them.

Request Ask to take a peak flow (and chest X-ray) of the patient. Say that you would like to have a look at the patient's oxygen saturations and temperature chart. Send any abnormally coloured sputum for microbiology (Gram and ZN stain), culture and cytology.

Different Colours of Sputum

Greyish white	Asthma
Black	Aspergillosis
Frothy pink specks	Acute pulmonary oedema
Bloodstained	(Haemoptysis) TB, bronchiectasis, pneumonia
Yellow, green	Viral and bacterial infection: pneumonia, bronchiectasis
Rusty golden	Pneumococcal pneumonia

▭▭▭ **Summarise** Check with the patient and deliver an appropriate summary.

EXAMINER'S EVALUATION

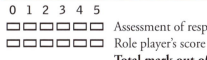

0 1 2 3 4 5

▭▭▭▭▭▭ Assessment of respiratory system
▭▭▭▭▭▭ Role player's score
Total mark out of 30

DIFFERENTIAL DIAGNOSIS

Cystic Fibrosis

The name 'cystic fibrosis' refers to the development of scar tissue (fibrosis) and cyst formation that takes place in the pancreas. This autosomal recessive condition affects 1 in 2500 live births with a carrier rate of 1 in 25 and is more common in Caucasians, particularly amongst Europeans and Ashkenazi Jews. It is a result of a mutation of the cystic fibrosis transmembrane conductance regulator (CFTR) gene on chromosome 7 that leads to viscous secretions through defective chloride transporters. Such transporters are located in epithelial cells of the respiratory tract and pancreas. It can be diagnosed through sweat testing which demonstrates a high sodium concentration (80–125 mmol/L). Respiratory symptoms include recurrent chest infections, failure to thrive, haemoptysis, bronchiectasis, pneumothorax, sinusitis and aspergillosis. On inspection, the child may use sputum pots to collect purulent sputum associated with a loose cough, may appear physically underdeveloped and have a portacath (a double lumened catheter) located by the nipple to administer regular antibiotics. Additionally, he may also have a gastrostomy or PEG (catheter port), emerging from the gastric area if his dietary requirements cannot be met. On examination, the child may have finger clubbing, a hyperinflated chest with coarse crepitations and with evident expiratory rhonchi and nasal polyps.

Features of Cystic Fibrosis
Mnemonic: 'CF PANCREAS'

Cough (chronic)	**C**lubbing, **C**hest infections
Failure to thrive	**R**ectal prolapse
Pancreatic insufficiency	**E**lectrolyte elevation in sweat, salty skin
Appetite decrease	**A**tresia of vas deferens (infertility)
Nasal polyps	**S**putum (*Staphylococcus, Pseudomonas*)

Asthma

The word 'asthma' is derived from the Greek word *aazein*, meaning 'to exhale with open mouth' or 'sharp breathing'. It is a chronic inflammatory disorder of the airways and is characterised by variable airway obstruction and hyper-reactivity. Exposure of the airway to environmental allergens results in persistent bronchospasm, bronchoconstriction, excessive mucus secretions and mucosal oedema. This leads to chronic airway narrowing and generates symptoms including wheeze, breathlessness, chest tightness a nocturnal cough or exercise-induced coughing. On examination, signs include a hyperinflated chest with prolonged expiratory phase, pectus carinatum and Harrison sulci, eczema (atopy), a generalised expiratory wheeze, tachypnoea, intercostal recessions and accessory muscle usage. Its severity can be gauged by a peak flow meter to assess the child's peak expiratory flow rate and diagnosis can be confirmed with reversibility and improvement in PEFR with a short course of a bronchodilator.

Features of Severe and Life-threatening Asthma

Severe	Child too breathless to speak or feed
	Respiratory rate >50 breaths per minute
	Heart rate >140 beats per minute
	Peak flow <50% of best predicted value
Life-threatening	Agitated (hypoxia) or reduced levels of consciousness (hypercapnia)
	Fatigued or exhausted
	Silent chest, cyanosed or poor respiratory effort
	Peak flow <33% of best predicted value

Bronchiolitis

Bronchiolitis is one of the commonest lower respiratory tract infections affecting infants under the age of 1. It is usually caused by a viral infection of the bronchioles – the respiratory syncytial virus (RSV) is implicated in 70% of cases. Other causes include adenovirus, influenza and the parainfluenza virus. A combination of increased mucus production and oedema results in the bronchioles becoming narrowed and obstructed. Bronchiolitis is predominantly seen in the winter months (from November to February). Symptoms include coryza preceding a cough, a low-grade fever, increasing shortness of breath, an audible wheeze, irritability and poor feeding. On examination, intercostal and subcostal recession, hyperinflated chest, widespread fine inspiratory crepitations and high-pitched wheeze can be ascertained.

Croup

Croup, otherwise known as laryngotracheobronchitis, is often caused by the para-influenza virus but RSV, adenovirus and influenza virus have also been implicated. It affects infants and young children between the ages of 3 months and 3 years with peak incidence at 2 years of age. Severe cases can result in inflammation of the subglottic region in an already narrowed developing trachea. Symptoms are generated by the narrowing of the airway, particularly of the larynx, trachea and bronchi. This is caused by an inflammatory response to the infection rather than the infection itself. Symptoms include a harsh barking cough (or seal-like bark which is pathognomonic), inspiratory stridor and hoarseness preceding a low-grade fever and coryza (**mnemonic** of croup symptoms: **Three S's** – **S**tridor, **S**ubglottic swelling, **S**eal-bark cough). Symptoms are often noted to be worse at night. Moderate and severe symptoms include sternal and suprasternal recession at rest, inspiratory and expiratory stridor, respiratory distress, agitation and drowsiness. An AP film can be performed to reveal the steeple sign (narrowing of the subglottic lumen by 1–1.5 cm producing an inverted 'V' configuration resembling a church's steeple). Croup should be differentiated from epiglottitis, which is a life-threatening emergency due to respiratory obstruction.

Epiglottitis	Croup
Affects (usually) 1 to 6 years of age	Affects (usually) 3 months to 3 years of age
Rapid onset (hours)	Slow onset (days)
Absent or weak cough	Barking (seal-like) cough
No preceding coryza	Preceding coryza
Drooling saliva	Able to swallow
Temperature >38.5°C	Temperature <38.5°C
Weak, whispering voice	Hoarse voice
Unable to eat or drink (painful throat)	Able to eat and drink
Soft continuous stridor, unwilling to speak	Harsh inspiratory stridor
Toxic, upright, mouth open, immobile	Appears unwell but communicative

Pneumonia

Pneumonia can be caused by a bacterial, viral or parasitic infection of the lung. It results in inflammation of the alveolar space with consolidation and a compromise in air exchange. Symptoms include fever, cough, lethargy, poor feeding, pleuritic chest pain and shortness of breath. On examination, signs of consolidation may be elicited, including reduced breath sounds over the affected area, dullness to percussion, bronchial breathing with increased vocal fremitus and crepitations on auscultation. A chest X-ray may reveal evidence of consolidation and a sputum or blood culture may disclose the causative organism.

Causative Organisms of Pneumonia in Children

Newborn	Group B beta haemolytic *Streptococcus*
	Escherichia coli (E. coli)
	Gram-negative bacilli
	Chlamydia trachomatis
Infancy	Respiratory syncytial virus (RSV)
	Streptococcus pneumoniae
	Haemophilus influenzae
	Staphylococcus aureus
Older children	*Mycoplasma pneumoniae*
All ages	Tuberculosis

PAEDIATRICS: **Abdomen Examination**

INSTRUCTIONS: You are a foundation year House Officer in paediatrics. Examine this child's abdominal system. Explain to the examiner what you are doing as you proceed and present your differential diagnosis.

NOTE: When conducting a paediatric examination, it is important to be opportunistic. Be prepared to tailor your examination to the child and be flexible in your approach.

EXAMINATION

0 1 2

☐☐☐ **Introduction**   Introduce yourself. Establish rapport with the child.

Explain   Explain the purpose of the examination and obtain consent from the parent (and child where appropriate) to expose and examine the child.

☐☐☐ **Position**   Lie the patient flat on the couch and expose the abdomen by lowering the child's clothes to the pubic symphysis.

INSPECTION

☐☐☐ **General**   Observe the patient from the edge of the bed. Check if the child's physical appearance is consistent with their age and comment on their nutritional status. Note the shape of the abdomen, evidence of distension or abnormal movements. Inspect for any visible organomegaly or any masses, commenting on site, size, overlying discolouration and cough impulse.

General Observations in the Abdomen Examination

Development	Height and weight for age (check against growth chart)
Stoma sites	Ileostomy, colostomy, gastrostomy, nephrostomy
Catheters/tubes	Nasogastric tube, central line (TPN), continuous ambulatory peritoneal dialysis or other dialysis catheters
Abdominal contour	Flat, scaphoid (sunken), protuberant (normal – young children)
Presence of scars	Roll the child onto their side in order to avoid missing any scars located on the back
Abdominal movements	Gastric peristalsis (pyloric stenosis, intestinal obstruction) or pulsations

Distension	Ascites (umbilical eversion), intestinal obstruction, faeces, hernias
Wasted buttocks	Coeliac disease (weight loss)

☐☐☐ **Hands** Feel the hands and inspect the nails. Look in the hands for:

Hand Signs in the Abdomen Examination
Clubbing	IBD, coeliac disease, biliary cirrhosis and billiary atresia
	Chronic active hepatitis, CF
Palmar erythema	Chronic liver disease
Leuconychia	Cirrhosis
Koilonychia	Iron deficiency (coeliac disease)

RH	Right Hypochondrium		RF	Right flank or lumbar area
RIF	Right iliac fossa		E	Epigastrium
UR	Umbilical region area		H	Hypogastric or suprapubic
LH	Left hypochondrium		LF	Left flank or lumbar area
LIF	Left iliac fossa			

☐☐☐ **Face** With patient looking down, lift one eyelid and look at the sclera for signs of jaundice and anaemia. Kayser-Fleischer rings in the periphery of the cornea appear in children with Wilson's disease, best seen under slitlamp examination. Look around the lips for brown freckles (Peutz–Jeghers syndrome). Inspect the mouth for:

Signs in the Tongue in the Abdomen Examination
Central cyanosis	Blue tongue
Macroglossis	Congenital hypothyroidism, Beckwith–Wiedemann syndrome

Atrophic glossitis	Iron, folate, B12 deficiency
Dry tongue	Dehydration
Ulcers	Crohn's, coeliac disease, Behcet's disease
Breath smell	Ketosis, foetor hepaticus

Body

Inspect the rest of the body for skin changes and visible manifestation of hepatic impairment including bruising, petechiae, spider naevi and caput medusa (dilated collateral veins around umbilicus).

PALPATION

☐☐☐ **Abdomen**

Enquire if the child has any tenderness in their abdomen by asking: '*Does your tummy hurt?*' Explain to the youngster in simple terms what you intend to do. If the child is young you may wish to demonstrate on a toy how you will be palpating his abdomen. Be cautious in being patronising when talking to an adolescent.

Distraction Techniques when Examining a Child
1 Play 'peek-a-boo' or blow 'raspberries' at infants
2 Permit toddlers to play with your instruments (stethoscope, ophthalmoscope)
3 Provide infants with something to hold (their favourite toy)
4 Engage them in conversation (discuss computer games, school, best friends)

Warm your hands and examine the child at their level by kneeling down. Look at the child's face for grimacing while palpating for signs of local tenderness. A toddler may initially resist you examining them. Employ distraction techniques if necessary. If unsuccessful, use the child's hand to guide yours around his abdomen.

☐☐☐ *Light Palpation*

Palpate all quadrants of the abdomen starting away from the site of the pain. Note any tenderness, rebound tenderness (greater pain felt on releasing pressure), guarding (reflex contraction of abdominal muscles) or rigidity.

Deep Palpation

Palpate all quadrants more deeply. Feel for masses and deep tenderness. If a mass is detected note its size, shape, edge, consistency, percussion note and the presence of bowel sounds or a thrill.

Liver

Palpate the liver from the right iliac fossa. Ask the child to take deep breaths in. During inspiration, press firmly inwards and upwards using the flat of your hand to palpate the liver. Allow the liver edge to slip under your fingertips as the liver descends. Progressively palpate towards the costal margin.

Feel for an enlarged liver describing its edge (smooth, irregular), size (in centimetres below costal margin), consistency (soft, firm, hard), nodularity and tenderness.

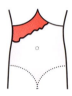

Causes of Hepatomegaly

The liver edge can be normally found 1–2 cm below the costal margin. However, the anterior border is hidden beneath the ribs but can be determined by percussion. It enlarges towards the RIF and moves with respiration

Infection	Hepatitis A B C, infectious mononucleosis, malaria
Malignancy	Leukaemia, lymphoma, neuroblastoma
Liver disease	Neonatal liver disease, chronic liver disease, polycystic disease
Metabolic	Reye's syndrome, glycogen storage disorders, galactosaemia, Wilson's disease, alpha-1 antitrypsin deficiency
Haematological	Haemolytic disease of newborn (sickle cell disease, thalassaemia)
Congestion	Heart failure, biliary atresia

Spleen

Palpate the spleen from the right iliac fossa towards the left hypochondrium using the same technique for the liver edge. The spleen should be found between the 9th and 11th ribs extending to the anterior axillary line in adolescents, but in infancy it can be felt on inspiration as a soft swelling as far as 1–2 cm below the costal margin. Feel for a notch, size, consistency and tenderness.

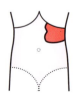

Causes of Splenomegaly

The spleen can normally be felt just below the costal margin. It has a smooth soft edge posteriorly with the anterior border hidden beneath the ribs. The spleen moves with respiration. During infancy, a 1–2 cm spleen tip is usually palpable

Infective	Malaria (massive splenomegaly, fever and rigors), SBE, infective endocarditis, typhoid, infectious mononucleosis, TB (fever, weight loss, CNS signs), toxoplasmosis
Haematological	Sickle cell disease

| Malignancy | Leukaemia (massive), lymphoma (lymphadenopathy, weight loss, CNS signs) |
| Congestion | Portal hypertension (portal vein obstruction, cirrhosis) |

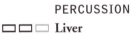 **Kidneys**

Ballot the kidneys on inspiration. Position one hand beneath the patient's lower rib cage and the other hand on the surface of the abdomen. Ask the patient to breath in deeply. Attempt to push the kidney with the lower hand onto the finger tips of the resting hand. Note any tenderness or enlargement.

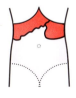

Causes of Enlarged Kidneys

The kidneys are usually not palpable after the neonatal period. They can be palpated by balloting bimanually. They also move with respiration

| Unilateral enlarged | Polycystic kidney disease, perinephric abscess, hydronephrosis, malignant (hypernephroma, nephroblastoma) |
| Bilateral enlarged | Polycystic kidney disease, hydronephrosis, nephroblastoma |

PERCUSSION

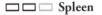 **Liver**

Inform the child that you wish to percuss their abdomen '*like a drum*'. Percuss the upper and lower liver borders to detect any enlargement. Note a change in percussion note from resonant to dull. The normal liver span varies with height and sex but is generally located between the 4th and 6th rib (mid-clavicular line) and the costal margin or up to 1–2 cm below the costal margin in children aged up to 3 years. The upper limit of normal for the liver span is 8 cm at 5 years and 13 cm by puberty onwards.

Causes of Hepatosplenomegaly

Hepatosplenomegaly is the concurrent enlargement of both the spleen and liver. There are usually other associated signs to support your diagnosis

Infective	Malaria, SBE, infectious mononucleosis
Haematological	Sickle cell disease, thalassaemia
Congestion	Portal hypertension (portal vein obstruction, cirrhosis)

Spleen

Percuss the spleen employing a similar technique as for the liver.

Splenomegaly	Left Kidney
Palpable in infants (not in older children)	Usually not palpable (after birth)
Notched edge	Smooth shape
Moves early in inspiration	Moves late in inspiration
Dull to percussion in Traub's space	Resonant to percussion
Cannot get above the spleen (ribs on top)	Possible to get above the kidney
Not ballotable	Manually ballotable
Enlarges towards RIF in older children but LIF in infants	Directed downwards

☐☐☐ **Ascites**

Examine the child for shifting dullness or fluid thrill.

Shifting Dullness

Percuss from the umbilicus towards the flanks while noting the point of dullness. Roll the child towards you keeping your finger over this point. Wait 30 seconds and percuss the marked point again to see if the dullness has shifted. Return the patient to the supine position and check if dullness has returned to this point.

Percuss from the midline down to the flank until percussion goes dull. Mark this level

Resonant

Dull

Roll the child and percuss the marked level

Resonant

Ascites

Fluid Thrill

To assess the presence of a fluid thrill, ask the young person or parent for assistance. Place the assistant's hand along the midline of the child's abdomen. Place your detecting hand in the flank area while softly flicking the surface of the skin on the opposite flank area with your index finger. The presence of a fluid thrill suggests severe ascites.

☐☐☐ **Bladder**

Percuss the suprapubic area for dullness (bladder distension).

AUSCULTATION

☐☐☐ **General**

Listen over the abdomen with a stethoscope for peristaltic bowel sounds. Listen for 30 seconds and establish the number of sounds heard (at least 2–3 in 30 seconds). Determine if they are hyperactive ('tinkling' – obstruction), hypoactive or absent (general peritonitis, paralytic ileus).

Renal Bruits   Listen over the renal arteries, approximately 2–3 cm superior and lateral to the umbilicus, for bruits (renal artery stenosis).

ADDITIONAL POINTS

☐☐☐ **Hernias**   Feel for a cough impulse over the hernial orifices as the patient coughs.

Nodes   Feel for inguinal lymph nodes.

☐☐☐ **Request**   For the purpose of completion, state that you would like to examine the external genitalia, inguinal and perianal regions, including a PR examination. However, you would not be expected to do this in the OSCE as it is likely to upset the child. Request to dipstick the urine.

☐☐☐ **Summarise**   Check with the patient and deliver an appropriate summary.

EXAMINER'S EVALUATION

0 1 2 3 4 5
☐☐☐☐☐☐ Assessment of abdomen examination
☐☐☐☐☐☐ Role player's score
Total mark out of 32

DIFFERENTIAL DIAGNOSIS
Coeliac Disease

The term 'coeliac' is derived from the Greek word *koiliakos*, which means 'suffering in the bowels'. It was first described by the Greek physician Aretaeus of Cappadocia, who wrote a chapter entitled 'The coeliac diathesis' where he described the symptoms of fatty diarrhoea (steatorrhoea), weight loss and pallor. Coeliac disease is an autoimmune disorder of the small bowel and is defined pathologically as a permanent gluten-sensitive enteropathy. It is caused by an intolerance reaction to gliadin found in dietary gluten (wheat, barley, rye), which results in villous atrophy. Its prevalence in the UK is 1 in 2000 but higher incidences are noted in Ireland (1 in 300). Classically, it presents in childhood between 6 months and 2 years. Symptoms include chronic diarrhoea, steatorrhoea (pale, bulky), failure to thrive, occasional vomiting, weight loss, constipation and abdominal distension. On examination, signs include short stature, distended abdomen and wasted buttocks. Patients often live a near-normal life with a life-long gluten-free diet.

Inflammatory Bowel Disease (IBD)

Inflammatory bowel disease comprises Crohn's disease and ulcerative colitis. Although it is uncommon in childhood, up to one-quarter of patients present with it in childhood or adolescence. Crohn's disease is a transmural chronic inflammatory disease that can affect any part of the gastrointestinal tract from the mouth to the anus (the distal ileum and proximal colon being most frequently affected). Ulcerative colitis is an ulcerating disease affecting only the mucous membrane of the large bowel. Presentations are not dissimilar to the adult form. Symptoms include abdominal pain, diarrhoea, rectal bleeding, growth failure and weight loss. Crohn's disease may also present with perianal tags, fissures and fistulae and with extra-intestinal symptoms such as arthritis, uveitis and erythema nodosum. Ulcerative colitis, on the other hand, may present with pyoderma gangrenosum, erythema nodosum, arthritis and spondylitis. Colonoscopy and biopsy are the most definitive tools to diagnose and differentiate between Crohn's disease and ulcerative colitis. In ulcerative colitis, inflammation with granular erythematous mucosa and absence of vascular markings is noted in the rectum and progresses proximally in a continuous fashion. Crohn's disease presents with aphthous ulceration sparing the rectal muscosa and with skip lesions (**mnemonic**: 'Crohn's has Cobblestones on endoscopy'). Visualisation of the terminal ileum (small bowel) is useful since inflammatory changes at this point would suggest Crohn's disease rather than a diagnosis of ulcerative colitis.

Features of Crohn's disease	
Mnemonic: 'CHRISTMAS'	
Cobblestones on endoscopy	Transmural (all layers, aphthous muscles)
High temp (fever)	Malabsorption
Reduced lumen	Abdominal pain
Intestinal fistulae	Submucosal fibrosis
Skip lesions	

Kidney Transplant

A common case in clinical examinations is an older child with a transplanted kidney for the treatment of end stage kidney disease. In children, by far the commonest cause of chronic renal failure (CRF) is a structural malformation (vesicoureteral reflux, obstruction – posterior urethral valves, pelviureteric or vesicoureteric junction obstruction), hypoplasia and dysplasia. Older children may also develop end stage renal failure secondary to glomerular disease such as chronic glomerulonephritis and tubulointerstitial disease. Cystic disease may also be responsible for the development of CRF, the most common being cystic renal dysplasia. CRF may also be seen in haemolytic–uraemic syndrome and tends to manifest as a triad of renal failure, thrombocytopenia and microangiopathic haemolytic anaemia; typically between the ages of 3 and 10 years. Hereditary nephropathies may also be implicated. For example the autosomal recessive polycystic kidney disease may present with enlarged kidneys during infancy and with the development of portal hypertension from hepatic fibrosis by mid-childhood. These children may therefore have signs of a transplanted kidney and a RIF scar, anaemia, osteomalacia and growth retardation that need to be picked up during physical examination.

PAEDIATRICS: Gait and Neurological Function

INSTRUCTIONS: You are a foundation year House Officer in paediatrics. Examine this child's gait and neurological system. Explain to the examiner what you are doing as you proceed and present your differential diagnosis.

4.8

NOTE: In the OSCE setting you will probably be expected to examine an adolescent teenager. However, it may be appropriate, particularly in the case of a young child, to ask a few questions of the parent regarding development and make general observations of the child at play before commencing your examination.

EXAMINATION

0 1 2

□ □ □ **Introduction**   Introduce yourself. Establish rapport. Ascertain the patient's name and age. If an adult is present, confirm their relationship to the child.

Explain   Explain the purpose of the examination and obtain consent from the parent to expose and examine the child. Check that the child is comfortable.

Exposure   Position and expose the child's arms and legs adequately and appropriately.

EXAMINING GAIT

□ □ □ **General**   Observe the child's limbs. Look for any wasting, fasciculation or hypertrophy.

□ □ □ **Sitting**   Observe the child while they are sitting. Look for any postural abnormality or instability.

□ □ □ **Rising**   Ask the child to stand up. Look specifically for Gower's sign whereby the child tries to elevate himself using his arms and hands to 'climb up' his body from squatting as a result of weak hip and thigh muscles (Duchenne muscular dystrophy).

Gower's Sign

When the child is asked to stand up from the floor, the child attempts to elevate himself by holding onto and pushing off his thighs (limb girdle weakness – DMD)

☐☐☐ **Walking**

Ask the child to walk to the end of the room, turn round and return. Observe each stage of their gait including the start, rate, type of gait, arm swinging and how they turn round.

Observing the Child's Gait

Wide base/ataxic	Cerebellar disease
Hemiplegic	Stroke, infection, trauma, tumour, hemiplegic cerebral palsy
Spastic diplegic	*(Little's disease)* Spastic cerebral palsy
Painful/antalgic	Causes of pain: arthritis, sepsis, trauma
Limp and lurch	Unilateral hip dislocation
Waddling gait	Bilateral hip dislocation, muscular dystrophy (DMD)

ASSESSING NEUROLOGICAL FUNCTION

☐☐☐ **Tone**

Assess tone in the arms by asking the child to relax their arms by making them go 'floppy'. Gently test tone by flexing and extending the wrists and elbows while supinating and pronating the forearm. Assess tone in the legs by asking the child to relax their legs while you gently roll them back and forth with your hands.

☐☐☐ **Power**

Carry out a formal assessment of power if (as is likely) the child is old enough to follow your instructions. Each muscle should be tested in isolation. Compare both sides. For younger children it may be sufficient to assess them playing, for example, throwing or kicking a ball or picking up a toy from the floor.

Upper Limbs

Ensure that the child is sat upright before the examination.

Instructions to Assess Power in the Upper Limb

Shoulder abduction	'Raise your elbows like wings; don't let me push them down'
Elbow flexion	'Bring your arms up like a boxer; pull towards you'
Elbow extension	'Push me away'
Long wrist extensors	'Make a fist with your hand and bend your wrist back; don't let me push it back down'
Finger extension	'Straighten your fingers and stop me from bending them when I push down'
Finger flexion	'Grab my fingers and squeeze them as hard as possible'

Finger abduction	'Spread your fingers wide apart and don't let me push them together'
Thumb abduction	'Raise your thumb to the ceiling and don't let me push it down'

Lower Limbs

Ensure that the child is lying flat when examining his lower limbs. Note that, if the child is very young, it is easier to observe their movements during physical activity and watch closely the relevant use of muscles against gravity.

Instructions to Assess Power in the Lower Limb

Hip flexion	Place hands on thigh. 'Push up against my hand'
Hip extension	Place hands under thigh. 'Push down against my hand'
Knee flexion	Bend child's knee and place a hand behind heel. 'Bring your heel to your bottom'
Knee extensors	Bend child's knee. 'Kick me away'
Ankle dorsiflexion	Hold child's medial and lateral malleoli with one hand. Place ulnar part of the other hand against the dorsal aspect of the foot. 'Push against my hand'
Ankle plantarflexion	Place ulnar part of hand against the plantar aspect of the foot. 'Push down against my hand'
Big toe extension	Place finger against the big toe. 'Push your toe against my finger'

□□□ **Reflexes**

Use a tendon hammer to elicit reflexes in the arms (biceps, supinator and triceps) and legs (knee and ankle). Exaggerated reflexes are suggestive of an upper motor neurone lesion. Reduced reflexes are indicative of lower motor neurone lesion. Indicate that you would not try and elicit a plantar response as the Babinski test is not reliable in children.

Common Nerve Roots
Mnemonic: Nerve roots ascend from 1–8

Ankle	S1, 2	Supinator	C5, 6	Triceps	C7, 8
Knee	L3, 4	Biceps	C5, 6		

□□□ **Coordination**

Test coordination in the upper and lower limbs. As with testing muscle power, a formal assessment is appropriate for children who can follow instructions effectively. Otherwise assess the child's coordination by asking the child to hop on one leg (lower limb) or to carry out a simple task like building blocks (upper limb).

Upper Limbs   Test finger-nose coordination by asking the child to move their index finger between your finger and their nose as fast as possible. Observe for past pointing and intention tremor. Test for dysdiadochokinesia by asking the child to clap their hand against their thigh alternating between dorsal and palmar surfaces (demonstrate this to the child).

Lower Limbs   Direct the child to move the heel of one foot and place it on the knee of the other leg. Next, ask them to run their heel down their shin and repeat the cycle again. Repeat the test on the other leg.

Sensation   A formal assessment of sensation is not usually required in an OSCE setting. However, do offer to perform a full sensory assessment.

☐☐☐ **Cranial Nerves**   A formal assessment of cranial nerve function is not usually required and is quite difficult to perform on an infant or toddler. Indicate to the examiner that you would like to carry out a full cranial nerve examination.

Assessing Cranial Nerves in an Infant or Child

I	**Smell**	Can be difficult to assess in a young child (try mint or vinegar)
II	**Acuity, pupils**	Can the child see? Perform visual test appropriate for age. Check direct and consensual light reflex as well as peripheral vision
III,IV,VI	**Eye movements**	Have the child follow your torch. Form an 'H' sign and observe the eye movements and ability to track your movements succinctly. Look for nystagmus
V	**Sensation**	Apply light touch to the child's face. Note a rooting reflex in a baby
VII	**Facial muscles**	Observe the child crying. Is there any facial asymmetry? Does the child close both eyes?
VIII	**Hearing**	Check the red book for formal hearing tests at birth. Consider distraction tests (infant) or audiometry tests
IX,X	**Swallowing**	Observe swallowing of water or bottle of milk

| XI | Trapezius | Observe neck movements or ask child to shrug shoulders |
| XII | Tongue | Observe tongue movements or ask child to move protruded tongue from side to side |

| **Request** | State that you would request investigations as appropriate (imaging, nerve conduction, etc.) in order to confirm and support your diagnosis. |
| □□□ **Summarise** | Check with the patient and deliver an appropriate summary. |

EXAMINER'S EVALUATION

0 1 2 3 4 5

□□□□□□ Assessment of neurological system

□□□□□□ Role player's score

Total mark out of 23

DIFFERENTIAL DIAGNOSIS

Duchenne Muscular Dystrophy

Duchenne muscular dystrophy (DMD) is an X-linked form of muscular dystrophy that occurs in around 1 in 3000 male births (although one-third of cases are spontaneous mutations). It results from mutations in the dystrophin gene, which is important for basic muscle function. It usually presents in the first 6 years of life with generalised symmetrical weakness of proximal muscles. This can manifest as delayed walking (18 months) with a waddling gait, frequent falls and impaired ability to climb stairs. Other features which may be elicited include muscle wasting, pseudohypertrophy of the calves (due to fatty infiltration) and Gower's sign. Later features include a more widespread pseudohypertrophy, loss of tendon reflexes and osteoporosis. Often, the diagnosis is clinical. Blood creatine phosphokinase (CPK-MM) can be measured in suspected individuals with an elevation of 100–200 times the normal level in those affected. In most cases affected individuals are wheelchair bound by the age of 12. The disease is usually fatal by the age of 20.

Cerebral Palsy

Cerebral palsy (CP) is the term used to describe a variety of persistent, non-progressive motor syndromes affecting children up to age of three. In most cases, the developmental abnormality occurs during pregnancy. Prevalence is approximately 1 in 1000 live births. It is usually categorised depending on the clinical picture: spastic (70% of cases), choreoathetoid (dyskinetic) (10%) and ataxic (10%). The remaining 10% of cases have a mixed picture. Known factors which increase the risk of CP include premature birth and low birth weight. Causes of CP include prenatal cerebral malformation (60% of cases), injury during or after birth, infections, brain hypoxia and metabolic abnormalities. Despite being described as 'non-progressive', the disorder can present differently in the early years as the child attains more developmental milestones. The infant may show early hand preference (within 1 year), be stiff on handling and may not meet expected developmental milestones. Symptoms and signs are diverse and largely depend on the type of CP, although in general they include spastic tone, unsteady gait, involuntary movements, abnormal posture (adducted shoulder, flexed elbow and wrist with clenched hand), impaired coordination and abnormal tendon reflexes. In patients who are able to walk, a scissor gait and walking on toes are common. There are also several associations with CP, including mental retardation, severe learning difficulties, visual and hearing impairment, speech disorders, behavioural disorders and epilepsy. There is no cure for CP and management is primarily based around improving the patient's quality of life and reducing symptoms through the use of physiotherapy, occupational and speech therapy. Associated conditions (e.g. epilepsy) are managed as necessary.

Myotonic Dystrophy

Myotonic dystrophy is an autosomal dominant inherited, chronic and progressive form of muscular dystrophy. The incidence of the disease is 5 per 100 000 and demonstrates a phenomenon called anticipation. This is when the illness presents earlier in successive generations and with increased severity. It can sometimes present at birth although it usually appears between the ages of 15 and 40. Presenting features often include muscle weakness, stiffness and fatigue. Other features and associations include frontal balding, myopathic facies ('fish face'), sternocleidomastoid wasting (causing a 'swan neck' appearance), cataract formation, heart conduction defects and hypogonadism. Characteristically, sufferers have distal muscle weakness and wasting, and are unable to release their hands after grasping an object. Diverse cognitive problems may also be present.

INSTRUCTIONS: You are leaving your busy paediatric outpatient clinic when you see a collapsed child in the waiting area. Nobody else is available for help. Assess the situation and commence resuscitation.

4.9

PROCEDURE

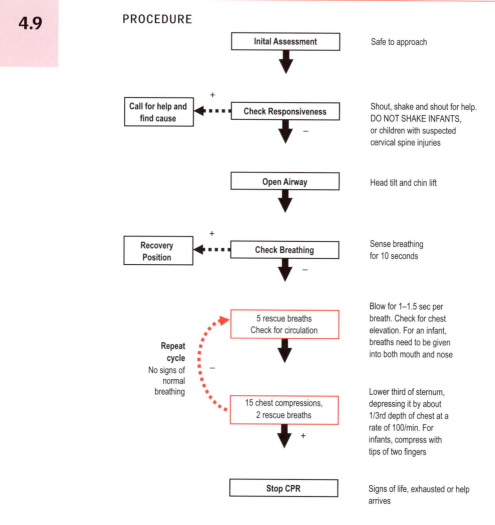

Inital Assessment	Safe to approach
Check Responsiveness / Call for help and find cause (+)	Shout, shake and shout for help. DO NOT SHAKE INFANTS, or children with suspected cervical spine injuries
Open Airway	Head tilt and chin lift
Check Breathing / Recovery Position (+)	Sense breathing for 10 seconds
5 rescue breaths / Check for circulation	Blow for 1–1.5 sec per breath. Check for chest elevation. For an infant, breaths need to be given into both mouth and nose
15 chest compressions, 2 rescue breaths	Lower third of sternum, depressing it by about 1/3rd depth of chest at a rate of 100/min. For infants, compress with tips of two fingers
Stop CPR	Signs of life, exhausted or help arrives

Repeat cycle
No signs of normal breathing

✱ Assessment *Mnemonic* – SSSS

0 1 2
☐ ☐ ☐ **Safe**   Ensure your own safety by confirming that it is safe to approach the patient. Check there is no immediate

danger from the surroundings such as electricity, gas or chemical spillage.

□□□ **Shout**   Check the responsiveness of the child by shouting, '*Are you all right?*'

□□□ **Shake**   Gently shake their shoulders to see if there is a physical response. Do not shake if the casualty is an infant (1 year old or less), or a child with a suspected cervical spine injury.

□□□ **Shout for Help**   If there is no response from the patient, shout for help.

Responsive   If the patient is responsive (replies or moves), leave them in the position you found them, ensuring that the surrounding environment poses no danger. Try and establish the cause of the patient's current state and try to obtain assistance. Reassess the patient regularly in case of deterioration.

✴ Airway

□□□ **Open Airway**   The patient should initially be left in the position they were found in. Open the airway by gently tilting the head back and lifting the chin. If you suspect a cervical spine injury then open the airway by jaw thrust only. The jaw thrust method may also be used if you encounter difficulty in opening the airway using the head-tilt, chin-lift method.

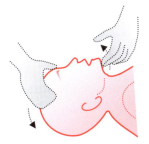

Airway Management
Open the patient's airway by placing your hand on his forehead and tilting the head backwards. Lift the chin by using your fingertips beneath it. In a suspected cervical spine injury perform a jaw thrust only

If you suspect that the neck has been injured, the airway should be opened using chin lift or jaw thrust alone. If in such a case the airway does not open, then the head should be tilted in small stages until the airway is opened.

✳ Breathing

☐☐☐ **Sense**

Keeping the airway open, bring your ear to the victim's mouth and sense for signs of breathing. Look for chest movements, listen for breath sounds and feel for breathing against your cheeks for no more than 10 seconds.

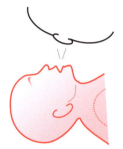

Assessing Breathing

Assess the patient's breathing by bringing your head to the patient's mouth and feeling for a breath against your cheek. Look for chest movements and listen for breath sounds for no more than 10 seconds. If in any doubt treat as if the patient's breathing is abnormal

Breathing

If the victim is breathing, reposition them into the recovery position and check for signs of continued breathing. Send for help or if alone seek assistance.

Not Breathing

If the child is not breathing normally, rescue breaths and assessment of circulation with subsequent chest compressions should be commenced before calling for help. In children and infants, five initial breaths should be given. Agonal gasps are infrequent, noisy breaths and should not be assumed to be evidence of normal breathing. This occurs in the proceeding minutes after a cardiac arrest and should be treated as abnormal breathing.

☐☐☐ **Technique**

Administer five rescue breaths appropriate for the child's age employing the correct technique if they are neither breathing nor have agonal gasps.

Child (>1 Year)

Maintain the airway by ensuring that the head is tilted and chin is lifted. Pinch the patient's nose and place your lips around the mouth forming a good seal. For each breath, blow steadily for 1–1.5 seconds making sure each breath causes the chest to rise and fall. Head tilt and chin lift must be maintained even when your mouth leaves the patient and you are watching for the chest to fall. If a face mask is available, apply it over the patient's mouth before providing rescue breaths.

Infant (<1 Year)	The head should be kept in a neutral position and chin lift should be applied. Take a deep breath and form a tight seal over the mouth and nasal apertures of the infant. Blow steadily for 1–1.5 seconds, making sure each breath causes the chest to rise and fall.
Difficulty	Difficulty may be encountered if the airway is obstructed. In this case, look for any visible obstruction in the child's mouth but do not attempt a blind finger sweep. Check that the neck is not over-extended. If head tilt and chin lift has not opened the airway, jaw thrust may be attempted.
Unsuccessful	Progress to chest compression if, after five attempts, you remain unsuccessful in achieving effective breaths.

✳ Circulation

☐☐☐ **Signs of Life** — Look for signs of movement, coughing or normal breathing. Agonal gasps do not count as signs of life.

☐☐☐ **Pulse** — Check the pulse for no more than 10 seconds. In a child check the carotid pulse; in an infant (<1 year) palpate the brachial pulse.

Circulation	If there are signs of circulation present, continue rescue breaths until the child starts breathing on their own effectively. At this point, put the child in the recovery position and check for breathing regularly.
No Circulation	If there is no pulse, a slow pulse (<60 bpm with poor perfusion) or if you are unsure about the pulse, chest compressions need to be started.

☐☐☐ **Technique** — Administer chest compressions appropriate for the child's age employing the correct technique if no signs of circulation are present.

All ages	In all children, compression of the upper abdomen needs to be avoided. The xiphisternum should therefore be located and compressions should be performed one finger's breadth above this. Avoid the child's ribs, upper abdomen or base of the sternum.
Children	For small children older than 1 year, adequate compressions can be achieved using the heel of one hand only. Ensure that you are positioned vertically

above the child's chest with your arm straightened, with your shoulder above your wrist and fingers lifted to avoid pressure over the ribs. Press down on the sternum, depressing the chest to about one-third of its depth, with the same duration taken for compression and release. If your hands and arms are too small or the child is too large for adequate compressions to be performed with one hand only, then both hands may be used with interlocked fingers. Take care not to apply pressure to the ribs.

Infants

For an infant, the tips of two fingers should be used rather than hands and arms, and ensure that the sternum is depressed by about one-third of the depth of the chest. If there are two or more rescuers, the 'encircling technique' can be employed. Place both thumbs flat, side by side, on the lower third of the sternum, with the tips pointing towards the infant's head. Encircle and support the infant's lower back with the rest of your fingers.

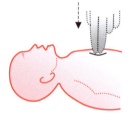

Two-finger Technique

Employ the two-finger technique on infants less than 1 year of age. Compress the chest by one-third of its depth with the tips of your index and middle finger over the sternum

Hand-encircling Technique

Place both thumbs flat, side by side, on the lower third of the sternum, with the tips pointing towards the infant's head. Encircle and support the infant's lower back with the rest of your fingers. Depress the chest by one-third of the depth of the chest

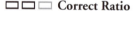 **Correct Ratio**

Two or more healthcare professionals should use a ratio of 15 compressions to two ventilations. Lay rescuers should use a ratio of 30 compressions to two ventilations. Maintain compressions at a rate of 100 per minute (just under two compressions per second). If assistance is available alternate chest compressors every two minutes to prevent exhaustion. Ensure the duration of the transitions is kept to a minimum.

Call for Help

One minute of CPR should be given before calling for help. Ask an individual to call the resuscitation team. If you are alone, leave the side of the victim and seek assistance by telephoning the emergency number. Dial 2222 (or equivalent).

'I am a foundation year House Officer in the paediatric outpatients' department. A child has collapsed in front of me and has no cardiac output. Please call the resuscitation team immediately.'

☐☐☐ **Repeat Cycle**
After completing 15 or 30 compressions (depending on whether you are a lone rescuer or not), give the patient two effective rescue breaths. After providing two rescue breaths, continue with chest compressions. Maintain compressions at a rate of 100 per minute. If assistance is available alternate chest compressors every 2 minutes to prevent exhaustion.

☐☐☐ **Stop CPR**
Continue resuscitating the patient until help arrives, the victim shows signs of life or you feel exhausted.

EXAMINER'S EVALUATION

0 1 2 3 4 5
☐☐☐☐☐☐ Assessment of performance of paediatric BLS
Total mark out of 24

PAEDIATRICS: **Explaining Asthma to a Child**

INSTRUCTIONS: You are a foundation year House Officer in general practice. Mr Durman and his 10-year-old son Thomas have attended clinic today for a follow up to review the persistent nighttime cough he has been experiencing for the past 2 months. Thomas has been diagnosed with asthma and Mr Durman is worried that it might affect his football. You will be marked on your communication skills and the information you provide.

4.10

HISTORY

0 1 2

☐☐☐ **Introduction** — Introduce yourself. Elicit the patient's name and age. Establish the adult's relationship to the child.

☐☐☐ **Ideas** — Explore parent and child's understanding of asthma.

'I understand that you have been complaining of a cough for the last 2 months and you have been told that you have asthma. Can you tell me what you understand by this?'

☐☐☐ **Concerns** — Elicit the parent and child's concerns about having asthma.

Expectations — Elicit patient's expectations of what they would like to achieve from the consultation today.

MEDICAL ADVICE

☐☐☐ **Explain** — Explain to the child what asthma is in a simple way, avoiding the use of jargon.

'When you breathe in, air passes from your mouth and into your lungs through a tube that looks like a big drinking straw. Your lungs are two big balloons filled up with lots of little tubes. In kids with asthma these tubes become smaller and tighter, making it hard for air to pass into your lungs. This is why you may cough, make a wheezy noise or find it hard to breathe.'

☐☐☐ **Treatment** — Establish the medication prescribed and explain the rationale behind the treatment of asthma.

'Your asthma medication makes it easier for you to breathe by opening up the tubes in the lungs. We normally use inhalers to treat asthma. These contain the medicine as a gas that you breathe into your lungs. There are two different types of inhalers, one blue and one brown. Normally we start you on the blue one, known as a reliever. This works by opening up the little tubes quickly and helps relieve your asthma straight away. The other type is the brown inhaler and is called a 'preventer'. This helps prevent your asthma from getting very bad and we normally give you this if you use your blue one too often.'

☐☐☐ **Monitoring**   Advise the patient when to attend the doctor for follow-up monitoring.

'It is important for your doctor to monitor your asthma regularly using a peak flow device, usually once or twice a year. However, there are particular occasions when you should visit your doctor; for example, if your asthma affects your school or sport activities; if it affects your sleep or if you find yourself using your inhaler three or more times a week. These situations may mean that your asthma is not well controlled and we may need to change your medication.'

☐☐☐ **Advice**   Offer appropriate advice to child and parent regarding cigarette smoke exposure at home, regular dusting and cleaning (anti-mite cover for mattresses and pillows) and avoid keeping any pets in the bedroom.

Precipitating Factors for an Acute Asthma Attack
Mnemonic: 'DIPLOMAT'

Drugs (aspirin, NSAIDs, beta blockers)	**O**esophageal reflux (nocturnal asthma)
Infections (URTI, LRTI)	**M**ites
Pollutants	**A**ctivity and exercise
Laughter (emotion)	**T**emperature (cold)

☐☐☐ **Reassurance**   Reassure any parental concerns about asthma.

'Asthma is very common and is something you may have to live with for the rest of your life. If we took three children suffering wih asthma, one child will ultimately grow out of it, the other may improve during their teen years only for the asthma to return in adulthood, and the last one will continue to be asthmatic. Even if you were to suffer with asthma for the rest of your life, you should be able to maintain a normal lifestyle. I understand that you have particular concerns about your son competing competitively in football tournaments. However, I would like to reassure you that there are a number of famous sport personalities who suffer with asthma, such as Paula Radcliffe and Paul Scholes, who continue to lead a successful and fruitful life.'

CLOSING

☐☐☐ **Understanding**   Confirm that the patient has understood what you have explained to them.

☐☐☐ **Questions**   Respond appropriately to the patient's questions.

	Leaflet	Offer to give them more information in the form of a handout. Advise that the leaflet contains much of the information you have mentioned.
☐☐☐	**Follow-up**	Offer the child and parent a follow-up appointment.

COMMUNICATION SKILLS

☐☐☐	**Rapport**	Maintain rapport and engage both the parent and the child throughout.
☐☐☐	**Fluency**	Speak fluently and do not use jargon.
☐☐☐	**Summarise**	Check with the patient and deliver an appropriate summary.

EXAMINER'S EVALUATION

0 1 2 3 4 5
☐☐☐☐☐☐ Overall assessment of explaining asthma to a child
☐☐☐☐☐☐ Role player's score
Total mark out of 28

INSTRUCTIONS: You are a foundation year House Officer in general practice. Mrs Wilson gave birth to a baby boy 3 days ago. She has attended the practice and wishes to speak to a doctor as the baby has developed jaundice over the past day. It is otherwise healthy and doing well. Explain the possible causes of the baby's jaundice and deal with the mother's concerns appropriately. You will be assessed on your communication skills and on the information that you provide.

INTRODUCTION

4.11

0 1 2

☐☐☐ **Introduction**   Introduce yourself and establish rapport. Elicit the name of the mother and the age of the child and confirm their relationship.

☐☐☐ **Ideas**   Explore the mother's ideas of what may be causing her son's jaundice.

☐☐☐ **Concerns**   Elicit the mother's concern about her son's condition.

☐☐☐ **Expectations**   Elicit the mother's expectations from the consultation.

EXPLAINING JAUNDICE

☐☐☐ **Jaundice**   Explain what jaundice is, its causes and its significance in newborn babies.

'The yellow tinge that you have noticed in your child's skin and eyes is called jaundice. It occurs in about half of newborn babies. This form of jaundice is called physiological jaundice and is quite safe. It usually appears 2–3 days after birth, peaking after 5 days before gradually resolving within a couple of weeks without the need for treatment.'

'When the baby is in the womb it needs a higher number of red blood cells to carry oxygen around the body. Once it is born it can breathe oxygen on its own and so does not need as many red blood cells. These cells eventually get broken down by the body. When they get broken down a yellow substance called bilirubin is released. Usually this is carried to the liver. Sometimes in newborn babies the liver is not fully developed and so cannot get rid of this excess bilirubin which builds up and causes the yellowish appearance of the skin and sometimes in the whites of the eyes (sclera).'

☐☐☐ **Prolonged**   Explain to the patient what prolonged jaundice is.

'Jaundice can sometimes be prolonged for more than 2–3 weeks and this can occur if the baby has an infection. Occasionally, breast milk

183

·jaundice can occur and this is perfectly normal. The baby is healthy but produces low level of jaundice from the mother's milk. This type of jaundice usually clears up within 6 weeks. In such cases the mother may be asked to stop breast-feeding for a few days. Most of the other causes of jaundice are quite rare but may be serious. In such cases your baby may exhibit other symptoms, such as poor sucking or feeding and sleepiness.'

Diagnosis   Explain to the mother that their child is likely to be suffering from breast milk jaundice.

EXPLAINING TREATMENT

□ □ □ **Feeding**   Explain that the mother should continue on with normal feeding.

'Since this form of jaundice is harmless to the baby, we advise you to continue breast-feeding or bottle feeding the baby.'

□ □ □ **Blood Test**   Explain when blood tests may be required.

'If the baby is unwell or not feeding, and if the jaundice does not improve within 2 weeks or begins to spread to include the arms or legs, or if the baby has pale stools and dark urine, you will need to bring him back to the GP. A blood test may be required to check the level of bilirubin in the blood.'

□ □ □ **Treatment**   Explain when phototherapy or exchange transfusion may be required.

'If the bilirubin level is found to be above a certain level (related to the child's age) the baby may require treatment. The main treatment of choice is known as phototherapy. This involves the baby lying naked with eyes covered, under a special ultraviolet lamp. The lamp produces a special light that converts the harmful pigment into a harmless form that is later excreted by the baby. In rare occasions where the bilirubin levels are very high an exchange transfusion may be required. This is where we need to take out some of the baby's blood containing the pigment and replace it with donor blood.'

□ □ □ **Other Causes**   Explain that there are other causes of jaundice in the newborn, and that treatment involves treating the cause.

'Other causes of jaundice in the newborn do exist but they are quite rare. They include infections, incompatibility between the baby's and mother's blood, metabolic abnormalities and liver disease or infection. I would like to reiterate that these causes are rare. If the jaundice is found to be due to such a cause, then treatment may involve medication or in some cases surgery.'

☐☐☐ **Complications** Explain that untreated persistent jaundice is potentially dangerous and should be treated.

'It is important to treat jaundice that is not mild and self-limiting, as in severe jaundice high levels of bilirubin can build up in the brain. If this is untreated, it can lead to brain damage and even death. I know that this sounds alarming but it is important to know that these complications (Kernicterus) can be avoided if the jaundice is treated.'

Warning Signs Explain to the mother that she should contact the GP or bring the baby in if the baby becomes ill or if the jaundice does not resolve.

'Please do not hesitate to bring your child in if he develops a fever, is not passing urine normally, or appears to be unwell, or if the jaundice does not resolve within 2 weeks.'

☐☐☐ **Acknowledge** Acknowledge and address the mother's concerns and reassure her.

'I appreciate your concerns and understand that there is a lot of information to take in. However I would like to reassure you again that jaundice is quite common in babies, and as your child is otherwise doing well I suggest that you keep an eye on him for the next two weeks. If you have any concerns during that time please do not hesitate to call again as we are here to help.'

CLOSING

☐☐☐ **Understanding** Confirm that the patient has understood what you have explained to them.

☐☐☐ **Questions** Respond appropriately to the patient's questions.

Leaflet Offer to give them more information in the form of a handout. Advise that the leaflet contains much of the information you have mentioned.

☐☐☐ **Follow-up** Offer the child and parent a follow-up appointment.

COMMUNICATION SKILLS

☐☐☐ **Rapport** Maintain rapport and engage both parent and child throughout.

☐☐☐ **Fluency** Speak fluently and do not use jargon.

☐☐☐ **Summarise** Check with the patient and deliver an appropriate summary.

185

0 1 2 3 4 5

☐☐☐☐☐☐ Assessment of explaining jaundice

☐☐☐☐☐☐ Role player's score

Total mark out of 30

DIFFERENTIAL DIAGNOSIS

Physiological

Physiological jaundice occurs in up to 50% of all infants. It reflects a temporary inadequacy of the immature liver in breaking down the erythrocytes following birth. Characteristically, jaundice is absent in the first 24 hours of life and often appears in the second or third day after birth. It occurs in a well child with serum bilirubin levels never reaching treatment levels. The condition completely resolves within 2 weeks of birth.

Prolonged Jaundice

Prolonged jaundice is considered to be jaundice lasting more than 14 days in full-term babies or more than 21 days in pre-term babies. Causes include physiological jaundice that has not resolved, breast milk, infection, hepatitis (neonatal), endocrine disease (hypothyroidism, hypopituitarism), choledochal cysts and an abnormal biliary tract (biliary atresia).

Early Neonatal Jaundice

Jaundice that is apparent in the first 24 hours of life is never physiological and is suggestive of haemolysis. Causes include haemolytic disease (ABO incompatibility, rhesus iso-immunisation), congenital infection (**mnemonic: TORCH – TO**xoplasmosis, **R**ubella, **C**MV, **H**erpes), haemolysis secondary to haematoma, Crigler–Najjar Syndrome, Dubin–Johnson Syndrome, Gilbert's Syndrome, transient familial hyperbilirubinaemia and maternal autoimmune haemolytic anaemia.

Conjugated Neonatal Jaundice

Conjugated neonatal jaundice occurs if conjugated bilirubin levels are more than 10% of total bilirubin or greater than 20µmol/L. It is always pathological. Causes include infection, sepsis, parenteral nutrition, cystic fibrosis, alpha-1 antitrypsin deficiency and endocrine and metabolic disease.

Kernicterus

The term 'kernicterus' is from the Greek words *kern* and *icterus* and literally means 'yellow kern' (deep nuclei). This refers to the high serum levels of unconjugated bilirubin that enter the nervous system and are deposited in the kern (basal ganglia, hippocampus, geniculate bodies and cranial nerve nuclei). This rare condition may result in death or severe brain damage. It is often secondary to haemolytic diseases of the newborn such as rhesus isoimmunisation and G6PD deficiency.

PAEDIATRICS: **Explaining Immunisations**

INSTRUCTIONS: You are a foundation year House Officer in general practice. Mrs Wakefield has come into the practice with her newborn baby boy. She is aware that her son will require a programme of vaccinations, but does not know anything about them or when they are due. Advise Mrs Wakefield appropriately. You will be assessed on your communication skills and on the information that you provide.

INTRODUCTION

4.12

0 1 2

☐☐☐ **Introduction**   Introduce yourself. Elicit the patient's name, age and occupation. Establish rapport.

☐☐☐ **Ideas**   Explore the mother's understanding of immunisations.

'Congratulations on the birth of your new baby. I understand that you have come in today to discuss your child's immunisations, which are now due. Can you tell me what you already know about immunisations?'

☐☐☐ **Concerns**   Elicit her concerns and explore them appropriately.

'Is there anything in particular that worries you about immunisations?'

Expectations   Elicit the mother's expectations of what she would like to achieve from the consultation today.

MEDICAL ADVICE

☐☐☐ **Immunisation**   Briefly explain what immunisations are and how vaccines work.

'Immunisations give our body the ability to fight certain diseases if we come into contact with them. This is done by injecting a vaccine, which contains a tiny part of a bacterium, virus or their products. This small substance is not enough to make you unwell. However, it does allow the body to prepare a defence response and recognise the disease. If the child were to come in contact with the real disease, the immune system would be prepared to fight against the infection by using small proteins called antibodies and thereby protect the child.'

☐☐☐ **Programme**   Explain the diseases that the childhood immunisation programme would protect against.

187

List of immunisations that are offered to children

Diphtheria	Whooping cough (pertussis)
Tetanus	Measles
Mumps	Rubella (German measles)
Meningitis C	Pneumococcal infection
Polio	*Haemophilus influenzae* type b (Hib)

☐☐☐ Timing

Explain the ages at which the vaccines should be given and the importance of giving them at the right time.

'The vaccination programme is started when the child is still young. This is because the diseases can be very serious in childhood. It is therefore necessary to provide them with protection as early as possible.

'The first immunisations are performed when the baby is aged 2 months. Further doses are given at the ages of 3 months and 4 months. Additional immunisations are given around the ages of 12 months and 13 months, as well as at preschool (3.5–5 years) and finally, during the teens.'

Childhood Immunisation Programme

Routine and non-routine immunisations offered to children

Routine:	Age	Vaccine
	2 months	DTaP/IPV/Hib and PCV
	3 months	DTaP/IPV/Hib and MenC
	4 months	DTaP/IPV/Hib, MenC and PCV
	12 months	Hib/MenC booster
	13 months	MMR and PCV booster
	3.5–5 years	DTaP/IPV and MMR
	13–18 years	Td/IPV

Non-routine:	At birth	BCG (Babies at high risk of coming into contact with TB)
	At birth	Hep B (if mothers are hepatitis B positive)

DTaP = diphtheria, tetanus and pertussis; IPV = inactivated polio vaccine; Hib = Haemophilus influenzae B; PCV = pneumococcal conjugate vaccine; MenC = meningitis C; Td = tetanus and diphtheria; BCG = Bacille Calmette-Guérin; Hep B = hepatitis B; MMR = measles, mumps and rubella

☐☐☐ Multiple Doses

Explain why multiple doses of certain vaccines are required.

'For adequate protection, your child's immune system needs to be fully prepared against the specific diseases that we are trying to protect against. This is why for most immunisations more than one dose is needed. For long-term protection, booster doses are given later on in life.'

☐☐☐ **Effectiveness**   Explain the effectiveness of the immunisation programme.

'The UK immunisation programme has been very successful at reducing the incidence of infectious diseases in children. Because of the immunisation programme, some serious diseases such as diphtheria have almost disappeared from this country. Even though these diseases are now uncommon in the UK, they cause serious illness and death in millions of children under the age of five around the world. In most cases these deaths can be prevented by immunisation. Nowadays, there is a lot of travelling to and from the UK and there is a risk that the disease may be brought into the UK. The vaccines protect against this risk.'

☐☐☐ **Side Effects**   Explain that the vaccination may cause mild side effects in some children.

'The vaccines may produce mild side effects. In most cases, the child may become a little irritable and feel unwell. Some redness and swelling may appear at the site of the injection. Some babies may also develop a fever. If your child does develop a fever, you may consider giving them paracetamol to reduce it.'

ADDRESS CONCERNS

☐☐☐ **Concerns**   Address the mother's concerns appropriately including the number of vaccines, allergies and drug safety issues.

Overloading   Explain to the mother that having multiple vaccines does not overload the child's immune system.

'There are hundreds of thousands of young children who have successfully gone through the UK childhood immunisation programme without any problems. Vaccines are designed to make the baby's immune system stronger, and there is no evidence that multiple vaccines overload the immune system. I would like to point out that the risk of serious harm resulting because of non-immunisation is far greater than any potential risk from having multiple vaccines.'

Allergies   Explain that common allergies are not a contraindication to vaccines. Mention that in only rare circumstances are vaccines withheld.

No Obligation   Mention that although it is highly recommended, in the UK, parents can decide not to have their child immunised. Reiterate that immunisation is the best choice as it protects against serious and potentially fatal diseases.

CLOSING

☐☐☐ **Understanding**   Confirm that the patient has understood what you have explained to them.

☐☐☐ **Questions**   Respond appropriately to the patient's questions.

Leaflet   Offer to give them more information in the form of a handout. Advise that the leaflet contains much of the information you have mentioned.

☐☐☐ **Follow-up**   State that appointments and an immunisation schedule will be made for the child and can be found in their red book. Arrange a follow-up, if appropriate.

COMMUNICATION SKILLS

☐☐☐ **Rapport**   Maintain rapport and engage both parent and child throughout.

☐☐☐ **Fluency**   Speak fluently and do not use jargon.

☐☐☐ **Summarise**   Check with the patient and deliver an appropriate summary.

EXAMINER'S EVALUATION

0 1 2 3 4 5
☐☐☐☐☐☐ Overall assessment of explaining immunisation
☐☐☐☐☐☐ Role player's score
Total mark out of 30

CHILDHOOD INFECTIONS
Diphtheria

Diphtheria is an upper respiratory tract illness caused by the anaerobic Gram-positive bacterium *Corynebacterium diphtheriae* and is spread by direct physical contact or breathing in the vapourised secretions of infected individuals. The incubation period lasts 2–5 days. It typically presents with an initial sore throat and generalised symptoms such as fever and rigors. These can worsen and cause severe breathing difficulties associated with lymphadenopathy. In serious cases it can cause cardiomyopathy, peripheral neuropathy and even death.

Pertussis (Whooping Cough)

Pertussis is characterised by long bouts of severe coughing followed by a prolonged intake of breath (whooping). It is caused by the Gram-negative bacterium *Bordetella pertussis*, which is spread airborne via droplet discharges from mucous membranes of infected people. It initially presents with a cough, sneezing and a runny nose following a 2-day incubation period. These initial symptoms form the catarrhal stage. The onset of the characteristic cough signals the arrival of the paroxysmal stage, where fits of coughing can be associated with vomiting and choking. Pertussis can last for up to 10 weeks and babies under 1-year old are more at risk. The disease also has several complications, including pulmonary hypertension and encephalitis.

Tetanus

Tetanus is a condition affecting skeletal muscle. The symptoms occur as a result of the release of a neurotoxin produced by the anaerobic Gram-positive bacterium *Clostridium tetani*. Incubation generally lasts from 3 days to 3 weeks. Spread is through wound contamination and following infection, classically, there are muscle spasms affecting the jaw that can result in a locked jaw. Generalised spasms affect the rest of the body and breathing difficulties can follow. As neurotransmission becomes affected, unopposed contraction of muscle and seizures can also occur. Death occurs in around 10% of reported cases.

Polio

Polio is a disease caused by infection with poliovirus. The spread is primarily faecal and oral and the incubation period is normally around 2–20 days before first symptoms present. In most cases it is asymptomatic or produces a minor illness such as a sore throat, fever, nausea and vomiting. In around 3% of cases the central nervous system becomes affected and this can lead to either non-paralytic aseptic meningitis (with signs and symptoms of meningism) or paralytic poliomyelitis of the spinal, bulbospinal or bulbar forms. It can therefore lead to paralysis, cardiac arrest and eventually death. Due to the success of the polio vaccine, the last case of natural polio infection in the UK was in 1984.

Hib (*Haemophilus influenzae* type B)

H. influenzae type B is a form of the non-motile Gram-negative *Haemophilus influenzae* bacterium. The type B form is encapsulated, thus enabling it to resist phagocytosis. In young children and infants it can lead to septicaemia, pneumonia and meningitis. If left untreated it can be fatal.

Pneumoccocus

Streptococcus pneumoniae is a Gram-positive bacterium and is the most common cause of bacterial meningitis in children and adults. It can also cause pneumonia, otitis media and many other types of infection. Pneumonia caused by this organism, pneumococcal pneumonia, is more common in young children and the elderly.

INSTRUCTIONS: You are a foundation year House Officer in general practice. Mrs Fleming has come into the General Practice with her 11-month old son. She is aware that her son is due for an MMR vaccine in the near future but is extremely worried as she has heard that it can have adverse effects on children. Advise the mother appropriately. You will be assessed on your communication skills and on the information that you provide.

4.13

INTRODUCTION

0 1 2

☐☐☐ **Introduction**   Introduce yourself. Elicit the patient's name, age and occupation. Establish rapport with her.

☐☐☐ **Ideas**   Explore the mother's understanding of the MMR vaccine.

'I understand that you have come today to discuss with me about the MMR vaccine that your child is due to have. Can you tell me what you already know about the MMR vaccine?'

☐☐☐ **Concerns**   Elicit concerns and explore them appropriately.

'Is there anything in particular that worries you about the MMR vaccine?'

Expectations   Elicit the patient's expectations of what they would like to achieve from the consultation today.

The MMR (Measles, Mumps and Rubella) Vaccine
The MMR vaccine is a three-in-one vaccine that is administered as a subcutaneous injection and contains live attenuated viruses. The nationwide immunisation of children was introduced in 1988 protecting against measles, mumps and German measles (Rubella). It is given to children at 12–15 months with a preschool booster given between the ages of 3 and 5 years.

MMR vaccine and the autism link
Concerns over the vaccine were sparked by a paper published by Dr Andrew Wakefield *et al.* in The Lancet in 1998. They reported that 12 children had developed bowel symptoms as well as autistic features soon after being inoculated with the MMR vaccine. It was later suggested by the author that it was safer to vaccinate with single vaccines instead of the triple vaccine. The consensus of the medical and scientific community states that there is no scientific evidence for a credible link between the MMR vaccine and autism and that the lack of confidence in MMR has damaged public health. Single separate vaccines instead of the MMR vaccine would not reduce the chance of adverse

effects but would rather increase the risk of children catching the disease due to the increased time waiting for full immunisation cover. Since the article, many parents have been dissuaded from taking the MMR vaccine with take-up rates standing at 83% (London 71%), well below the 95% required to make the programme effective

MEDICAL ADVICE

▢▢▢ **Immunisation**   Briefly explain what immunisation is.

'Immunisation gives our body the ability to fight certain diseases if we were to come into contact with them. This is done by injecting a vaccine, which is a small part of the virus. This enables the body to recognise it and primes it, ready to protect against it in the future if necessary.'

▢▢▢ **MMR Vaccine**   Appropriately explain the MMR vaccine and its purpose.

'The MMR vaccine contains measles, mumps and rubella viruses that have been modified so that they no longer cause disease symptoms. It enables the body to produce an immune response which is strong enough to protect against the real disease.

'The MMR programme of vaccination started in the UK in 1988. In the year before it was introduced 86,000 children caught measles and 16 died. Because of the MMR vaccine, only one child has died from acute measles since 1992. We are close to completely eradicating rubella and mumps in children in the UK. Even though these diseases are rare, they remain common in many parts of the world. If we stopped giving these vaccines then the diseases would slowly return in the future.'

▢▢▢ **Diseases**   Briefly explain measles, mumps and rubella.

'Measles, mumps and rubella (also known as German measles) are diseases that are caused by viruses. They are often mild illnesses but can be serious and even fatal. Measles can cause a child to become very ill with a fever, rash and irritability to light. Of every 1000 people who get measles, between one and two die. Mumps causes swollen glands with a fever and headache and can cause meningitis (5% of cases), which can lead to permanent hearing loss. It can cause sterility in boys. Rubella can badly damage the baby if the mother catches it whilst pregnant.'

▢▢▢ **Timing**   Explain when the MMR vaccine is given.

'The first dose is given by injection at around 13 months. The second dose is given by injection between 3.5–5 years as part of a preschool booster programme.'

□□□ **Concerns**   Address the mother's concerns appropriately, including the autism and IBD link with triple vaccines.

Autism IBD Link   Explain to the patient that there is no proven association between the MMR vaccine and autism or inflammatory bowel disease (IBD).

'I should like to reassure you that there is no proven link between the MMR vaccine and autism. However, in 1998 a few doctors wrote an article suggesting that there was an association between taking the MMR vaccine and bowel disease. Although these scientists never claimed there was a direct link between MMR and developing autism, unfortunately that was how the media portrayed the article.

'The number of children diagnosed with conditions related to autism has been increasing for many years. Some people have taken this as an indication that the increase is caused by or linked to the MMR vaccine. In Japan a similar scare took place and the MMR was changed to single vaccines. However, this did not alter the number of children suffering from autism, therefore supporting the absence of any link.

'The World Health Organisation, one of the most respected international health organisations, has conducted extensive research into this issue and has categorically stated that there is no link between the vaccine and autism. Research has also been carried out in the USA, Sweden, Finland and Denmark. No link has yet been found.'

□□□ **Single Vaccine**   Explain why single vaccines are not recommended.

'Some people seem to believe that the MMR vaccine overloads the baby's immune system as it is three vaccines in one. In fact, the opposite is true and in most cases an excellent response is produced. If single vaccines were used there would be a time gap between the three vaccines that could potentially put the child at risk of these diseases. In addition, not all children would complete the prolonged programme, which would also result in a higher number of cases of the disease.'

CLOSING

□□□ **Understanding**   Confirm that the patient has understood what you have explained to them.

□□□ **Questions**   Respond appropriately to the patient's questions.

	Leaflet	Offer to give them more information in the form of a handout. Advise that the leaflet contains much of the information you have mentioned.
□□□	**Follow-up**	State that appointments and an immunisation schedule will be made for the child and can be found in their red book. Arrange a follow-up if appropriate.

COMMUNICATION SKILLS

□□□	**Rapport**	Maintain rapport and engage both parent and child throughout.
□□□	**Fluency**	Speak fluently and do not use jargon.
□□□	**Summarise**	Check with the patient and deliver an appropriate summary.

EXAMINER'S EVALUATION

0 1 2 3 4 5

□□□□□□ Overall assessment of explaining MMR vaccine

□□□□□□ Role player's score

Total mark out of 31

CHILDHOOD INFECTIONS

Measles

Measles is an infectious disease transmitted primarily via the respiratory spread of airborne droplets and is caused by a paramyxovirus. Following a 1–2-week incubation period, affected individuals present with a prodrome of general malaise, high fever and **C**ough, **C**oryza and **C**onjunctivitis (**mnemonic: three Cs**). During this time they may also develop Koplik spots – small, irregular buccal and lingual mucosal lesions that are pathognomic. A maculopapular rash is characteristic of the next stage that begins a few days later and the disease is considered to be infectious for up to a week following its onset. The itchy rash begins on the head and behind the ears and over the next 3 days spreads throughout the rest of the body before fading away. Diagnosis is clinical. In most cases the disease is self-limiting and treatment is supportive, with appropriate analgesia and fluids. Secondary complications (e.g. pneumonia and other systemic illness) need to be treated appropriately. Due to its infectious nature, the illness is classified as a notifiable disease in the UK.

Complications of Measles
Mnemonic: 'MEASLES COMPlication'

Myocarditis	**C**orneal ulcer
Encephalitis	**O**tis media
Appendicitis	**M**esenteric lymphadenitis

Subacute sclerosing panencephalitis   Pneumonia (bronchiolitis, bronchitis, croup)

Laryngitis
Early death
Shits (diarrhoea)

Mumps

Mumps is a viral illness which characteristically causes parotitis. It is caused by a paramyxovirus and has an incubation period of between 14 to 25 days. In around 30% of cases it is asymptomatic. It is infectious 3 days prior to symptoms starting until 10 days after onset. Transmission is via airborne droplet spread following sneezing or coughing from an infected individual. Initial symptoms can include fever, general malaise, a sore throat, a dry mouth, myalgia, fatigue and headaches. Parotid inflammation occurs in most symptomatic cases of mumps and can last for up to a week. Meningitis occurs in 15–20% of individuals with mumps although it is not usually serious. Orchitis is another manifestation of the illness and is commoner in post-pubescent individuals. As with measles, diagnosis is clinical although laboratory investigations can be used in difficult cases. Treatment is supportive although complications require specific management. This is a notifiable disease in the UK.

Rubella (German Measles)

Rubella is a disease caused by a togavirus and is often mild in nature, with a general increase in severity of symptoms with age. The incubation period is 2–3 weeks following airborne droplet transmission. After this a prodromal phase may present and can include general malaise, fever and headache. A pink macular rash may follow over the next couple of days, starting on the face, spreading to the trunk and limbs and then slowly fading away over the next few days. Characteristically there is cervical lymph node enlargement, particularly of the sub-occipital and post-auricular nodes. Forchheimer's sign refers to discrete rose-coloured petechiae on the soft palate although this is not specific to rubella. Infectivity is greatest just prior to the onset of symptoms. Diagnosis is by confirmation of the presence of rubella IgM along with the presence of a characteristic rash. Treatment is supportive and also involves appropriate isolation for children (i.e. keeping them away from school) and, for adults, enquiring if they have had contact with pregnant women. The major concern associated with rubella is congenital rubella syndrome (CRS) which is an illness affecting the neonates of mothers infected with rubella during pregnancy, particularly during the first trimester. CRS can lead to major birth defects, including deafness, congenital heart disease and mental retardation.

Dermatology

DERMATOLOGY: **Dermatological History**

You are a foundation year House Officer in dermatology. You are asked to see Miss Catteo, a 30-year-old woman, in the clinic. Take a full dermatology history, present your findings and give differential diagnoses to the examiner.

INTRODUCTION

0 1 2

□□□ **Introduction** — Introduce yourself appropriately and establish rapport with the patient.

□□□ **Name & Age** — Elicit the patient's name and age.

□□□ **Occupation** — Enquire about the patient's occupation.

FOCUSED HISTORY

□□□ **Skin Problem** — What seems to be the problem? Can you describe your skin problem? Where is it? When did it first start? Has it changed over time? Has it spread to other areas?

□□□ **Exag./relieving** — Does anything make it better or worse (cream, sunlight, heat, soaps)?

□□□ **Assoc. Sympt.** — Are there any associated symptoms (itching, pain, exuding, blistering, bleeding)? Have you noticed any problems with your nails, joints, scalp or hair?

□□□ **Medical History** — Have you had any similar episodes of this in the past? Have you had any other skin problems in the past? Do you have any allergies? Do you suffer from asthma, hayfever or eczema? Do you have any other medical conditions?

□□□ **Family History** — Do you have a family history of any skin conditions such as psoriasis, eczema or skin cancers?

□□□ **Drug History** — Have you tried any medication or creams for your skin problem? Do you use cosmetics or moisturising creams? Do you have any skin (nickel) or drug allergies?

Drug Induced Skin Reactions

Exanthematous reactions	Allopurinol, furosemide, phenytoin
Fixed drug eruption	Tetracycline, ibuprofen, sulphonamide, barbiturates
Urticaria/angiooedema	Penicillin, codeine, aspirin, anti-epileptics

5.1

Psoriasiform eruptions	ACE inhibitors, beta blockers, tetracycline, lithium
Purpura	Aspirin, quinine, sulphonamides, atropine, penicillin
Vasculitis	Allopurinol, carbamazepine, NSAIDs, thiazides
Erythema multiforme	Co-trimoxazole, lamotrigine, macrolides
Photosensitivity	Amiodarone, thiazide, tetracyclines, sulphonylurea
Alopecia	Antidepressants, cimetidine, lithium, valproate, warfarin
Nail disorders	Chloramphenicol, chlorpromazine, phenytoin

☐☐☐ **Social History** Does your skin problem have any relationship to your work? What does your job actually involve you doing? Do you have any particular hobbies? Do you come into contact with animals? Do you travel extensively? Do you get a lot of sun exposure? Do you smoke or drink alcohol?

☐☐☐ **Idea** What do you think may be causing this skin problem? Are there any particular concerns?

☐☐☐ **Impact on Life** How has this problem affected your life?

COMMUNICATION SKILLS

☐☐☐ **Rapport** Establish and maintain rapport with the patient and demonstrate listening skills.

☐☐☐ **Response** React positively to and acknowledge the patient's emotions.

☐☐☐ **Fluency** Speak fluently and do not use jargon.

☐☐☐ **Summarise** Check with the patient and deliver an appropriate summary.

'This is Miss Catteo, a 30-year-old fashion model, who presents with a history of a spot on her cheek that has slowly increased in size. She mentions that the lesion is getting redder, is ulcerative and has a shiny appearance. Although she was born in London, she spent most of her adult life in Australia where she worked as a fashion model. She states that she is fond of skin salons and in particular sun beds. There is no history of skin cancer in the family nor does she have any medical complaints (renal transplant, immunosuppression). She is extremely concerned that her skin problem is cancerous and may require an operation and that she may subsequently lose her job. In view of her history, I suspect that she may be suffering from a basal cell carcinoma (BCC). I would like to perform a biopsy to exclude other differentials such as actinic keratosis, Bowen's disease, squamous cell carcinoma and eczema.'

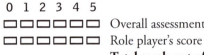

Overall assessment of dermatology history
Role player's score
Total mark out of 29

DIFFERENTIAL DIAGNOSIS
Acne Vulgaris
The term 'acne' is derived from the Greek word *acne*, which means 'skin eruption'. It is a very common skin condition (>85%) that affects male and female teenagers equally. Peak incidence is at 18 years of age, however, it usually begins prior to the onset of puberty when the adrenal gland begins to produce and release more androgen hormones. It is characterised by papules, open and closed comedones (blackheads and whiteheads), pustules, nodules and scars in the sebaceous gland distribution such as the face, neck, back and chest. Abscesses and sinuses with scaring (conglobate acne) are seen only in the most severe presentations. It is believed that androgen hormones act as the initial trigger resulting in increased sebum production and oily skin, which causes the blockage of pilosebaceous ducts giving rise to comedones. The ducts become colonised with *Propionibacterium acnes* bacteria that release a number of inflammatory markers. The body's hypersensitive response to *P. acnes* gives rise to inflammatory acne. Rarer external causes include endocrine disorders (PCOS, Cushing's, congenital adrenal hyperplasia), cosmetic agents and drugs (lithium, steroids and androgens).

Pityriasis Rosea
Pityriasis rosea is derived from the Greek word *pityron*, meaning 'bran', referring to its fine scaly appearance. Rosea, on the other hand, is derived from Latin and means 'pink'. It is a skin disease of unknown cause that commonly affects teenagers and young adults. It initially presents as a pink and flaky oval-shaped herald patch between 2 and 5 cm in diameter. Several days later, smaller cluster patches develop over the trunk, upper arms and thighs in a triangular pattern, like a Christmas tree. A severe itch often precedes the rash. The condition is self-limiting.

Pityriasis (Tinea) Versicolor
Pityriasis (tinea) versicolor is a common, benign fungal infection of the skin caused by *Pityrosporum orbiculare*. It is more frequent in humid tropical conditions such as Western Samoa (50% prevalence) and rarer in colder climates (Sweden). It often occurs in young teenagers with abnormal pigmentation. As the name suggests ('versicolor' in Latin means 'of many colours'), the lesion presents with varying colours and shapes. It manifests as a macular rash of different pigmentation to the patient's skin, with

well-defined margins. The lesions are often finely scaly, brownish pink in colour and oval or round on untanned skin. In darker skin, the lesions are more evident with a hypopigmented quality. However, each individual's lesions are evenly pigmented and lack any of the erythema or central clearing that is commonly seen in most fungal infections. They tend to collect on the trunk but can spread to the proximal limbs.

Lichen Planus

Lichen planus is derived from the Greek word *leichen*, meaning 'tree moss', and the Latin word *planus*, meaning 'flat'. The name was coined from its resemblance to tree moss although it has no known pathophysiological link with moss. It affects men and women equally but is more common in middle-aged adults. It presents as shiny itchy flat-topped (2–5 mm) polygonal lesions over flexor surfaces including the palm, soles, mucous membranes and genitalia. It is often characterised by its violaceous (violet, bluish purple) colour. Oral lichen planus is the most common presentation and manifests as lacy streaks called Wickham's striae. The condition is often self-limiting but steroids can be used to reduce the effects of inflammation.

Characteristics of Lichen Planus
Mnemonic: '5 Ps of Planus'

Peripheral (palm, soles)	**P**ruritic in nature
Polygonal (2–5 mm)	**P**urple (violaceous)
Plane (flat topped)	

Pemphigus and Pemphigoid

Pemphigus is derived from the Greek word *pemphix*, meaning 'bubble'. It comprises a group of rare autoimmune disorders that cause blistering of the skin and mucous membranes. It is more common in the middle-aged adult and presents as sores in the mouth that make eating and chewing painful. It manifests later on the skin as widespread flaccid superficial bullae particularly affecting the scalp, chest, back and face. The blisters may burst to form crusted erosions. Pemphigoid, on the other hand, is an autoimmune blistering skin disease that rarely involves the mucous membranes. It is the commoner of the two conditions, affecting predominately the elderly (a peak incidence at 65 years of age). It presents as an urticarial reaction with significant pruritus that rapidly develops into large tender, tense dome-shaped bullae ranging from 1–6 cm affecting the flexor surfaces and trunk. It is characterised by periods of exacerbation and remission with episodes lasting 1–5 years. Future recurrences are often mild and less severe.

Basal Cell Carcinoma (BCC)

Basal cell carcinoma, sometimes also called a 'rodent ulcer', is the most common malignancy of the skin. It is a slow-growing, locally invasive, but rarely metastasizing, tumour that arises from a subset of the basal cells in the epidermis. The main cause of BCC is prolonged ultraviolet exposure such that these tumours are more common in fair-skinned people living near the equator. BCC is seen typically on the face (commonly around the nose, the inner canthus of the eyelids and the temples) in elderly or middle-aged subjects. Aside from the face, BCC occurs on other sun-exposed sites, in the hair-bearing scalp, behind the ear and on the trunk. There are a number of clinical variants of BCC, the nodular type being by far the most common variety. This type of BCC usually presents as a nodule with a pearly, rolled edge and telangiectatic vessels on the surface.

DERMATOLOGY: **Dermatological Examination**

INSTRUCTIONS: You are a foundation year House Officer in dermatology. You are asked to see Mr Bowen, a 55-year-old man, in the clinic. Carry out a full dermatology examination. Present your findings and give a differential diagnosis to the examiner.

INTRODUCTION

0 1 2

☐☐☐ **Introduction**   Introduce yourself appropriately and establish rapport with the patient.

☐☐☐ **Name & Age**   Elicit the patient's name and age.

☐☐☐ **Occupation**   Enquire about the patient's occupation.

5.2

EXAMINATION

Consent   Explain the examination to the patient and obtain his consent.

☐☐☐ **Prepare**   Ensure that there is adequate illumination (skin needs to be examined in good light – preferably natural). Adequately expose the patient (ideally the patient should be undressed to his undergarments). Ask the patient if there is any pain or tenderness before commencing your examination.

★ Inspection

☐☐☐ **Observe**   Observe the skin and determine what type of lesions there are, their site, distribution, size, shape and colour.

Inspection in Dermatological Examination

Site	Describe the exact position(s) of the skin lesion(s): Flexor/extensor surfaces, ventral/dorsal surfaces Proximal/distal to nearest bony landmark
Location	Face/trunk/limbs/buttocks/scalp/ears/neck/nape/ axillae/groins/arms/forearms/legs/thighs/palms/ soles/knees/ankles/wrists/elbows/cubital fossae/ popliteal fossae
Hands/feet	Palmar/dorsal surface of hands, plantar/dorsal surface of feet
Distribution	Single/multiple, unilateral/bilateral, symmetrical/ asymmetrical Discrete/confluent/localised/grouped/generalised/ scattered/diffuse

	Dermatomal/photo-distribution (sun-exposed areas)
Size	Measure exact dimensions using a ruler: small/large/varying sizes
Shape	Spherical/hemispherical
	Oval/circular/annular (ring-like)/nummular (coin-like)/discoid (disc-like)
	Irregular/polygonal (multisided)/monomorphic (one form)/polymorphic (varying)
	Linear/curvilinear/arcuate (curved), reticular (net-like)/serpiginous (serpent-like)
Colour	Flesh-coloured (normal skin colour)
	Hyper-pigmented (darker than normal)/hypo-pigmented (paler than normal)
	Erythematous (red)/violaceous (violet)/purpuric (purple)
	White/yellow/orange/pink/pearly/translucent/brown/black

✳ Palpation
☐☐☐ Skin Lesion

Gently palpate the skin to assess the type of lesion present. Consider wearing gloves if you are examining an erosion or ulceration.

Macule

Flat, non-palpable, circumscribed area of skin discolouration.

Common Differentials of a Macular Rash

Drug reaction	History of drugs (antibiotics, thiazide), fever, affects trunk and limbs
	Distribution morbilliform (measles-like), urticarial or erythema multiforme
Freckles	Facial, small, light brown macules, darken in sun, common in redheads
Pityriasis rosea	Adolescent, generalised eruption preceded by herald patch (large 2–5 cm oval lesion), lesions are oval, pink, scaly, itchy
Pity. versicolor	Fungal (*Pityrosporum orbiculare*), adolescents, hypo-pigmented patches in darker skin, affects trunk and proximal limbs
Vitiligo	Well-defined white macules, no melanocytes, hands, face (eyes and mouth)
Café au lait spots	Neurofibromatosis, oval-shaped creamy brown patches

Plaque

Solid, palpable, flat-topped, area of skin elevation >5 mm diameter.

Psoriasis	Well-defined, erythematous coloured waxy disc-shaped plaques with silver scales, extensor surfaces and scalp, itchy
Eczema	History of asthma or hay fever, itchy, dry skin, excoriation, flexor surfaces
Fungal (tinea)	Affects trunk or limbs (corporis), groin (cruris), feet (pedis), scalp (capitis) Singular/multiple annular-shaped erythematous scaly plaques, defined margins, clear centrally. Alopecia if it affects the scalp

Papule Solid, raised, palpable skin lesion <5 mm diameter.

Common Differentials of Papules

Acne Vulgaris	Puberty, comedogenic areas (face, back, chest), greasy skin, blackheads and whiteheads, papules, pustules, cysts and scars
Scabies	Mite (*Sarcoptes scabiei*), intense itch, burrow (tortuous small ridge – 1 cm), affects fingers, wrists, nipples, does not occur above neck
Moll. Contagiosum	Viral (pox virus), pearly pink, 1–3 mm diameter, umbilicated papules, contain cheesy material, itchy, grouped lesions on truck, face, neck
Guttate Psoriasis	Adolescent, history of throat infection (beta haemolytic streptococcus), widespread raindrop-shaped pink papules over trunk or limbs
Lichen Planus	Itchy, shiny, polygonal, flat-topped (2–5 mm), white streaks (Wickham's striae), red papules turn violaceous, flexor surfaces, palm, soles, mucous membrane
Milia	Children, small white raised spots on face (upper cheeks and eyelids)
Urticaria	Superficial itchy pink swelling (wheals) with some papules, deep swelling (angiooedema) of tongue or lips, food (peanut) or drug (penicillin) reaction

Nodule Solid, raised, palpable skin lesion >5 mm diameter.

Common Differentials of Nodules

Sebaceous cyst	Firm smooth oval shaped, intradermal, visible punctum
Keloid scar	Proliferation of connective tissue, firm smooth nodules, history of trauma
Seborrhoeic wart	Papillary surface with keratin plug, defined margin, 'stuck on' appearance, pedunculated and protuberant, affects face, neck or trunk

Lipoma	Benign tumour of fat, soft masses, multiple, trunk, neck, upper extremities
Dermatofibroma	Firm nodule, commonly lower legs, history of trauma or insect bite
BCC	Pearly nodules, reddish colour, ulcer with rolled edge, sun-exposed areas
SCC	>55 yrs, actinic keratosis progresses to ulcerate and crust, sun-exposed areas
Keratoacanthoma	Rapidly growing nodule, keratin plug or crater, sun-exposed areas

Vesicle Fluid-filled (serous), raised, palpable skin lesion <5 mm diameter.

Bulla Fluid-filled (serous), raised, palpable skin lesion >5 mm diameter.

Common Differentials for Blisters (Vesicle and Bulla)

Insect bites	Depending on the insect, a blister, papules or urticarial wheal can occur
Herpes simplex	Itchy and tender clusters of tense vesicles with erythematous base, yellow crust formation, recurrent infections
Chickenpox	Prodromal illness (fever and pain), erythematous lesions develop into vesicles, pustules and dry crusts, crops of blisters affect trunk, face, limbs, scalp
Shingles (HZV)	Unilateral groups of vesicles in a dermatome with late scabs, very tender
Der. Herpetiformis	Coeliac disease, symmetrical, trunk and extensor surface, itchy vesicular rash
Pemphigus	Seen in the middle-aged, widespread flaccid superficial bullae, blisters and erosions, mucous membrane, Nikolsky sign
Pemphigoid	Seen in the elderly, urticarial reaction rapidly develops into tense bullae, flexor surfaces and trunk, recurrent and more common than pemphigus

Pustule Vesicle or bulla containing purulent fluid.

Common Differentials of Pustules

Impetigo	*S. aureus*, thin-walled blisters rupture forming yellow crust lesions, contagious
Boil, carbuncle	*S. aureus* infection of hair follicle, hard tender red nodule, increase in size, pus
Pustular psoriasis	Unwell, fever, small yellow pustules on erythematous base, commonly over palmar and plantar aspects, rapid spread
Acne vulgaris	As described as above

| | Rosacea | Erythema, telangiectasia, pustules, papules and oedema, affects cheeks, nose and forehead, rhinophyma (bulbous appearance of nose) |

| | *Erosion* | Area of skin denuded by partial or complete loss of epidermis |

Fissure
Slit in epidermis

Ulcer
Area of skin denuded by loss of epidermis and loss of underlying dermis

Wheal
Elevated area of cutaneous oedema with pale centre and pink rim

Petechia
Pinhead-sized macule of blood in skin that blanches on pressure

Purpura
Larger macule/papule of blood in skin that does not blanch on pressure

Ecchymosis
Larger extravasation of blood in skin (bruise)

Telangiectasia
Visible dilatation of small cutaneous blood vessels

☐☐☐ **Edge**
Describe the edge as well-circumscribed, ill-defined or irregular.

☐☐☐ **Surface**
Describe the surface of the skin lesion.

Palpation in a Dermatological Examination

| Surface | Smooth/rough/hard/soft/xerotic (dry)/wet/exudative Excoriation (superficial abrasion due to scratching) Atrophic (thinning of skin)/indurated (hardening of skin) Scaly (flakes due to shedding of epidermal cells)/crusted (dried exudate) Maceration (softening/disintegration of skin following prolonged wetting) Lichenification (increased epidermal thickness with accentuated skin markings) Flat-topped/umbilicated (central depression)/acuminate (pointed, spire-like) Pedunculated (with a stalk)/sessile (without a stalk)/verrucous (warty) |

☐☐☐ **2° Sites**
Look for associated features. In psoriasis, check for involvement of scalp, nails (pitting, onycholysis) and distal interphalangeal joints of the hands (arthropathy). In lichen planus, check for

involvement of the oral mucosa (Wickham's striae), hair (scarring alopecia) and nails (nail dystrophy).

Common Causes of Hair, Sweat Gland Problems and Nail Changes

Alopecia	Hair loss can be diffuse or localised
Diffuse	Genetic, hypothyroidism, malnutrition, iron deficiency, drug induced
Localised	Alopecia areata, tinea capitis (ringworm), SLE, trauma, secondary syphilis
Hirsutism	Excess hair in androgenic distribution. Idiopathic, drugs (phenytoin, corticosteroids), PCOS, menopause, Cushing's syndrome, ovarian cancer
Hypertrichosis	Excess hair in non-androgenic distribution (face and trunk)
	Drugs (phenytoin), malnutrition, anorexia nervosa, porphyria
Hyperhidrosis	Excess sweating. Physiological, menopause, malaria, thyrotoxicosis
Onycholysis	Separation of nail from nail bed. Psoriasis, fungal, thyrotoxicosis, trauma
Koilonychia	Spoon-shaped nails. Iron deficiency anaemia, lichen planus
Pitting	Psoriasis, eczema, lichen planus

☐☐☐ **Lymph Nodes**   In suspected skin malignancy, examine the regional lymph nodes for lymphadenopathy. Check as well for hepatomegaly and splenomegaly.

☐☐☐ **Summarise**   Summarise your findings to the examiner.

'This is Mr Bowen, a 55-year-old builder, who has been suffering from a red/silver scaly lesion on both extensor surfaces of his elbows. The right lesion measures 7 cm by 4 cm while the left measures 4 cm by 3 cm. Both lesions are oval in shape and are scaly in appearance. He also complains of nail changes. On examination, he was found to have widespread pitting and onycholysis. On direct questioning, he mentioned that the lesions were initially small but got worse when he started taking beta blockers for his angina. In view of the examination, I suspect Mr Frank suffers from psoriasis, however, I would like to rule out atopic dermatitis and eczema.'

EXAMINER'S EVALUATION

0 1 2 3 4 5
☐☐☐☐☐☐ Overall assessment of dermatology examination
☐☐☐☐☐☐ Role player's score
Total mark out of 27

DIFFERENTIAL DIAGNOSIS

Psoriasis

Psoriasis is a chronic skin condition characterised by inflamed, red, raised areas that develop as silvery scales on the scalp, elbows, knees and lower back. Around 2% of the population have psoriasis. Alcohol, beta blockers, lithium, NSAIDs and anti-malarials can exacerbate the condition. The most common form is called discoid or plaque psoriasis. Symptoms include salmon-coloured plaques with silver-white scales on the extensor surfaces as well as the scalp that are often itchy in nature. Other types include guttate and pustular psoriasis. Guttate psoriasis affects mostly teenagers and presents with multiple drop-like lesions that occur after a streptococcal throat infection. Pustular psoriasis presents with small pustules (pus-containing blisters) that can appear all over the body or on just the palms, soles and other small areas. Psoriasis can also involve the nails (in 50% of cases) as well as the joints (7%). Nail features include pitting, ridging, onycholysis (separation of distal nail from the nail bed) and hyperkeratosis (build up of keratin below the nail bed).

Eczema

Eczema is a term used for many types of skin inflammation (dermatitis) including atopic (the commonest), contact, allergic, seborrhoeic and stasis dermatitis. 'Atopic' refers to a collection of diseases that are hereditary including asthma, hay fever and atopic dermatitis. Atopic dermatitis (eczema) is a chronic skin disease characterised by an itchy, dry, inflamed skin causing redness, cracking, weeping, crusting, excoriations and sometimes lichenification. Atopic dermatitis occurs most often in infants and children and its onset decreases substantially with age. Although infantile eczema is common, the condition frequently improves or enters into permanent remission in the early teens; however, many are still affected throughout their life. In infants, eczema usually presents after 6 weeks of life, commonly affecting the face, forehead, chest and extensor surfaces of the extremities. In children it usually affects the flexor surfaces, such as the antecubital and popliteal areas, as well as the face, neck, back, ankles and wrists. Eczema is associated with an increased incidence of contact dermatitis, molluscum, warts and herpetic viral infections. Primary eczema lesions can be infected by secondary staphylococcus and candida infections.

Moles and Melanomas

Malignant melanoma is an invasive malignant tumour of melanocytes. Most cases occur in white adults over the age of 30, with a predominance in women. It is the most lethal form of skin cancer. The cause is not known, but exposure to ultraviolet radiation is thought to be involved. The incidence of malignant melanoma is rising rapidly. The highest incidence of melanoma occurs in countries with the most sunshine throughout the year. However, skin type and regularity of exposure to sun are also important. Malignant melanomas may occur de novo or may develop from a pre-existing melanocytic naevus (mole). Pre-existing moles can be screened for the possible development of malignant melanomas using the ABCDE system and/or the Glasgow 7-point checklist. According to the **ABCDE** system, **A**symmetry, **B**order irregularity, **C**olour variation, **D**iameter exceeding 6 mm or **E**levation of a mole warrants further investigation. The Glasgow 7-point checklist comprises three major signs (a change in the size, shape or colour of a mole) and four minor signs (diameter exceeding 6 mm, any crusting/bleeding, inflammation or altered sensation). Patients with lesions with one major and one or more minor signs should be considered for a diagnostic excision biopsy. The only treatment of proven benefit for a malignant melanoma is surgery. An excision biopsy is recommended for all suspicious lesions. If the histology confirms the diagnosis of malignant melanoma, then a wide local excision should be performed as soon as possible. When performing a wide local excision of the malignant melanoma, a 1 cm margin of normal skin around the melanoma is removed for every millimetre of thickness up to a maximum radius of 3 cm, whereby no extra benefit is achieved. Tissue is removed down to, but not including, the deep fascia. Histology can also be used to assess prognosis in malignant melanoma with the Breslow thickness used to calculate prognosis.

Breslow Thickness Predictive of Prognosis

The Breslow thickness is a valuable indicator when calculating the prognosis of malignant melanomas with no metastases. This is the vertical distance in millimetres from the granular cell layer of the epidermis to the deepest part of the tumour. Prognosis is calculated for 5-year survival and is dependent on the thickness of the melanoma. Overall prognosis is 62%

Thickness in mm	Prognosis (%)
<1.5 mm	93 (low risk)
1.5–3.49 mm	67 (intermediate risk)
>3.5 mm	37 (high risk)

DERMATOLOGY: **Advice on Sun Protection**

INSTRUCTIONS: You are a foundation year House Officer in General Practice. Mrs Cook, a 20-year-old Caucasian woman, is planning to settle in the Bahamas and work as a tourist guide. A friend of hers has recently been diagnosed with skin cancer. Counsel this patient and provide advice on sun protection and sunscreens.

INTRODUCTION

0 1 2

□□□ **Introduction** Introduce yourself. Elicit the patient's name, age and occupation. Establish rapport with the patient.

□□□ **Ideas** Elicit the patient's ideas and concerns regarding skin cancer.

'I am sorry to hear that a close friend of yours has recently been diagnosed with skin cancer. Can you tell me what you know about skin cancers?'

□□□ **Concerns** Elicit patient's concerns and explore them appropriately.

'Do you have any particular worries about skin cancer? Do you have any concerns about your new job and your chance of developing skin cancer?'

□□□ **Understanding** Check the patient's understanding of the risk of skin cancer associated with excessive sun exposure.

'What are your views on sunbathing and suntans? Do you know that too much sun exposure is not good for you? Are you aware that too much sun exposure has been linked to skin cancer? Do you know how you can protect yourself from the harmful effects of the sun?'

MEDICAL ADVICE

□□□ **Sunlight** Explain that excessive sun exposure can cause skin cancer.

'Some sunshine can be good for us, as it helps the body produce vitamin D which strengthens the bones. Sunlight has also been shown to make many of us have a feeling of well-being. However, too much sun exposure can lead to a number of skin problems, such as dryness, aging of the skin and sunburn. Sunlight is made up of different forms of energy. One in particular, ultraviolet or UV radiation, can damage the skin cells and lead to skin cancer.'

Ultraviolet light has a shorter wavelength than visible light and cannot be seen with the naked eye. It derives its name (Latin: *ultra* – 'beyond') from the position it holds on the electromagnetic spectrum, which is adjacent to the colour violet. It is a form of radiation that is emitted from the sun and is largely divided into three bands, UVA (long wave), UVB (medium wave) and UVC (short wave). The shorter the wavelength, the more damaging it is to the skin. The Earth's atmosphere blocks all UVC and most UVB rays. In fact, almost all radiation that penetrates through is UVA (98.7%). UVA radiation causes photo-aging whilst UVB rays cause sunburn (**mnemonic**: UV**A** – **A**ging, UV**B** – **B**urning). Both forms of radiation contribute towards the development of skin cancer

☐☐☐ **Measures**

Explain simple measures to reduce the risk of skin cancer.

Avoidance

'Most cases of skin cancer can be prevented by protecting our skin from the harmful effects of the sun. This is simple and need not be expensive. You should try and avoid sunbathing, sun beds and tanning lamps. When you choose to go out try and avoid the sun during its peak (from 11 am to 3 pm) when the sun's rays are strongest. If you are out in sun, avoid being out for long stretches and try and seek shade as much as possible.'

Clothing

'Ensure that you wear long sleeves and trousers rather than short sleeves and shorts. Use tightly woven clothing that will block UV radiation. Wear a wide-brimmed hat to protect your face, neck and ears. Wear a pair of UV protective sunglasses to help protect your eyes from the sun.'

☐☐☐ **Sunscreens**

Explain the role of sunscreen and the SPF and UVA system of labelling.

'Sunscreens play an important role in protecting your skin from damage by the sun's rays. However, they should not be viewed as an alternative to clothing and shade, but only as offering additional protection. It is important to note that no sunscreen will provide total protection against the sun. In addition, you should not use sunscreens to help you stay out in the sun for longer.

'Sunscreens work by blocking out both UVA and UVB radiation so it cannot reach the skin. Sunscreens with a high level of UVA protection help defend the skin against photo-aging and potentially against skin cancer, while sunscreens with a high level of UVB protection help prevent sunburn and the skin damage that can cause skin cancer. Sunscreens that offer both UVA and UVB protection are sometimes called "broad spectrum".'

☐☐☐ *SPF*

'In the UK there are two systems of labelling sun protection products, SPF and UVA star rating. SPF stands for the sun protection factor. This indicates the amount of protection against sunburn that the sunscreen provides. The SPF system primarily shows the level of protection against UVB, not the protection against UVA. For example, using an SPF of 20 means you will receive 20 times the protection against burning, compared to not using anything.'

☐☐☐ *UVA System*

'The UVA star system ranges from zero to five stars. This informs people how effective the sunscreen is against UVA rays. The best sunscreen products will block UVA and UVB rays equally and hence will get five stars. Lower star ratings indicate that less UVA radiation is blocked in relation to UVB.'

UV Rating Star System

There is no official internationally recognised standard to measure UVA absorbance. However, in the UK, a local industry recognised standard is employed known as the UVA star rating system

Star Rating	Mean UVA : UVB ratio	Description
No stars	0.0–0.2	No sun protection offered
★	0.2–0.4	Minimum sun protection
★★	0.4–0.6	Moderate sun protection
★★★	0.6–0.8	Good sun protection
★★★★	0.8–0.9	Superior sun protection
★★★★★	>0.9	Ultra sun protection

Recommend

Advise the patient on general characteristics of a recommended sun-cream product.

'When purchasing a sunscreen, always choose one that is broad spectrum with an SPF of 15 or above and has a UVA star rating of three stars or more.'

☐☐☐ **Application**

Explain to the patient how to apply the sunscreen.

'It is important to apply sunscreen thickly and evenly over all sun-exposed areas, in particular the ears, neck, any bald patches, hands and feet. Apply sunscreen up to 30 minutes before going out in the sun, and reapply at regular intervals throughout the day.'

Forecast

Recommend the patent to view weather forecasts before going out.

'It is important to take note of any weather reports on news bulletins. They often give a UV sunburn forecast which gives you a good guide as to how strong the sun rays will be on a particular day and the level of protection required.'

Ultraviolet (UV) Index

The UV index is a standardised method to measure the strength of UV (ultraviolet) radiation from the sun on a particular day. It is a scale that is used by weather forecasters to give the general public an idea of how much precaution and protection they should take against the sun's rays

UV index	Colour	Description
0–2	Green	No danger. Wear sunglasses
3–5	Yellow	Little risk. Sunscreen and hat
6–7	Orange	High risk. Sunscreen (SPF 15+), avoid peak hours
8–10	Red	Very high risk. Take extra precautions
>10	Violet	Extreme risk. Take all precautions

EVALUATION

☐☐☐ **Understanding** Confirm that the patient has understood what you have explained to them.

☐☐☐ **Questions** Respond appropriately to the patient's questions.

☐☐☐ **Leaflet** Offer to give them more information in the form of a handout. Advise that the leaflet contains much of the information you have mentioned.

COMMUNICATION SKILLS

☐☐☐ **Rapport** Attempt to establish rapport with the patient through the use of appropriate eye contact.

☐☐☐ **Fluency** Speak fluently and do not use jargon.

☐☐☐ **Summarise** Give a brief summary to the patient about what has been discussed. Thank the patient. Conclude the consultation.

EXAMINER'S EVALUATION

0 1 2 3 4 5

☐☐☐☐☐☐ Overall assessment of sun protection advice
☐☐☐☐☐☐ Role player's score

Total mark out of 30

INSTRUCTIONS: You are a foundation year House Officer in General Practice. Mrs Charles is planning to go on holiday to Spain with her family and would like to know more about sunscreen and how to apply it correctly. She is particularly worried about her two young children. Explain the correct way to apply sunscreen and deal appropriately with her concerns.

INTRODUCTION

0 1 2

☐ ☐ ☐ **Introduction**   Introduce yourself. Elicit the patient's name, age and occupation. Establish rapport with the patient.

☐ ☐ ☐ **Ideas**   Elicit the patient's ideas and concerns regarding sunscreen.

'I understand that you are going on holiday and would like to know a bit more about sunscreen lotion. Can you tell me what you know about sunscreens?'

☐ ☐ ☐ **Concerns**   Elicit the patient's concerns, i.e. not knowing the correct technique of applying sunscreen and confusion over the sunscreen grading system.

'Do you have any particular concerns about applying sunscreen?'

☐ ☐ ☐ **Expectations**   Elicit the patient's expectations.

'Is there anything in particular that you would like to learn about today?'

MEDICAL ADVICE

  ✻ Sunscreens

☐ ☐ ☐ **UV Light**   Explain the dangers of excessive sun exposure.

'The sun can emit ultraviolet (UV) radiation which can potentially harm the skin and that is why it is necessary to take precautions. The types of UV light are UVA, which can damage deeper layers of the skin and cause aging and wrinkles, and UVB, which causes tanning but also burning. UVB can damage the DNA of skin cells which can lead to skin cancer. However it is possible to achieve good protection against it by taking precautions when going out in the sun.'

☐ ☐ ☐ **Precautions**   Explain the necessary precautions to avoid excessive sun exposure such as avoiding peak hours, appropriate clothing, staying in shade where possible.

5.4

'There are some simple precautions that you and your children can take from the sun. Keep yourself inside or under the shade when the sun is at its strongest, between 11 am and 3 pm. Other things you can do to protect yourself are to wear hats with long brims, loose fitting baggy clothes, neck protectors for children and sunglasses for UV protection. Sunscreen is an additional tool in protecting your skin from the sun's harmful rays.'

❑❑❑ Grade System

Briefly explain the sun protection factor (SPF) and the UV star rating system.

'In the UK there are two systems of labelling sun protection products, SPF and UVA star rating. SPF stands for sun protection factor. The SPF system primarily shows the level of protection against UVB, not the protection against UVA. For example, using a cream with an SPF of 20 means you will receive 20 times the protection against burning, compared to using nothing. The UVA star system ranges from 0 to 5 stars. This informs people how effective the sunscreen is against UVA rays. The best sunscreen products will block UVA and UVB rays equally and hence will get five stars. Lower star ratings indicate that less UVA radiation is being blocked in relation to UVB.'

★ Application

❑❑❑ Pre-exposure

Give advice regarding pre-exposure application.

'Make sure that before applying the cream the skin is clean and dry. Try and apply it at least 15 minutes to half an hour before going out into the sun.'

❑❑❑ Application

Explain the importance in applying sufficient quantities of cream.

'Most people who use sunscreen do not apply enough of it for adequate protection. This leads to increased risk of skin damage. When applying the cream, apply generous amounts to the trunk, arms, legs and face. You must also be sure not to miss out the hands, feet, neck, around the eyes, ears, lips and the head if it is shaved or bald.'

❑❑❑ Rule of Nines

Explain the rule of nines principle to provide adequate coverage.

'In order to achieve full protection according to the sun protection factor stated on the cream, it is important to apply sufficient quantities of cream to the various parts of the body. This is easy if you follow the simple rule of nines. This means that the total surface area of skin is split up into 11 sections with each section representing 9% of the total. For each of these areas you must apply the same amount of cream equally. You can do this by squeezing out two strips of sunscreen cream from the palm crease of your hand to the tips of your index and middle fingers.'

The Rule of Nines

Most people fail to apply sufficient sunscreen on their body to ensure that the proper sun protection factor (SPF) is achieved. On average, due to their poor technique, people obtain only about one-third or one-quarter of the SPF stated on the product. 'The rule of nine' (a tool also used to assess skin burns) can be used to ensure adequate sun protection is applied. The body is divided into 11 areas, each area representing 9% of the total body surface area. Two strips of sun cream should be applied to the index and middle fingers and applied to each region. This will achieve an ideal thickness of sun cream over the body (2 mm thickness per every 1 cm^2 of skin).

Eleven areas of the body

1 Head, neck and face	7 Front abdomen
2 Left arm	8 Left upper leg and thigh
3 Right arm	9 Right upper leg and thigh
4 Upper back	10 Left lower leg and foot
5 Lower back	11 Right lower leg and foot
6 Front chest	

☐☐☐ **Rubbing In**

Explain that the sunscreen should remain visible after rubbing in.

'Rub in the cream only lightly. The cream should remain visible even after rubbing.'

☐☐☐ **Reapply**

Explain that sunscreen should be reapplied regularly, particularly to the areas that are uncovered.

'It is important to reapply the sunscreen regularly, at 2-hour intervals to ensure adequate protection. You must always reapply it after swimming, towelling, sweating or playing in the sand. However, for children it is important to reapply every hour. Focus on the areas that are exposed such as the neck, face, ears and arms and do not hesitate to use generous amounts.'

☐☐☐ **Warn**

Warn that sunscreen should never be used to spend longer in the sun.

'No sunscreen will provide 100% protection against the sun. In addition, you should not believe that sunscreens will help you stay out in the sun for longer.'

Storage	Explain that sunscreen should not be stored in very hot places (above 25°C) and should not be used past its expiry date.

EVALUATION

☐☐☐ **Understanding** Confirm that the patient has understood what you have explained to them.

☐☐☐ **Questions** Respond appropriately to the patient's questions.

☐☐☐ **Leaflet** Offer to give them more information in the form of a handout. Advise that the leaflet contains much of the information you have mentioned.

COMMUNICATION SKILLS

☐☐☐ **Rapport** Attempt to establish rapport with the patient through the use of appropriate eye contact.

☐☐☐ **Fluency** Speak fluently and do not use jargon.

☐☐☐ **Summarise** Give a brief summary to the patient about what has been discussed. Thank the patient. Conclude the consultation.

EXAMINER'S EVALUATION

0 1 2 3 4 5

☐☐☐☐☐☐ Overall assessment of explaining sunscreen application

☐☐☐☐☐☐ Role player's score

Total mark out of 35

Rheumatology

RHEUMATOLOGY: **Rheumatological History**

INSTRUCTIONS: You are a foundation year House Officer in rheumatology. Please elicit a full history relevant for this patient's complaints. You will have 10 minutes to complete this.

INTRODUCTION

0 1 2

☐☐☐ **Introduction** — Introduce yourself and establish rapport with the patient.

☐☐☐ **Name & Age** — Elicit the patient's name and age.

☐☐☐ **Occupation** — Enquire about the patient's present occupation.

6.1

HISTORY

☐☐☐ **Complaint** — Elicit all the patient's presenting complaints.

History — When did it/they first start? What did you first notice? Is it getting better or worse? Have you ever had it before? Any recent trauma or infection?

☐☐☐ *Pain* — Where is the pain? When does it start? Did it start suddenly or gradually? Does the pain move anywhere? What does the pain feel like? How severe is the pain? What makes it worse? Is the pain worse after activity? What makes it better? Is the pain better on resting? Are there any other symptoms?

☐☐☐ *Stiffness* — When do you notice stiffness in your joints? Did it start suddenly or gradually? Is it there all the time? Does it come and go? What makes it worse? What makes it better? Is it worse first thing in the morning or later on in the day? Do you find difficulty starting an action or maintaining an action?

☐☐☐ *Swelling* — When did you notice the swelling of your joints? Is it there all the time? Does it come and go? What makes it worse? What makes it better?

Distribution — How many joints are affected with the above symptoms, only one joint (monoarticular), less than four joints (oligoarticular) or five or more joints (polyarticular)? Are the problems on one side only (asymmetrical distribution) or on both sides (symmetrical)?

☐☐☐ **Concerns**	Do you have any particular concerns or worries about the symptoms you are experiencing? Do you know what may be causing them?
☐☐☐ **Impact**	How have these symptoms affected your life? And your family?
☐☐☐ **Function**	Are you able to dress yourself? Can you comb your hair? Are you able to feed yourself or hold a knife and spoon? Are you able to cook for yourself? Are you able to walk up the stairs or do the cooking? Are you able to work?

ASSOCIATED HISTORY

☐☐☐ **Medical history**	Do you suffer from any medical illnesses? Do you have any of the following; (**mnemonic: G R O S S** – **G**out/**R**heumatoid arthritis/**O**steoarthritis/**S**LE/**S**arcoidosis) or tuberculosis/hypertension/high cholesterol/rheumatic fever/epilepsy/asthma/angina/diabetes? Have you ever been admitted to hospital?
☐☐☐ **Drug History**	Are you on any medications? Are you taking diuretics (gout) or hydralazine (SLE-like symptoms)? Are you taking any over-the-counter preparations? Do you have any drug allergies?
☐☐☐ **Family History**	Has anyone in your family had similar troubles? Are there any inherited family disorders? Do any of your family members suffer from psoriasis?
Social History	Do you smoke? How many a day and how long for? Do you drink alcohol? How many units a week do you drink?
☐☐☐ *Home*	Do you live in a house or a flat? Do you have stairs? Does anyone else live with you? Are they helping to care for you? Do you have any carers?
Travel	Have you recently returned from travel? Which countries did you visit or stop over at? Did you take any vaccines?
☐☐☐ **System Review**	Perform a wide scoping systemic review including constitutional and extra-articular symptoms.
Constitutional	Have you lost any weight? How is your appetite? Do you have any night sweats? Any recent fevers? Do you have any lumps on your body?

Extra-articular Have you noticed your fingers change colour and go white in the cold (Raynaud's)? Have you noticed any dry eyes (Sjögren's disease)? Or have your eyes gone red (conjunctivitis – RA, sarcoid)? Have you noticed any bloody diarrhoea (IBD)? Have you noticed any urethral discharge (Reiter's)? Have you noticed any rash (SLE)?

Systems Review in Rheumatology
Mnemonic: 'The CNS'
Temporal artery tenderness, Headaches, Cognitive disturbance, Neuropathy, Seizures

---

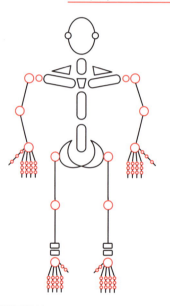

Extra-Articular Features

Mood, cognitive disturbances, alopecia
Red eyes (Conjunctivitis – Reiter's, RA)
Fatigue, butterfly rash, photosensitivity (SLE)
Heliotrope rash on face (dermatomyositis)
Dry eyes and dry mouth (Sjögren's), ulcers

Pericarditis

Back pain, trauma / surgery
Muscle aches and pain, psoriasis

Weight loss, altered bowel habit/IBS

Paraesthesiae, cold sensitivity (Raynaud's)

Genital/oral ulcers (Behcet's disease), STDs

Preceding gastroenteritis/urethritis (Reiter's)

Thrombosis, purpura

EVALUATION

☐☐☐ **Rapport** Establish and maintain rapport with the patient and demonstrate listening skills.

☐☐☐ **Questions** Respond appropriately to the patient's questions.

☐☐☐ **Summarise** Check with the patient and deliver an appropriate summary.

'This is Mr Hughes, a 25-year-old man, who is complaining of a 3-week history of joint pains. He states that the joint pains started after recovering from the 'flu. The pain is described as an ache affecting both knees. There is also slight swelling and stiffness in the joints. He is also complaining of itchy red eyes and painful urethral discharge. He has not had any sexual relationship within the last 6 months and does not suffer from any previous medical problems. He has tried simple analgesia over the counter with some symptomatic relief. In view of his history, I suspect he is suffering from reactive arthritis (Reiter's Syndrome). I would like to exclude other differentials such as rheumatoid arthritis, gout and septic arthritis.'

0 1 2 3 4 5

☐ ☐ ☐ ☐ ☐ ☐ Overall assessment of rheumatological history
☐ ☐ ☐ ☐ ☐ ☐ Role player's score

Total mark out of 34

DIFFERENTIAL DIAGNOSIS

Gout and Pseudogout

The word 'gout' originates from the Latin word *gutta*, meaning 'drop.' The disease was initially believed to have been caused by drops of viscous humours seeping from the blood into the joints. Gout is an arthritic condition caused by abnormal uric acid metabolism. Excessive amounts of urate or uric acid in the bloodstream deposit as crystals on the articular cartilage of joints, tendons and surrounding tissues. This results in an inflammatory response causing swelling and tenderness of the affected joints. The deposits eventually rupture through to the skin and form urate deposits called tophi. The condition affects about 1 in 200 people and men aged between 40 and 60 are the most commonly affected. It also occurs more frequently in alcoholics and in patients on thiazide diuretics. Symptoms include a sudden onset of an excruciating burning pain with redness, warmth and stiffness in one of the joints, commonly the metatarsophalangeal joint of the big toe (podagra). Other joints that are less commonly affected include the ankle, heel, knee, wrist, elbow and fingers. The tophi produce firm, irregular nodules that can be palpated in the pinna of the ear. The symptoms usually occur in 'attacks' and may resolve independently after a period of time. Subsequent attacks may increase in frequency and duration if left untreated. Diagnosis can be confirmed with hyperuricaemia in the blood, joint fluid aspirate showing urate crystals that are negatively birefringent under polarised light consisting of long needle-shaped crystals under microscopy. This condition should be differentiated from pseudogout, which is the deposition of calcium pyrophosphate crystals in the joints (**mnemonic: P**seudogout crystals are **P**ositively birefringent and **P**olygon shaped). It occurs commonly in elderly women and usually affects the knee. A synovial fluid examination will reveal brick-shaped pyrophosphate crystals that are positively birefringent to polarised light.

Precipitants, Causes and Symptoms of Gout
Mnemonic: 'DARK' (acute symptoms most often occur at night)
Diuretics, **A**lcohol, **R**enal disease, **K**icked (trauma)

223

Mnemonic: 'drugs are FACT, foods are SALTS'
FACT: Furosemide, Aspirin or Alcohol, Cytotoxic drugs, Thiazide diuretics
SALTS: Shellfish, Anchovies, Liver and kidney, Turkey, Sardines
Mnemonic: 'GOUT'
Great toe, One joint (75% monoarticular), Uric acid increased, Tophi

Systemic Lupus Erythematosus (SLE)

Systemic lupus erythematosus (SLE) is a complex autoimmune rheumatic disease that is characterised by inflammation involving multiple organ systems. It is defined clinically and associated with antibodies directed against cell nuclei. It commonly affects the skin and musculoskeletal systems; however, it can affect any organ including the kidney, heart, lung and central nervous system. It is up to 10 times more common in women than men, particularly between the ages of 15 and 40, and has a higher prevalence in Afro–Caribbean and Asian people and those of Chinese descent. SLE has a multiplicity of presentations and tends to present with an insidious onset in adolescence. Some features include a classical photosensitive butterfly rash over the nasal bridge and malar bones, profound tiredness, Raynaud's phenomenon affecting hands and feet, profound lethargy and tiredness, arthralgia (polyarticular, symmetrical, episodic, morning stiffness) and non-scarring alopecia. Less common features include oral mucosal ulcers, pericarditis and pleuritis, renal involvement and CNS involvement (migraine headaches, psychosis and depression).

ARA Revised Criteria for the Classification of SLE

Patients need to fulfil four of 11 criteria to reach a diagnosis of SLE:

1	Malar flush	
2	Discoid rash	
3	Photosensitivity	
4	Oral ulcers	
5	Arthritis	
6	Serositis	Pericarditis or pleuritis
7	Renal disorder	Persistent proteinuria >0.5 g/24 hr or cellular casts
8	Neuro. disorder	Seizures or psychosis (after excluded other causes)
9	Haemo. disorder	Haemolytic anaemia or leucopenia of <4.0 × 10^9/L on two or more occasions
		Lymphopenia or <1.5 × 10^9/L on two or more occasions
		Thrombocytopenia <100 × 10^9/L
10	Immunological	Raised anti-native DNA (antibodies to genetic material in cells)
		Anti-Sm antibody (Sm is a protein found in the cell nucleus)
		Positive antiphospholipid antibodies
11	Antibody	Antinuclear antibody in raised titre (autoantibodies to cell nuclei)

Reactive Arthritis (Reiter's Syndrome)

Reiter's Syndrome was named after Hans Reiter in 1916. It describes a classical triad of arthritis, non-gonococcal urethritis and conjunctivitis. It is an autoimmune disease that occurs as a reaction to an infection. Triggers include enteric (gastroenteritis – shigella, salmonella), urogenital (urethritis – chlamydia) or viral infections. In 25% of cases no trigger is found. It commonly affects white men between 20 and 40 years of age and is associated with the gene HLA-B27. Symptoms appear within 2 weeks of the initial infection, often after the initial infection has subsided. Symptoms include urinary symptoms (dysuria, frequency, polyuria, prostatitis or cervicitis), arthritis (large joints – knee, ankle, stiffness, swelling) and eye involvement (conjunctivitis, uveitis). Dermatological features include keratoderma blenorrhagicum, circinate balanitis, nail thickening and ridging and superficial oral ulcers.

Features of Reiter's Syndrome

Mnemonic: 'Can't see (conjunctivitis and uveitis), Can't pee (urethritis), Can't bend my knee (arthritis)'

INSTRUCTIONS: Examine this patient who developed sudden onset back pain while gardening. Report your findings to the examiner as you go along, and make an appropriate diagnosis.

NOTE: The acronym 'GALS' stands for the 'gait, arms, legs and spine' examination. It represents the screening assessment for each system. If an abnormal finding is elicited, a more thorough and detailed regional examination and review will be required. The sequence of the four elements does not have to be performed in this order. A preferred order of G-S-A-L may be undertaken to reduce inconvenience to the patient.

HISTORY

0 1 2

6.2

☐ ☐ ☐ **Introduction** — Introduce yourself. Elicit the patient's name, age and occupation. Establish rapport with the patient.

★ Screening Questions

☐ ☐ ☐ **Pain/stiffness** — Do you suffer from any pain or stiffness in your muscles, joints or back? Where is it (in the back, neck, arms, legs)? Is it better or worse during the day?

☐ ☐ ☐ **Mobility** — Can you walk up and down the stairs without any problems?

☐ ☐ ☐ **Impact on Life** — Do you have any difficulties dressing yourself? How has it affected your life?

EXAMINATION

Consent — Explain the examination to the patient and seek their consent.

☐ ☐ ☐ **Expose** — Ask the patient if they can undress to their undergarments.

★ Gait

☐ ☐ ☐ **Walk** — Ask to examine their gait. Ask the patient if they could walk to the end of the room and return.

Signs to Observe in Gait	
Use of a walking aid	Sticks, frames
Speed	Rhythm, presence of a limp
Phases of walking	Heel strike, stance, push off and swing
Stride length	Reduced, limited
Arm swing	Present, absent

★ Spine

□□□ Look

Inspect with the patient standing. Observe the skin, shape and posture.

Signs to Observe in the Back Examination

Skin		Scars, sinus, pigmentation, abnormal hair, unusual skin creases
Muscle		Wasting (paraspinal, gluteal, shoulder), fasciculations
Posture		**Observe from the back:**
	List	Lateral deviation of the spine
	Scoliosis	Lateral curvature of the spine
		Observe from the side:
	Kyphosis	Undue bending of the spine
	Kyphos	Sharp bend of the spine
	Spondylolisthesis	Loss of lumbar lordosis
Asymmetry		Limb alignment, spine alignment, level iliac crests

Feel

Palpate over mid-supraspinatus for tenderness to test for signs of hyperalgesia or fibromyalgia.

Move

Ask the patient to replicate your movements. Note for any limited range of movement or the citing of pain during a movement.

□□□ *Neck*

Ask the patient to bring their ear towards their shoulder to assess lateral flexion of the neck. Repeat on the other side.

□□□ *Spine*

Assess the patient's spinal flexion. Stand behind the patient and ask them to touch their toes while keeping their knees straight.

□□□ *Mod. Schober's*

Perform the modified Schober's test. Mark two bony spinal processes on the patient's back keeping your fingers 10 cm apart. Ask the patient to flex their back and reassess the gap between the two bony points. The difference should be greater than 5 cm.

★ Arms

□□□ Look

Inspect with the patient sitting down on the couch. Examine both surfaces of the hands outstretched. Look for muscle wasting, swellings or deformities.

Signs to Observe in the Hands during GALS

Hand	*Skin*	Rheumatoid nodules
	Muscle	Wasting (1st dorsal interossei, thenar, hypothenar eminences),

Joints	Swellings: Heberden's nodes (DIPJ) and Bouchard's nodes (PIPJ)
	Deformity: Swan neck, Boutonniere's deformity, z-shaped thumb

☐☐☐ **Feel** — Gently squeeze the patient's hands at the metacarpal joints assessing for tenderness and swelling of bone or soft tissue.

Move — Assess range of movements in the hand, wrist, elbow and shoulder. Check both sides and note any limitation of movement.

☐☐☐ *Hands* — Assess the power grip by asking the patient to make a fist. Test grip strength by asking the patient to grab and squeeze your middle and index fingers. Check precision grip by asking the patient to oppose their thumb to their index finger and then attempt to break it with your index finger.

☐☐☐ *Wrists* — Ask the patient to perform wrist flexion, by forming the praying position and wrist dorsiflexion by taking the reverse praying position.

Elbows — Check elbow extension by asking the patient to have their hands by their sides and arms straight.

Shoulders — Ask the patient to put their hands behind their head (internal rotation) and then to touch their back between their shoulder blades (external rotation). Check shoulder abduction by requesting the patient to raise their arms sideways above their head.

★ **Leg**

☐☐☐ **Look** — Inspect with the patient lying on the couch. Note any nodules or callosities especially in the foot. Look for wasting and fasciculation particularly in the quadriceps muscle. Observe for any asymmetry or swelling in the hip, knee or foot. Check for joint deformities such as pes cavus or high arched foot.

☐☐☐ **Feel** — Squeeze the metatarsal bones assessing for tenderness and swelling. Slide your hand down the thigh to empty the suprapatellar pouch forcing any effusion behind the patella. Perform the patellar tap test by tapping on the patella checking for the presence of an effusion. Next perform the bulge test.

Move		Assess range of movements in the hip, knee and ankle. Check both sides and note any limitation of movement.
□ □ □	*Flexion*	Check for active and passive flexion in the hip and knee by asking the patient to bring their heel to their bottom.
	Extension	While extending the knee feel for crepitus in the joint.
□ □ □	*Hip rotation*	With the knee held at 90 degrees, gently internally rotate the hip by steering the foot outwards.
	Ankle	Briefly test ankle dorsiflexion and plantar flexion.

CLOSING

□ □ □	**Examination**	Elicit any signs or symptoms in the GALS screening assessment. Ask to perform a more detailed regional examination of an affected system.
	Investigations	Ask for any relevant investigations such as blood tests and X-rays of affected areas.
	Summarise	Thank the patient and offer to assist them to put on their clothes. Acknowledge the patient's concerns. Summarise your findings to the examiner.
□ □ □	**Document**	Ask to record both positive and negative findings in the notes in the form of a table. Briefly summarise any abnormal findings.

Documenting findings of GALS examination		
	Appearance	Movement
Gait	√	
Arms	√	√
Legs	X	X
Spine	√	√

Swelling and effusion in the right knee with positive patellar tap test

EXAMINER'S EVALUATION

0 1 2 3 4 5

□ □ □ □ □ □ Overall assessment of GAL examination

□ □ □ □ □ □ Role player's score

Total mark out of 34

RHEUMATOLOGY: **Hand Examination**

INSTRUCTIONS: This patient has been complaining of pain and swelling of his hands. Take a brief history and examine the swelling, reporting your findings to the examiner as you go along.

HISTORY

0 1 2

☐☐☐ **Introduction** Introduce yourself. Elicit the patient's name, age and occupation. Establish rapport with the patient.

★ Nature of Pain

☐☐☐ **Site** Where exactly is the pain (small joints, thumb, wrist)?

Onset When does it come on? First thing in the morning or after exercise?

☐☐☐ **Character** What does the pain feel like? Is it a dull ache or a sharp pain?

Exag./relieving What makes the pain worse? What makes it better?

★ Nature of Stiffness

☐☐☐ **Stiffness** Do you notice any stiffness in your joints?

Onset When do you feel stiff? First thing in the morning or after exercise?

Duration How long does the stiffness last for?

★ Associated Symptoms

☐☐☐ **Swelling** Do you have any swelling in any of your joints?

☐☐☐ **Tingling** Have you noticed any tingling or change in sensation in your hand?

★ Impact on Life

☐☐☐ **Fine Movement** Ask about fine movements such as holding a pen or undoing buttons.

☐☐☐ **Daily Activities** Ask about their ability to comb their hair, feed, wash, dress and bathe.

☐☐☐ **Daily Tasks** Ask about their ability to shop, carry, cook and clean.

★ Causal Factors

☐☐☐ **Medical History** Previous rheumatoid/osteoarthritis or trauma.

Social History Is there anyone at home who can help you?

6.3

EXAMINATION

Consent
Explain the examination to the patient and seek consent.

☐☐☐ **Expose**
Ask the patient to expose their arms to above their elbows.

Pillow
Place a pillow on the patient's lap and ask them to rest their hands on it.

☐☐☐ **Pain**
Ask the patient before beginning the examination if they are in any pain. Do not shake the patient's hand as this might cause them undue pain.

★ Look

☐☐☐ **Inspect**
Examine both the dorsal and palmar surfaces of the hands and then examine them from the side with the patient's hands outstretched. Look for a rash, swelling or joint deformity. Next inspect the hands in the prayer position. Finally, ask the patient to elevate their arms to the boxing position in order to inspect the elbows.

Signs to Observe in the Hand Examination

Hands	*Nails*	Nail fold infarcts, clubbing, psoriatic changes (pitting, onycholysis)
	Skin	Palmar erythema, Dupuytren's contracture, rheumatoid nodules, shiny skin (sclerosis), violaceous papules MCP/PIPJ (dermatomyositis)
	Muscle	Wasting (1st dorsal interossei, thenar, hypothenar eminences)
	Joints	Swellings: Heberden's nodes (DIPJ) and Bouchard's nodes (PIPJ), synovitis (soft boggy swelling around joint)
		Deformity: Swan neck, Boutonniere's deformity, z-shaped thumb
Wrists	Swelling, ganglion, vertical carpal scars	
Elbows	Psoriatic plaques, gouty tophi, rheumatoid nodules	

★ Feel

☐☐☐ **Skin**
Run the back of your hands over the patient's forearm, hands and fingers to assess the temperature.

☐☐☐ **Joints**
Squeeze patient's hand at the carpal and metacarpal joints and then each and every MCP and IP joint assessing for tenderness and swelling of bone or soft tissue. Check for tenderness in the anatomical

snuffbox (scaphoid fracture), the tip of the styloid process (de Quervain's disease) and the head of ulna (extensor carpi ulnaris tendinitis).

✶ Move
☐☐☐ **Fingers**

Hold each joint (MCP and IP) between your thumb and finger; flex and extend each joint in isolation. Assess for any limited range of movements. Ask the patient to make a precision grip by opposing their thumb to their index finger then attempt to break it with your finger. Next test grip strength by asking the patient to grab and squeeze your middle and index fingers. Compare grip strength on both sides.

☐☐☐ **Thumb**

Have the hand flat with the palms facing upwards. Test thumb abduction by asking the patient to point their thumbs to the ceiling and to hold it in position against the resistance of your finger. Test opposition by requesting the patient to make a ring with the tip of their little finger maintaining it against resistance. Finally, ask the patient to firmly place their thumb against their palm for adduction and to stretch out their thumb to the opposite side for extension.

Wrist

Ask the patient to make a fist and passively move the wrist joint through flexion and dorsiflexion. If possible, test for radial and ulnar deviation as well as pronation and supination.

✶ Function
☐☐☐ **Daily Tasks**

Assess function by asking the patient to carry out everyday daily tasks such as undoing buttons, holding a pen or a cup.

✶ Special Tests
☐☐☐ **Froment's Sign**

Ask the patient to clutch a piece of paper between their thumb and index finger. Attempt to pull the paper away from the clasp of the patient. If the thumb adductor is weak then the patient can only hold onto the card by flexing the interphalangeal joints of the thumb and is unable to hold the thumb straight (ulnar nerve compression).

Summarise	Thank the patient. Acknowledge the patient's concerns. Restore the patient's clothing. Summarise your findings to the examiner.

'This is Mrs Freeman, a 77-year-old former typist, complaining of chronic stiffness and swelling of the joints of the hand that is worse in the mornings. For the past 6 months she has noticed that the stiffness has worsened to the extent she finds it very difficult to hold a cup or undo buttons. Recently she has been increasingly reliant on her neighbour to prepare meals as she cannot cook. On examination, there are apparent bilateral ulnar deviations of the wrist joint with swan neck and Boutonniere's deformity of the joints. There are swellings in the PIP joints as well tenderness in the MCP joints. She is unable to do up her buttons or write with a pen. In conclusion, I suspect that this patient is suffering from rheumatoid arthritis of the hands. I would like to carry out a full examination to exclude systemic involvement.'

EXAMINER'S EVALUATION

0 1 2 3 4 5

☐☐☐☐☐☐ Overall assessment of rheumatological hand exam

☐☐☐☐☐☐ Role player's score

Total mark out of 30

DIFFERENTIAL DIAGNOSIS

Rheumatoid Arthritis of the Hand

Rheumatoid arthritis is an autoimmune disease that causes a chronic symmetrical polyarthritis. It is considered a systemic disease but in the early stages is restricted to articular involvement, with the systemic extra-articular manifestations not developing until later on. It affects 1–3% of the population with peak age of onset at 35–45 years with women being affected three times more than their male counterparts. Symptoms include pain and stiffness following periods of inactivity. There is usually morning stiffness which improves as the day draws on. On examination, there may be swelling and tenderness at the MCP and PIP joints. Symmetrical involvement of both hands is common. Hand deformities, which manifest later as the disease progresses, include Boutonniere's deformity (PIP flexion and DIP hyperextension), swan-neck deformity (flexion contracture of MCP with PIP hyperextension and DIP flexion), ulnar/lateral deviation of fingers and MCP and wrist subluxation. If these deformities become fixed then the patient may need assistance with daily activities involving fine finger movements, e.g. washing, dressing and feeding. Other less common hand features include nail fold infarcts, palmar erythema and carpal tunnel or other compression syndromes.

Osteoarthritis of the Hand

Osteoarthritis of the hand and wrist is more common in post-menopausal women. It presents as pain and stiffness which is made worse by movement but relieved by rest. On examination there is arthritis of joints which mainly affects the DIP joints of the hands as well as the base of the thumb (first carpometacarpal joints). It also can affect the weight-bearing joints including the hip, knees and vertebrae as well as the feet. Arthritis is commonly asymmetrical in distribution. Hand deformities include bony thickening around the DIP joints (Heberden's nodes) and PIP joints (Bouchard's nodes).

Psoriatic Arthritis

Psoriatic arthritis is a seronegative arthritis that affects approximately 5% of patients with psoriasis. It usually occurs between the ages of 30 and 50 but can occur at almost any age. Unlike rheumatoid arthritis, it affects men and women equally. It has several patterns of presentation, including asymmetrical oligoarticular arthritis (affecting small joints in hands and feet, 'sausage' appearance (dactylitis)), symmetrical polyarthritis (affects hands, wrists, ankles, and feet – similar to RA), distal interphalangeal arthropathy (involves DIP with nail changes), arthritis mutilans (destructive polyarthritis) and associated with ankylosing spondylitis.

Orthopaedics

ORTHOPAEDICS: **Back Examination**

INSTRUCTIONS: Examine this patient who is complaining of sudden onset back pain whilst gardening. Report your findings to the examiner as you go along, and make an appropriate diagnosis.

HISTORY

0 1 2

☐☐☐ **Introduction** — Introduce yourself. Elicit the patient's name, age and occupation. Establish rapport with the patient.

★ **History of Presenting Complaint**

History — When did it first start? Have you had this problem in the past? Have you ever fallen or injured your back before? Were you carrying or lifting anything heavy at the time?

☐☐☐ **Pain** — Where is the pain located? Does the pain move? How severe is the pain graded out of 10? Did it come on suddenly or gradually? What does the pain feel like?

Severe pain radiating to a well-defined area with motor, sensory and reflex impairment is suggestive of a prolapsed disc. A radiating pain that is vague, diffuse and with an ill-defined distribution is most likely referred pain.

☐☐☐ **Stiffness** — Do you have any stiffness? Is it worse in the morning or evening? Does it come on suddenly or gradually?

Deformity — Have you noticed a change in the shape of your back or neck?

☐☐☐ **Neurology** — Do you have weakness in your arms or legs (saddle anaesthesia – cauda equina)? Have you noticed any tingling or numbness in your toes or fingers? Have you noticed any problems with your bladder or bowel (urinary incontinence – spinal cord compression, retention/bowel incontinence – cauda equina lesion)?

☐☐☐ **General Health** — How is your general health? Do you have any malaise, fever or weight loss?

☐☐☐ **Impact on Life** — How has your back problem affected your daily activities and/or mobility?

7.1

EXAMINATION

Consent

Explain the examination to the patient and seek their consent.

□□□ **Expose**

Ask the patient if they can undress to their undergarments.

★ Gait

□□□ **Walk**

Ask to examine the patient's gait. Ask the patient if they could walk to the end of the room and return.

Signs to Look for in Gait	
Use of a walking aid	Sticks, frames
Speed	Rhythm, presence of a limp
Phases of walking	Heel strike, stance, push off and swing
Stride length	Reduced, limited
Arm swing	Present, absent

★ Look

□□□ **Inspect**

Inspect the patient's back while they are standing. Observe the skin, shape and posture.

Signs to Observe in the Back Examination		
Skin	Scars, sinus, pigmentation, abnormal hair (spina bifida), unusual skin creases	
Muscle	Wasting (paravertebral, gluteal muscles), fasciculations	
Posture	**Observe from the back:**	
	List	Lateral deviation of the spine
	Scoliosis	Lateral curvature of the spine
	Observe from the side:	
	Kyphosis	Undue bending of the spine
	Kyphos	Sharp bend of the spine
	Spondylolisthesis	Loss of lumbar lordosis
	Hyperlordosis	Hollowing of the lumbar spine
Asymmetry	Chest, trunk or pelvis (may appear with patient leaning forwards)	

★ Feel

□□□ **Palpate**

Palpate the full length of the spine over the spinous processes, paravertebral muscles and interspinous ligaments for any tenderness. Establish the site of the pain.

✱ Move

Movement	Ask the patient to replicate your movements. Note any limited range of movement or the citing of pain during a movement.
Extension	Stand behind the patient and ask them to lean backwards as far as they can.
☐☐☐ *Flexion*	Ask the patient to touch their toes while keeping their knees straight.
☐☐☐ *Lateral Flexion*	Ask the patient to slide their right hand down their right leg. Repeat on the other side.
☐☐☐ *Rotation*	Fix the patient's pelvis with your hands and then ask them to rotate their chest from side to side.
Expansion	Assess chest expansion by measuring chest circumference in full expiration and then in full inspiration. Normal expansion is around 7 cm; less than 5 cm suggests ankylosing spondylitis.

✱ Special Tests

☐☐☐ **Schober's Test**	Make a mark at the level of the dimples of Venus. Next make another mark 10 cm above and 5 cm below this level (a total distance of 15 cm). Ask the patent to flex their back and measure the distance from the initial top point down to the bottom point. The total distance should be greater than 20 cm (an increase of less than 5 cm is abnormal).

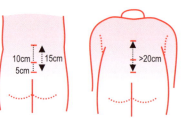

Schober's test

Make a mark at the level of dimple of Venus. Place one finger 5 cm below this mark and another finger 10 cm above this mark. Instruct the patient to flex their back. Note an increase in distance between the two fingers. An increase less than 5 cm is suggestive of a limitation of lumbar flexion

☐☐☐ **SLR Test**	Offer assistance to get the patient onto the couch to carry out this test. Ask the patient to lie on their back keeping their legs straight. Raise the patient's leg off the couch until the patient experiences pain. Pain is commonly experienced in the thigh, buttock or back (back pain suggestive of central disc prolapse, leg pain lateral disc prolapse). Note the angle at which this occurs and then repeat the test for both legs. Normal

range of movement for hip flexion is about 90°
(however, 70–120° is acceptable).

The test is positive if the patient experiences pain
on the affected side within the sciatic distribution
between 30° and 70° of passive flexion. Pain elicited
before 30° is not due to disc prolapse as the lumbar
nerve roots are only brought to tension between 30°
and 70°. Severe impingement (large disc herniation,
central disc prolapse with cauda equina) is suggested
if the patient complains of pain on the affected side
when the SLR test is performed on the opposite
unaffected leg (crossed sciatic reflex).

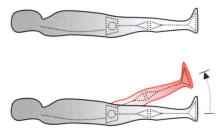

Normal

Ask the patient to lie completely flat on
their back with their legs straight

Sciatic Stretch test

Patient is unable to raise their leg
beyond a certain angle due to the
tension on the root by the prolapsed disc

Bragard's Test

If the straight-leg-raising test is positive, lower the
leg on the affected side until the pain is diminished
and then dorsiflex the patient's foot. If the pain is
regenerated, this suggests sciatic neuritis.

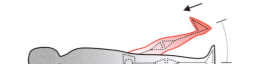

Bragard's Test

Determine the angle of hip flexion where
the patient feels pain and paraesthesia.
Lower the leg until the pain disappears
and then gently dorsiflex the foot
increasing the tension on the nerve root

Lasegue's Test

Ascertain the limit of straight leg raising that
generates the pain. Next flex the knee to reduce the
pressure on the sciatic nerve root which should in
turn reduce the pain. Now continue to flex the hip
with the knee flexed. Slowly and gently extend the
knee until the pain is reproduced.

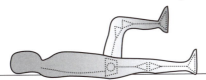

Reduce root tension

With the knee flexed, the hip is able to
be elevated to a higher angle compared
with the straight-leg-raising test without
the pain being reproduced

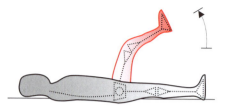

Lasegue's test

From the above position, extending the knee reproduces the sciatic pain caused by the prolapsed disc

Bowstring Test   Ask permission to perform the bowstring test. Once again, ascertain the angle of hip flexion required to generate the pain. Flex the knee slightly to relieve the pain. Next, apply firm pressure to the popliteal fossa behind the lateral hamstrings over the stretched common peroneal nerve. Induction of pain suggests nerve root irritation.

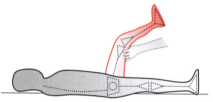

Bowstring test

Note the angle of hip flexion that causes pain. Flex the knee slightly to reduce the pain. Apply pressure with your thumb in the popliteal fossa to regenerate pain

Femoral Stretch   Ask permission to perform the femoral stretch test. Ask the patient to lie on their front. Lift the patient's leg flexing the patient's knee whilst extending the hip. A positive test suggests ipsilateral irritation of L2, L3, L4 due to a prolapsed disc.

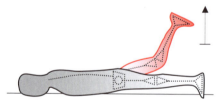

Femoral Stretch test

Ask the patient to lie prone. Flex the knee to put tension on the femoral roots and to replicate the pain. If there is no pain, slowly extend the hip with the knee flexed

Sacroiliac Joint   Ask permission to perform the Gaenslen's test and FABER test to assess sacroiliac joint involvement (sacroiliitis – ankylosing spondylitis).

Gaenslen's Test   Have the patient lying on their back with one leg hanging off the edge of the examining couch. The opposite knee should be flexed towards the patient's chest. Push apart the patient's knees by pushing the flexed knee towards the patient's chest and the contralateral knee towards the floor. With one hip joint flexed maximally and the opposite hip joint extended, both sacroiliac joints are stressed simultaneously. Pain represents a positive test and suggests sacroiliitis.

FABER Test

Flex the hip and knee and then abduct and externally rotate the hip as far as possible so that the legs form a figure '4' shape. Next apply firm downward pressure on the protruding knee. Pain generated in the back suggests sacroiliitis.

The FABER test
Mnemonic: Flexion, Abduction, External Rotation of the hip

☐☐☐ **Neurovascular**

Check capillary refill time on both feet. Check for the presence of peripheral pulses (femoral, popliteal, post tibial and dorsalis pedis). Assess power, light touch and tendon reflexes of the legs comparing both sides.

☐☐☐ **Request**

State that you would like to carry out a full examination of the lower limbs (neurovascular and orthopaedic) and that you would like to examine the upper limbs including the neck, shoulder and wrist.

☐☐☐ **Summarise**

Thank the patient and offer to assist them to put on their clothes. Acknowledge the patient's concerns. Summarise your findings to the examiner.

'Mr Farmer is a 57-year-old builder who was working in his garden carrying some compost. He felt a sudden sharp pain in his back that radiated to his big toe. He is complaining of persistent lower back pain worse on lifting and bending. There are no red flag features. On examination, he has an antalgic gait and was unable to weight bear fully on the right side. His back was tender on palpation at the L5/S1 level. He also was found to have limited forward flexion and a positive SLR on the right side. Both Bragard's and Lasegue's test were positive. There were no neurovascular signs. In conclusion, I suspect that this is a case of sciatica. However, I would like to exclude malignancy or mechanical back pain.'

EXAMINER'S EVALUATION

0 1 2 3 4 5
☐☐☐☐☐☐ Overall assessment of back examination
☐☐☐☐☐☐ Role player's score
Total mark out of 32

DIFFERENTIAL DIAGNOSIS
Ankylosing Spondylitis

Ankylosing spondylitis is derived from the Greek word *ankylos*, meaning 'stiffening of a joint' and *spondylos*, meaning 'vertebra'. It is a generalised chronic inflammatory disease that affects predominantly the sites of insertion of ligaments and tendons in bones. It often affects the spine and sacroiliac joints but may also involve the hip, knees and smaller joints. It typically affects young males (5:1) with peak onset between 15 to 30 years but is rarely seen to develop beyond the age of 40. It has a strong genetic component with familial inheritance and a strong association with the HLA-B27 genotype. The presenting complaint is often lower back pain and stiffness that may radiate to the buttocks. Rest does not resolve the pain but exercise and activity may improve it. The pain is noted to be worst in the morning but improves throughout the day. On examination, there is tenderness over the sacroiliac joints (sacroiliitis), loss of lumbar lordosis, increased kyphosis, reduced spinal flexion, fixed flexion of the hips and limitations in chest expansion. This often forms a classical appearance of ankylosing spondylitis. Other features include Achilles tendonitis and plantar fasciitis. Non-articular features include iritis, aortic incompetence and apical lung fibrosis.

Features of Ankylosing Spondylitis
Mnemonic: 7 As for Ankylosing Spondylitis

Achilles tendonitis	**A**pical lung fibrosis
Atlantoaxial subluxation	**A**nterior uveitis
Aortic regurgitation	Ig**A** nephropathy
Arthritis	

Prolapsed Disc

A prolapsed disc is a common cause of severe lower back pain. The prolapsed disc often presses upon a nerve root which causes the pain and symptoms in the lower leg. The most common sites include the L4/5 and L5/S1 disc areas. The patient may complain of back pain when he or she lifts a heavy object while being unable to straighten their back thereafter. This can be accompanied with sciatic leg pain (sciatica) characterised by severe pain localised in the lumbar region or pain that radiates from the lower spine down the back of either leg. Both the back pain as well as sciatica can be reproduced by coughing, sneezing or straining. Other features include the presence of a list to one side, a limitation of spinal forward flexion and extension of the back with tenderness of the lower vertebrae and paravertebral muscles. The straight-leg-raising test is an important test in checking for a prolapsed disc and is limited on the affected side. Both Bragard's test and Lasegue's test can be used to confirm the diagnosis of a prolapsed disc. There are a number of neurological signs that, if identified, permit the examiner to localise the level of the prolapsed disc. Weakness of the hallux extension with loss of sensation on the outer aspect of the leg and the dorsum of the foot suggests an L4/L5 level prolapse. Pain in the calf, weakness of plantar flexion and eversion of the foot, loss of sensation over the lateral aspect of the foot and a depressed ankle reflex suggests an L5/S1 level prolapse.

Scoliosis

Scoliosis is defined as a lateral curvature of the spine, the presence of which is abnormal. The most common type of spinal curvature is idiopathic scoliosis. Idiopathic scoliosis may either be of early onset, arising before the age of seven, or late onset, after the age of seven. As much as 80% of late onset idiopathic scoliosis occurs in girls while 80% of this group have their rib prominence on the right-hand side. The spinal curvature can bend towards either side of the body and at any place. Scoliosis can be subdivided by the location where the spine bends, i.e. in the chest area (thoracic scoliosis), in the lower part of the back (lumbar), or above and below these areas (thoraco-lumbar). If there are two bends present in the spine it will cause an S-shaped curve (double curvature). Such an arrangement may be unnoticeable since the two curves may appear to counteract each other leading to the appearance that the patient's back is straight and normal.

Kyphosis

Kyphosis is derived from the Greek word *kyphos*, meaning 'a hump'. It is used to describe the normal curvature of the upper spine as well as being used to describe excessive dorsal curvature. Scheuermann's disease is a form of kyphosis that occurs predominantly in teenagers. It is caused by a growth disorder of the spine whereby the vertebrae become irregular and wedge shaped and can herniate over at least three adjacent levels. Consequently the deformity is fixed and cannot be compensated for by changes in posture as in postural kyphosis. Clinical features include fatigability and backache which can be aggravated by strenuous exercise and long periods of sitting or standing.

ORTHOPAEDICS: **Shoulder Examination**

INSTRUCTIONS: Please examine this patient with shoulder pain. Report your findings to the examiner as you go along, and make an appropriate diagnosis.

HISTORY

0 1 2

☐☐☐ **Introduction**   Introduce yourself. Elicit the patient's name, age and occupation. Establish rapport with the patient.

★ **History of Presenting Complaint**

☐☐☐ **Pain**   Where is the pain located? Does the pain move anywhere? What does the pain feel like? How severe is the pain graded out of ten? What were you doing at the time it started?

Stiffness   Do you have any stiffness? Did it come on progressively or suddenly? Is it worse in the morning or the evening?

Swelling   Have you noticed any swelling? Did it occur after an injury?

☐☐☐ **Impact on Life**   How has your shoulder problem affected your daily activities? Do you have any difficulties with dressing or grooming?

EXAMINATION

Consent   Obtain consent before beginning the examination.

☐☐☐ **Expose**   Ask the patient if they can remove their outer garments to expose their upper body.

★ **Look**

☐☐☐ **Inspect**   Inspect the patient from the front, behind and sides. Observe the shoulder for any obvious abnormal posture, deformity or wasting.

Signs to Inspect for in the Shoulder Examination

Alignment	Asymmetry of the shoulders, winging of the scapula
Position	Internal rotation of the arm (posterior dislocation of shoulder)
Bones	Bony prominences of the acromioclavicular joints (ACJ) and the sternoclavicular joints (SCJ), deformity of clavicle (old fracture)
Skin	Colour (bruising), sinuses, scars

7.2

244

Muscles	Wasting of deltoids (axillary nerve palsy), supra and infraspinatus, pectoral muscles
Axilla	Lumps (lymph), large joint effusions

✳ Feel

Skin

Run the back surface of your fingers over the patient's shoulder to assess the temperature. Compare both sides.

▭▭▭ **Joints**

Palpate the shoulder for tenderness and effusions. Begin at the sternoclavicular joint then move along the clavicle towards the acromioclavicular joint ending at the acromion. Palpate the greater and lesser tuberosities and also the glenohumeral joint. Note any tender sites.

▭▭▭ **Tendons**

Have the patient sitting with their arms straightened. Ask the patient to flex their arm, contracting the biceps muscles. Palpate the biceps tendon within the bicipital groove in an attempt to elicit pain which may suggest biceps tendonitis.

✳ Move

Active

Request the patient to perform a number of active movements including abduction, adduction, flexion, extension and rotation. Note any limited range of movements or the reporting of pain.

▭▭▭ *Abduction*

Ask the patient to raise both arms starting from their sides and meeting above their head in the midline (180°).

If pain is present, establish the angle when it begins within the painful arc. If pain occurs in the mid-range

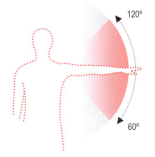

Painful Shoulder Arc

The 'painful arc' lies between 60 and 120 degrees of shoulder abduction. Pain noted in this arc suggests supraspinatus tendonitis or a partial rotator cuff tear

of the arc it suggests supraspinatus tendonitis or a partial rotator cuff tear. If the pain is established at the end of the arc it may suggest acromioclavicular joint arthritis.

Causes of Painful Shoulder Arc

Partial tear of supraspinatus tendon	Supraspinatus tendonitis
Calcified deposits in supraspinatus tendon	Subacromial bursitis
Fracture of greater tuberosity of humerus	

☐☐☐ *Adduction*

Ask the patient to move their arms inwards towards the midline and across their chest (50°).

☐☐☐ *Flexion*

Ask the patient to raise their arms forward (165°).

☐☐☐ *Extension*

Ask the patient to swing their arms backwards (65°).

☐☐☐ *Rotation*

To test for external rotation, have the elbows flexed at 90° and placed firmly against their sides with their hands facing forwards. Externally rotate the shoulder by turning the arms laterally as far as possible (normal range 60°).

☐☐☐ **Scratch Test**

Perform Apley's scratch test by asking the patient to scratch their scapula with their fingers by reaching behind their back (internal rotation with adduction) and behind their neck (external rotation with abduction).

Passive

Stand behind the patient, rest one hand on their shoulder and move their arm in all planes. Observe for crepitus, pain and limitation of movement.

★ **Neurology**

☐☐☐ **Power**

Test the deltoid muscles by asking the patient to raise their arms like wings and to hold them in position against resistance (C5/6, axillary nerve). Pectoralis major can be tested by requesting the patient to push their hands against their waist. Test the biceps by asking the patient to flex the elbow against resistance. Ask the patient to push against the wall as hard as possible to test for serratus anterior muscle (long thoracic nerve C5–7). Observe from behind for winging of the scapula.

☐☐☐ **Sensation**

Test light touch and proprioception on the upper limbs. Note any sensation loss or paraesthesia over the shoulder particularly over the deltoid muscle which could indicate an anterior dislocation of the shoulder.

★ Special Tests

□□□ **Apprehension**

The apprehension test assesses for anterior dislocation of the shoulder and can be tested in a number of ways. Have the patient in the supine position, with the arm abducted 90° and hanging off the bed. Grasp their elbow in your hand and gently rotate the shoulder externally by pushing the forearm posteriorly. At the same time push the head of the humerus anteriorly with your other hand. Instability will give the sense that the humeral head is about to slip out anteriorly and the patient resists further movement.

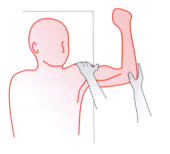

Apprehension Test

Have the patient's arm abducted to 90 degrees while lying on the edge of a couch. Hold the elbow and gently push the forearm posteriorly. Gently push the head of the humerus anteriorly with your other hand. The patient will sense that his shoulder will dislocate and resist further movement.

Alternatively, stand behind the patient with the elbow at 90°. Slowly abduct, externally rotate and extend the shoulder with one hand while applying pressure over the head of the humerus (from behind) with the opposite thumb. The patient will apprehend that their shoulder may dislocate and resist further movement.

□□□ **Neer's Test**

Have the patient seated before performing Neer's impingement test. Place one hand on the patient's scapula, and grasp their forearm with your other. Internally rotate the arm with the thumb facing downwards and gently abduct and forward flex the arm. If impingement is present, the patient will experience pain as the arm is abducted. A positive test suggests subacromial impingement.

Request

State that you would also like to perform a full neck, back and elbow orthopaedic examination.

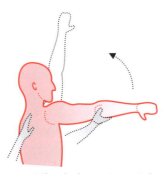

Neer's Impingement Test

Place a hand on the patient's scapula while holding their forearm with the other. Have the arm internally rotated so that the thumb is pointing downward. Next, gently forward-flex the arm up to the vertical position. A positive test is noted if the patient complains of pain.

□ □ □ **Summarise**   Thank the patient. Acknowledge the patient's concerns. Restore the patient's clothing. Summarise your findings to the examiner.

'This is Mr Patel, a grocery shop manager, who is complaining of shoulder pain with stiffness for the last 4 months. The pain initially began after he fell off his stepladder while he was stacking shelves. The pain gradually worsened over the last few months and now he is unable to work. On examination, there is diffuse tenderness around the glenohumeral joint, and generalised reduced movement in the elbow with limited abduction and external rotation. I suspect that this patient suffers from a frozen shoulder.'

EXAMINER'S EVALUATION

0 1 2 3 4 5
□ □ □ □ □ □   Overall assessment of shoulder examination
□ □ □ □ □ □   Role player's score
Total mark out of 31

DIFFERENTIAL DIAGNOSIS
Chronic Tendinitis (Impingement Syndrome)

Impingement syndrome is a condition that affects the rotator cuff causing shoulder pain. Impingement of the rotator cuff muscles against the coracoacromial ligament is believed to be the cause of this condition. Impingement occurs due to repetitive overhead activities such as swimming, skiing, tennis or jobs involving reaching high up. Symptoms include, pain and weakness. Pain originates in the shoulder and over the deltoid muscle and is exacerbated by above the head activities. A frequent complaint is night pain, often disturbing sleep, particularly when the patient lies on the affected shoulder. Weakness and loss of motion are associated symptoms. On examination the impingement tests described above are invariably positive. There is a painful arc between 60° and 120° of abduction; however, is usually absolved if the patient repeats abduction with the arm in full external rotation.

Cervical Radiculopathy

Cervical radiculopathy is nerve root dysfunction in the cervical spine in which symptoms are generated from nerve root compression. It is often caused by a herniated disc (young), degenerative disc disease (old) or acute injury (whiplash). Most commonly C6 and C7 are affected. Symptoms include pain, numbness and weakness affecting different areas depending on the involvement of the nerve root. Patients often describe a diffuse shoulder pain that ranges from a dull ache to a burning pain. As the condition progresses, the pain may radiate to the medial border of the scapula, occiput, arm or hand. Neck pain is frequently absent. On examination, there is reduced range of movement in the neck, with extension and neck rotation generating the pain. There is loss of sensation, muscle weakness and absent reflexes corresponding to nerve root level. A positive Spurling test is elicited where the patient's neck is extended and rotated whilst a downward pressure is applied to the head. Pain is noted to radiate down the ipsilateral limb towards the side to which the patient's head was rotated. Lhermitte's sign is negative in pure cervical radiculopathy (when the neck is flexed, the patient describes an electric shock sensation radiating down spine and into limbs, suggestive of cervical cord involvement).

Examination Findings for Cervical Radiculopathy	
C5 radiculopathy	(Spondylosis, brachial neuritis) Weakness of biceps, spinati (infraspinatus, supraspinatus) and deltoid. Numbness over deltoid area. Absent biceps reflex
C6 radiculopathy	(Spondylosis, disc herniation) Weakness of the biceps and brachioradialis muscles. Numbness over thumb and index finger. Absent supinator jerk
C7 radiculopathy	(Disc herniation) Weakness of triceps muscle with numbness over middle finger. Absent triceps reflex
C8-T1 radiculopathy	(Pancoast tumour, thoracic outlet syndrome) Weakness of small muscles of hand with atrophy. Numbness of little finger (C8)

Rotator Cuff Tears

Tears to the rotator cuff (supraspinatus, infraspinatus, subscapularis) are often due to chronic tendinitis (partial tears) or a sudden strain caused by a fall (complete tear). Partial tears present with a sustained painful arc in the absence of limitation of the range of movement, whilst complete tears restrict shoulder abduction to just 60° with a characteristic shrug when attempting to abduct beyond this. Full range of passive movements are present. When the arm is passively assisted above 90° of abduction, the patient is able to hold it in place and continue active abduction by utilising their deltoid muscles. However, on lowering their arm below 90° of abduction, the arm will suddenly drop (drop arm sign). Tenderness can be elicited under the acromion process. Partial and complete tears can be differentiated by infiltrating local anaesthetic into the shoulder joint, thereby eliminating pain and recovering full active abduction in a partial tear.

The Rotator Cuff Muscles
Mnemonic: The 'SITS' muscles

Supraspinatus	Teres minor
Infraspinatus	Subscapularis

Frozen Shoulder (Adhesive Capsulitis)

Frozen shoulder (adhesive capsulitis) is a disorder characterised by pain, loss of motion and stiffness in the shoulder. The process involves thickening and contracture of the capsule surrounding the shoulder joint. It is more common in women between 40 and 60 years of age. In the elderly, it is normally preceded by a history of minor injury followed by progressively worsening pain in the shoulder that prevents the patient from sleeping on the affected side. The pain may subside after 9 months with stiffness intensifying and persisting over this time, limiting the range of movements of the shoulder. It is usually greater with internal rotation of the shoulder than with external rotation. Restriction of movement is often severe with almost no glenohumeral movements possible. Stiffness begins to subside usually after 12 months with a return to full range of movement after 18 months.

Anterior Instability (Shoulder Dislocation)

Up to 95% of all shoulder dislocations occur anteriorly, commonly affecting men aged 18 to 25 years. This usually occurs when the arm is forced into abduction, external rotation and extension, i.e. when falling backward onto an outstretched hand. A patient with anterior dislocation presents holding the arm in slight abduction and internal rotation and reports pain with any attempt to rotate the arm. A mass may be palpable over the anterior shoulder. Occasionally, axillary nerve injury occurs with anterior dislocations manifesting as loss of sensation over the lateral deltoid as well as decreased strength of the deltoid muscle. Diagnosis is made by a positive apprehension test (see above).

ORTHOPAEDICS: **Elbow Examination**

INSTRUCTIONS: Examine this patient who is complaining of pain in his elbow. Report your findings to the examiner as you go along, and make an appropriate diagnosis.

HISTORY

0 1 2

☐☐☐ **Introduction**   Introduce yourself. Elicit the patient's name, age and occupation. Establish rapport with the patient.

★ History of Presenting Complaint

☐☐☐ **Pain**   Where is the pain located? Does the pain move anywhere? What does the pain feel like? How severe is the pain, graded out of ten? What were you doing at the time it started?

☐☐☐ **Stiffness**   Do you have any stiffness in your elbow?

Swelling   Have you noticed any swelling? Did it occur after an injury?

☐☐☐ **Neurology**   Have you noticed any tingling or numbness in your fingers? Do you have any weakness in your hands (ulnar nerve symptoms)?

EXAMINATION

Consent   Explain the examination to the patient and seek consent.

☐☐☐ **Expose**   Ask the patient to remove their upper garments in order to expose their elbows.

★ Look

☐☐☐ **Inspect**   Inspect the elbows with the patient's arms by his sides. Look from the front, back and sides of the patient. Observe the skin, muscle and alignment.

7.3

Signs to Observe in the Elbow Examination

Skin	Scars, psoriatic plaques, rheumatoid nodules
Muscle	Wasting and fasciculation (biceps, triceps and brachioradialis)
Joints	Effusions (olecranon bursitis), gouty tophi
Alignment	Varus deformity (cubitus varus – supracondylar fracture)
	Valgus deformity (cubitus valgus – non-union of fractured lateral condyle)

✱ Feel

□□□ **Palpate**

Ascertain if the elbow is painful. Ask the patient to locate the pain before palpating. Palpate the epicondyles and olecranon. Feel for any joint effusions or tenderness along the joint margin.

Signs to Palpate in the Elbow Examination	
Skin	Temperature (infections, inflammation), subcutaneous nodules
Joints	Effusions, olecranon bursitis, synovial thickening, gouty tophi
Bones	Tenderness in the medial epicondyle (golfer's elbow) or lateral epicondyle (tennis elbow)

✱ Move

□□□ **Movement**

Have the arms by the side of the patient. Assess the range of movement of the elbow during active and passive flexion (flexion deformity) and extension. Next check pronation (palms facing downwards) and supination (palms facing upwards) of the radioulnar joints with the elbows close to the patient's sides and flexed to 90°. Feel for crepitus during passive movements.

Difference between Supination and Pronation	
Mnemonic:	SUPinated is the position of the forearm when carrying a bowl of SOUP
Mnemonic:	PROnation is to turn your arm with the palm facing down as if you are POURing a jug of water

✱ Function

Function

Ask the patient to put on a jacket or pour a glass of water.

□□□ **Neurovascular**

State that you would like to check for the presence of any distal neurovascular deficits. Check for presence of a radial and brachial pulse. Also test sensation and proprioception in the hand comparing both sides (ulnar nerve compression).

□□□ **Summarise**

Thank the patient and offer to assist them to put on their clothes. Acknowledge the patient's concerns. Summarise your findings to the examiner.

'This is Mr Bob, a 35-year-old carpenter. He is right handed, and has been complaining of pain in his right elbow which has been affecting his work. He recently started work on a building site fitting doors and noted the pain getting worse after this. On examination, both elbows appear normal with a full range of movements. However, on palpation there was significant tenderness over the right lateral epicondyle. The pain is reproduced on forced dorsiflexion of the wrist. In view of his history and examination, I believe that he suffers from tennis elbow.'

EXAMINER'S EVALUATION

0 1 2 3 4 5

☐ ☐ ☐ ☐ ☐ ☐ Overall assessment of elbow examination

☐ ☐ ☐ ☐ ☐ ☐ Role player's score

Total mark out of 24

DIFFERENTIAL DIAGNOSIS

Elbow Deformities

Cubitus varus (Gunstock deformity) is a common complication of a supracondylar fracture. It describes an inward angulation of the distal segment of bone. The deformity is best seen with the elbow extended and arm elevated. Cubitus valgus is a common sequel of a disunited fractured lateral condyle. It is a deformity in which the elbow is turned out and a bony protrusion can be felt in the medial aspect of the joint. Possible complications include a delayed presentation of an ulnar nerve palsy which should be excluded.

Lateral Epicondylitis (Tennis Elbow)

Tennis elbow is an inflammatory condition of the wrist extensor tendons, particularly the extensor carpi radialis brevis which attaches to the lateral epicondyle. It was termed 'tennis elbow' due to its association with athletes in racquet sports. However, most individuals who suffer from this condition sustain the injury at work, such as carpenters or house painters, by engaging in repetitive movements and unaccustomed strenuous activity involving the wrist. Peak incidence occurs between the ages of 30 and 50 years. Symptoms include pain of the lateral aspect of the elbow that is often severe and burning in nature and which gradually worsens over weeks or months. It is often aggravated by gripping, lifting or movements that involve extending the wrist such as pouring out a glass of water, turning a door handle or lifting a cup of coffee. On examination, tenderness is localised to the lateral epicondyle and can be reproduced by passively extending the wrist with the elbow held straight or when the patient resists forced dorsiflexion of the wrist.

Medial Epicondylitis (Golfer's Elbow)

Golfer's elbow, or medial epicondylitis, is similar to tennis elbow in presentation and pathology. It is due to inflammation of the wrist flexor tendon that attaches at the medial epicondyle. It is called 'golfer's elbow' due to its frequency in golfers, although individuals who have never played golf can develop the condition. The most common cause is overuse or repetitive stress of the flexor muscles involved in flexing the fingers and thumb, clenching the fist or supinating the wrist. These actions are often re-enacted as golfers take their swing but can also occur in other professions such as carpentry. On examination, tenderness is noted in the medial epicondyle which is reproducible when the patient resists forced flexion of the wrist.

Olecranon Bursitis

Olecranon bursitis is inflammation of the olecranon bursa as a result of direct trauma, prolonged pressure from leaning on a surface over a long duration, infection, or underlying medical conditions such as gout or rheumatoid arthritis. It presents as an impalpable small fluid-filled sac located at the tip of the elbow. It facilitates movement of the joint by permitting the skin to glide over the underlying bone. On examination, a tender, inflamed swelling is noted over the proximal end of the ulna. In the presence of infection, the overlying skin may become red and warm.

ORTHOPAEDICS: **Hand Examination**

INSTRUCTIONS: This patient has noticed pains in their hand. Examine the hand and report your findings to the examiner as you go along, and make an appropriate diagnosis.

HISTORY

0 1 2

□□□ **Introduction** — Introduce yourself. Elicit the patient's name, age and occupation. Establish rapport with the patient.

★ **History of Presenting Complaint**

History — When did it first start, have you had this problem in the past, have you ever fallen, injured or fractured your hand before?

□□□ **Pain** — Where is the pain located? Describe the nature of the pain. What makes it better or worse? Do you suffer from night pains?

□□□ **Stiffness** — Do you suffer from stiffness in your joints? How long does it last for? Is it worse in the morning or the evening?

Swelling — Do you have any swelling in your joints?

□□□ **Sensation** — Have you noticed any numbness or tingling in your hands?

EXAMINATION

Consent — Obtain consent before beginning the examination.

□□□ **Expose** — Ask the patient to expose their arms to above their elbows.

Pillow — Place a pillow on the patient's lap and ask them to rest their hands on it.

□□□ **Pain** — Ask the patient before beginning the examination if they are in any pain. Do not shake the patient's hand as this might cause undue pain.

★ **Look**

□□□ **Inspect** — Examine both the dorsal and palmar surfaces of the hands and then examine them from the side with the patient's hands outstretched. Next inspect the hands in the praying position. Finally ask the patient to

7.4

elevate their arms in the boxing position in order to inspect their elbows.

Signs to Observe in the Hand Examination

Hand	*Nails*	Nail fold infarcts, clubbing, psoriatic changes (pitting, onycholysis)
	Skin	Palmer erythema, Dupuytren's contracture, rheumatoid nodules
	Muscle	Wasting (1st dorsal interossei, thenar, hypothenar eminences),
	Joints	Swellings: Heberden's nodes (DIPJ) and Bouchard's nodes (PIPJ)
		Deformity: Swan neck, Boutonniere's deformity, z-shaped thumb
Wrists		Swelling, ganglion, vertical carpal scars
Elbows		Psoriatic plaques, gouty tophi, rheumatoid nodules

★ Feel

□□□ **Palpate**

Palpate the skin assessing for temperature and joints for tenderness.

Skin

Run the back of your hand over the patient's forearm, hands and fingers to assess the temperature.

□□□ *Joints*

Squeeze the patient's hands at the carpal and metacarpal joints and then each and every MCP and IP joint assessing for tenderness and swelling of bone or soft tissue. Check for tenderness in the anatomical snuffbox (scaphoid fracture), the tip of the styloid process (de Quervain's disease) and the head of ulna (extensor carpi ulnaris tendinitis).

★ Move

□□□ **Movement**

Move each joint in the hand in turn noting any reduced movements.

Fingers

Hold each joint (MCP and IP) between your thumb and finger; flex and extend each joint in isolation. Assess for any limited range of movements. Ask the patient to make a precision grip by opposing their thumb to their index finger then attempt to break it with your index finger. Next, test grip strength by asking the patient to grab and squeeze your middle and index fingers. Compare grip strength on both sides.

□□□ *Thumb*   Have the hands flat with the palms facing upwards. Test thumb abduction by asking the patient to point their thumbs to the ceiling and to hold it in position against the resistance of your finger. Test opposition by requesting the patient to make a ring with the tip of their little finger, maintaining it against resistance. Finally, ask the patient to place their thumb firmly against their palm for adduction and to stretch out their thumb to the opposite side for extension.

□□□ *Wrist*   Ask the patient to perform wrist flexion (80°) and wrist dorsiflexion (80°). If possible, test for radial (40°) and ulnar deviation (10°) as well as pronation and supination.

Nerve Supply to Muscles in the Hand

Mnemonic: 'LOAF'

Median nerve (ape hand)	Lateral two Lumbricals, Opponens pollicis, Abductor pollicis brevis, Flexor pollicis brevis

Mnemonic: 'BESTS'

Radial nerve (wrist drop)	Brachioradialis, Extensors of wrist, Supinator, Triceps, loss of Sensation over the anatomical snuffbox

Mnemonic: 'MAFIA'

Ulnar nerve (claw hand)	Medial lumbricals, Adductor pollicis (pincer grip), First dorsal interossei, Interossei, Abductor digiti minimi

---

✻ Sensation

□□□ **Neurology**   Assess sensation in the hand by testing light touch. Touch a wisp of cotton over the little finger (ulnar nerve), index finger (median nerve) and the lateral aspect of the thumb or anatomical snuff box (radial nerve). Ask permission to formally assess pain sensation using a neurological pin. Test both sides and compare.

✻ Function

□□□ **Daily Tasks**   Assess function by asking the patient to carry out everyday tasks such as undoing buttons and writing a sentence using a pen or holding a cup.

✱ Special Tests

☐☐☐ **Tinel's Sign**   Tap over the median nerve (carpal tunnel) at the wrist to reproduce symptoms of pain or tingling in the distribution of the median nerve.

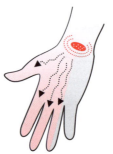

Tinel's sign

Tap over the median nerve at the wrist to reproduce symptoms in the fingers and thumb

☐☐☐ **Phalen's Test**   Hold the wrists fully hyperflexed for 1–2 minutes to reproduce symptoms of pain or tingling in the distribution of the median nerve.

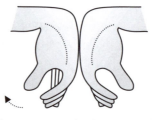

Phalen's test

Have the wrists fully hyperflexed for one minute to reproduce symptoms in the fingers and thumb

☐☐☐ **Fromen's Sign**   Ask the patient to clutch a piece of paper between their thumb and index finger. Attempt to pull the paper away from the clasp of the patient. If the thumb adductor is weak then the patient can only hold onto the paper by flexing the interphalangeal joints of the thumb and is unable to hold the thumb straight (ulnar nerve compression).

☐☐☐ **Flexor Digitorum Profundus**

Ask the patient to flex the distal interphalangeal joint while holding the finger in extension at the proximal interphalangeal joint.

☐☐☐ **Flexor Digitorum Superficialis**

Hold all the fingers in full extension except for the finger being tested. Ask the patient to flex the remaining finger at the proximal interphalangeal joint.

Anatomy of the Flexor Digitorum Muscles
Mnemonic: 'Superficialis splits in two, to permit profundus passing through'

☐☐☐ **Summarise**

Thank the patient. Acknowledge the patient's concerns. Restore the patient's clothing. Summarise your findings to the examiner.

'This is Mrs Susan Gregory, a 40-year-old pregnant woman. She is complaining of hand pains that are worse during the night. She has to shake her hands in order to relieve the pain. The pain is described as a burning sensation. On examination, the patient has pain and burning in the median nerve distribution. Her power and joint movements were normal. However, Tinel's and Phalen's test were positive. From the history and examination findings, I believe that this patient has carpal tunnel syndrome. I would like to perform a nerve conduction test to confirm my suspicions.'

EXAMINER'S EVALUATION

0 1 2 3 4 5
☐☐☐☐☐☐ Overall assessment of hand examination
☐☐☐☐☐☐ Role player's score
Total mark out of 33

DIFFERENTIAL DIAGNOSIS
Carpal Tunnel Syndrome

Carpal tunnel syndrome is caused by the entrapment of the median nerve in the carpal tunnel due to pressure. It usually affects patients aged between 40–50 years of age and is eight times more frequent in women than in men. It can be due to hypothyroidism, diabetes mellitus, pregnancy, obesity, rheumatoid arthritis and acromegaly; however, in most cases the cause is unknown. Symptoms include burning pain and tingling felt in the distribution of the median nerve (thumb, index, middle and lateral half of the ring finger). The pain is usually worse at night but can be relieved by shaking the wrist. On examination there is loss of sensation in the median nerve distribution, wasting of the thenar eminence and weakness of the abductor pollicis brevis. The diagnosis can be confirmed with a positive Phalen's and Tinel's test.

Treatment of Carpal Tunnel Syndrome
Mnemonic: 'WRIST'
Wear splints at night, **R**est, **I**nject steroid, **S**urgical decompression, **T**ake diuretics

Trigger Finger (Stenosing Tenovaginitis)

The flexor tendons extend from the wrist to the fingers. Occasionally a flexor tendon may become trapped in the opening of its sheath due to nodules or a thickening of the tendon sheath. Trigger finger can affect any finger, but the middle and ring fingers are most commonly affected. Patients note a clicking noise when the finger is flexed with the affected finger remaining bent when the others are extended. With some effort the tendon can be suddenly freed ("triggering") and the finger snaps back into place.

Mallet's Finger

Mallet's finger, otherwise known as 'baseball finger' is a deformity of the finger where the distal interphalangeal joint is held in the flexed position. It is a common sports injury and occurs when a ball strikes the tip of the finger or thumb causing either rupture to the extensor tendon or an avulsion fracture. As a result the patient is unable to extend and straighten the distal joint of the finger.

De Quervain's Disease (Stenosing Tenovaginitis)

Repetitive abduction and adduction of the thumb can irritate the tendons of the extensor pollicis brevis and abductor pollicis longus muscles which can become inflamed and thickened. This can occur from repetitive actions which require much force, such as pruning a hedge. When this occurs, any movement of the thumb (in particular, gripping) may cause pain at the radial side of the wrist. On examination, there may be swelling overlying the tendons of the thumb. Tenderness can be located at the tip of the radial styloid where the tendons of the extensor pollicis brevis and longus cross. Passive stretching of the tendons as well as abduction of the thumb against resistance and passive adduction are extremely painful. The diagnosis can be confirmed with a positive Finkelstein test. The Finkelstein test consists of flexing the thumb across the palm inside a clenched fist and placing the wrist in ulnar deviation. This stretches the inflamed tendons over the radial styloid, reproducing the patient's pain.

Finkelstein Test

Clench the thumb inside a closed fist and tilt the hand into forward flexion. Note a sharp pain over the radial styloid suggesting De Quervain's tenosynovitis

Tenderness in the styloid process

Forward flexion of the wrist generates pain

INSTRUCTIONS: Please examine this patient, who is complaining of pain and stiffness in the hip. Report your findings to the examiner as you go along, and make an appropriate diagnosis.

HISTORY

0 1 2

☐☐☐ **Introduction** Introduce yourself. Elicit the patient's name, age and occupation. Establish rapport with the patient.

✴ **History of Presenting Complaint**

History When did it first start? Have you had this problem in the past? Have you ever fallen, injured or fractured your hip before?

☐☐☐ **Pain** Where is the pain located? Does the pain move anywhere? How severe is the pain, graded out of 10? What does the pain feel like?

7.5

Pain in the hip may be felt in the groin or inner thigh. It often radiates to the knee. Hip pain is often made worse by exercise or walking.

Stiffness Do you have any stiffness in your hip? Is it worse in the morning or evening? Does it come on suddenly or gradually?

General Health How is your general health? Do you have any malaise, fever or weight loss?

☐☐☐ **Impact on Life** How has your hip problem affected your daily activities and/or mobility?

EXAMINATION

Consent Obtain consent before beginning the examination.

☐☐☐ **Expose** Ask the patient if they can undress to their undergarments.

✴ **Look**

☐☐☐ **General** With the patient standing, look for alignment of the shoulders, hips and patella and ensure that the ASISs (anterior superior iliac spine) are aligned and at the same level to one other. Inspect from behind for scoliosis and gluteal wasting. Inspect from the side for increased lumbar lordosis (fixed flexion deformity).

☐☐☐ Gait

Observe their gait. Ask the patient if they can walk to the end of the room and return.

Signs to Look for in Gait

Use of a walking aid	Sticks, frames
Speed	Rhythm, presence of a limp
Phases of walking	Heel strike, stance, push off and swing
Stride length	Reduced, limited
Arm swing	Present, absent
Types of gait	Such as Trendelenburg's and antalgic gait
Trendelenburg's gait	Ineffective hip abduction results in the pelvis dropping during the weight-bearing stance phase and the body leaning to the unaffected side
Antalgic gait	Pain in the hip causing a shortening of the stance phase and the body leaning to the affected side. Most common cause is osteoarthritis

☐☐☐ Trendelenburg

The Trendelenburg test is used to assess hip stability. Instruct the patient to stand upon the sound limb while raising the opposite foot by bending it at the knee. Carefully observe, or palpate with a hand on the iliac crest, for pelvic tilting and noting which side it drops towards. Repeat the test but on the opposite leg.

Interpreting Trendelenburg's Test

Negative test	Pelvis rises on the opposite, unsupported side
Positive test	Pelvis drops on the opposite, unsupported side
Causes	Dislocation of the hip, weakness of the abductor muscles, shortening of femoral neck, pain in the hip

In general, when standing on one leg the weight-bearing hip is held stable by the abductor muscles

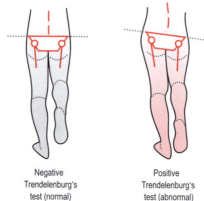

Negative Trendelenburg's test (normal)

Positive Trendelenburg's test (abnormal)

Trendelenburg's test

Ask the patient to stand on one leg while flexing the opposite leg at the knee keeping their foot off the ground. Normally, the hip is held stable by the abductor muscles contracting in the supporting leg. A positive Trendelenburg's sign is noted if the pelvis drops on the unsupported side

which contract, elevating the pelvis on the unsupported side. However, if the hip is unstable, abduction of the hip does not occur and the pelvis drops on the unsupported side.

☐☐☐ **Observe** Inspect the hip with the patient lying on the couch.

Signs to Look for in the Hip Examination

Skin	Scars, sinus, pigmentation, unusual skin creases	
Muscle	Wasting, fasciculations	
Swelling	Look for effusion in hip or knee (effusions in knee joint – OA)	
Position	*Shortened limb*	Ankle misalignment with pelvic tilting
	Limb rotation	Externally (#NOF, femoral shaft) or internally
	Fixed flexion deformity	Excessive lordosis

☐☐☐ **Measure** Before measuring the length of the limbs, square the pelvis by ensuring that the iliac crests are aligned and on the same level. Inability to square the pelvis indicates possible fixed adduction or abduction deformity of the hip.

Measure the apparent limb length by measuring the distance from the xiphisternum to the medial malleolus on each side. Then measure the distance between the ASIS to the medial malleolus on each side to assess the true limb length. Compare the two values.

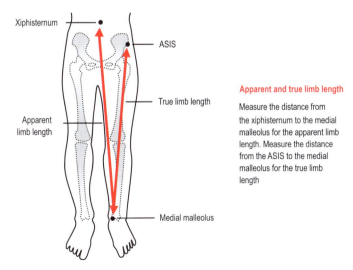

Xiphisternum

ASIS

True limb length

Apparent limb length

Medial malleolus

Apparent and true limb length

Measure the distance from the xiphisternum to the medial malleolus for the apparent limb length. Measure the distance from the ASIS to the medial malleolus for the true limb length

If the apparent limb lengths appear unequal but with no disparity between the true limb lengths, this could be due to a fixed adduction deformity of the hip. If the true limb length measurements appear unequal then there is true limb shortening.

Causes of Limb Length Inequality

True shortening	Perthes' disease, slipped femoral epiphysis, avascular necrosis, arthritis, hip dislocation
Apparent shortening	Fixed adduction deformity of hip (arthritis)

★ Feel
☐☐☐ **Palpate**

Palpate the hip with the patient still lying on the couch. Feel the hip for temperature, effusions and bony landmarks.

Signs to Palpate in the Hip Examination

Skin	Temperature (infections, inflammation), soft tissue contours
Joints	Effusion in the hip
Bones	Palpate for tenderness over the greater trochanter (bursitis), lesser trochanter (tears of the iliopsoas), ischial tuberosity (tears of the hamstrings), feel for bony landmarks – (greater trochanter, ASIS)

★ Move

Note any limited range of movements or the reporting of pain. Examine each joint actively first by asking the patient to perform the movement independently. Re-examine the joint passively by helping the patient move the joint.

☐☐☐ **Flexion**

Have the patient flex their knees and move their hip joint into the flexed position as far as possible (normal range 130°).

☐☐☐ **Thomas' Test**

Keep one hand flat on the examining table under the patient's lumbar spine. Have both hips flexed then ask the patient to hold on to his sound knee (sound hip is flexed to limit) while straightening the suspect leg. If the limb is elevated off the examining table and is unable to fully straighten there is a fixed flexion deformity of the hip on the affected side. The angle through which the thigh is raised from the couch is the angle of fixed flexion. Repeat the test for the other hip.

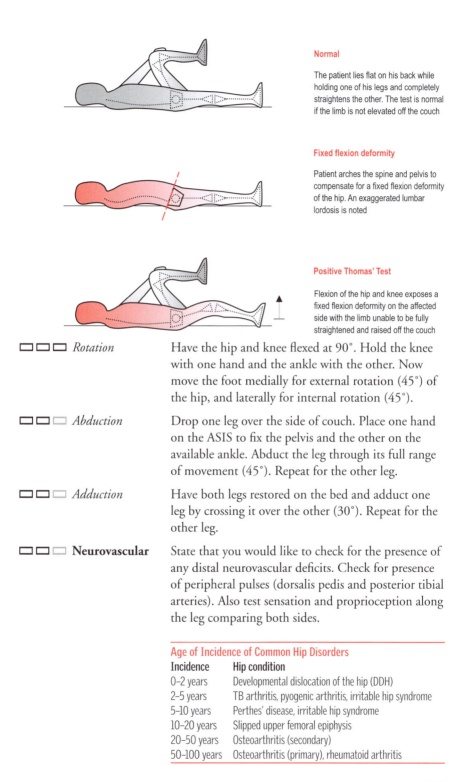

Normal

The patient lies flat on his back while holding one of his legs and completely straightens the other. The test is normal if the limb is not elevated off the couch

Fixed flexion deformity

Patient arches the spine and pelvis to compensate for a fixed flexion deformity of the hip. An exaggerated lumbar lordosis is noted

Positive Thomas' Test

Flexion of the hip and knee exposes a fixed flexion deformity on the affected side with the limb unable to be fully straightened and raised off the couch

☐☐☐ *Rotation*

Have the hip and knee flexed at 90°. Hold the knee with one hand and the ankle with the other. Now move the foot medially for external rotation (45°) of the hip, and laterally for internal rotation (45°).

☐☐☐ *Abduction*

Drop one leg over the side of couch. Place one hand on the ASIS to fix the pelvis and the other on the available ankle. Abduct the leg through its full range of movement (45°). Repeat for the other leg.

☐☐☐ *Adduction*

Have both legs restored on the bed and adduct one leg by crossing it over the other (30°). Repeat for the other leg.

☐☐☐ **Neurovascular**

State that you would like to check for the presence of any distal neurovascular deficits. Check for presence of peripheral pulses (dorsalis pedis and posterior tibial arteries). Also test sensation and proprioception along the leg comparing both sides.

Age of Incidence of Common Hip Disorders

Incidence	Hip condition
0–2 years	Developmental dislocation of the hip (DDH)
2–5 years	TB arthritis, pyogenic arthritis, irritable hip syndrome
5–10 years	Perthes' disease, irritable hip syndrome
10–20 years	Slipped upper femoral epiphysis
20–50 years	Osteoarthritis (secondary)
50–100 years	Osteoarthritis (primary), rheumatoid arthritis

□ □ □ **Summarise**   Thank the patient and offer to assist them to put on their clothes. Acknowledge the patient's concerns. Summarise your findings to the examiner.

'This is Mrs Smith, a 60-year-old widower who has been complaining of hip pain for a number of years. She states the pain is getting worse, particularly at end of the day and during periods of activity. The pain radiates to her thigh and is not controlled by her usual analgesia. On examination, there is an antalgic gait with a positive Trendelenburg's test, reduced generalised movement of the hip and a positive Thomas' test. In view of these findings, I believe that Mrs Smith suffers from osteoarthritis. However, I would like to perform an X-ray to exclude other causes (rheumatoid arthritis, neck of femur fracture).'

EXAMINER'S EVALUATION

0 1 2 3 4 5
□ □ □ □ □ □   Overall assessment of hip examination
□ □ □ □ □ □   Role player's score
Total mark out of 33

DIFFERENTIAL DIAGNOSIS
Osteoarthritis of the Hip

Osteoarthritis in the hip can be primary in nature or secondary to Perthes' diseases (in the young), rheumatoid arthritis and Paget's (in the elderly). Symptoms include pain and stiffness in the hip. Symptoms progress slowly over time (years) with pain precipitated by lesser activity (shorter distances walked) as the disease worsens. Osteoarthritis tends to occur in patients over the age of 50 since the risk of wear and tear on the joint increases with age. The pain originates in the groin and may radiate to the knee. Pain usually occurs after a period of activity while stiffness occurs after periods of rest. On examination, the patient may reveal a positive Trendelenburg's sign with a limp in the gait. The affected leg is held externally rotated and in adduction appearing short in limb length, whilst the Thomas' test may expose the presence of a fixed flexion deformity. There is also a general restriction in limb movements.

Slipped Femoral Epiphysis

Slipped upper femoral epiphysis is a disease of adolescence where the upper femoral epiphysis slips downwards from its normal position on the femoral neck, causing a coxa vara deformity. It is a common cause of hip and knee pain in those aged between 10 and 20 and is the most common hip disorder in adolescence. It is three times more common in boys than girls and commonly affects the left hip more than the right, though bilateral slips do occur. The condition is linked with overweight (obesity) from endocrine disorders (hypothyroidism, hypopituitarism, growth hormone deficiency) and occasionally there is a history of preceding trauma. The patient may complain of pain in the hip or knee and walks with a limp. In the acute setting weight bearing is impossible. On examination, there is a loss of motion in the hip joint, particularly internal rotation, and abduction of the affected hip. Forceful examination of the restricted movements will exacerbate the pain. The limb is externally rotated with true shortening of the leg causing an inequality in limb length.

Trochanteric Bursitis

The trochanteric bursa is found overlying the greater trochanter of the femur. Inflammation can occur from either acute trauma, such as a fall or a football tackle, or more commonly from repetitive, cumulative trauma. Classically, there is pain over the greater trochanteric region of the lateral hip. The pain is made worse when the patient lies on the affected bursa and can awaken the patient at night. Symptoms tend to get worse with walking. On examination, the range of motion is generally preserved. Tenderness can be elicited on direct palpation over the bursa.

INSTRUCTIONS: Please examine this patient who is complaining of pain and stiffness in the knee. Report your findings to the examiner as you go along, and make an appropriate diagnosis.

HISTORY

0 1 2

☐☐☐ **Introduction** — Introduce yourself. Elicit the patient's name, age and occupation. Establish rapport with the patient.

★ History of Presenting Complaint

History — When did it first start? Have you had this problem in the past? Have you ever fallen, injured or fractured your knee before?

☐☐☐ **Pain** — Where is the pain located? Does the pain move anywhere? How severe is the pain, graded out of 10? What does the pain feel like?

7.6

☐☐☐ **Stiffness** — Do you have any stiffness? Is it worse in the morning or the evening?

Swelling — Have you noticed any swelling? Did it occur after an injury? How long after did it occur (immediately – haemarthrosis, some hours after – torn meniscus)?

☐☐☐ **Locking** — Have you noticed that you are unable to fully straighten your leg when you walk (torn meniscus)?

☐☐☐ **Giving Way** — Have you ever felt that your knee was about to give way (torn meniscus, torn ligament, patella dislocation)?

☐☐☐ **Impact on Life** — How has your knee problem affected your daily activities and/or mobility?

EXAMINATION

Consent — Obtain consent before beginning the examination.

☐☐☐ **Expose** — Ask the patient if they can undress to their undergarments.

★ Look

Gait — Assess the patient's gait by asking the patient if they could walk to the end of the room and return. Observe the phases of gait, the presence of a limp and for restriction of movement.

☐☐☐ **General**　　Inspect the patient standing, then lying on the couch in the supine position. Look at the posture, position and alignment of the knees. Measure the quadriceps girth 10 cm above the patella for wasting on both legs.

Signs to Look for in the Knee Examination

Observe with the patient standing

Posture	Alignment of shoulder, hips and patella
Joint	Inspect the popliteal fossa from the back for a Baker's cyst
Position	Neutral, valgus (knock knee), varus (bow leg) deformity, Fixed flexion deformity/attitude, recurvatum (hyperextension)

Observe with the patient lying on the couch

Skin	Colour, sinuses, scars (arthroscopic)
Muscle	Wasting (quadriceps – vastus medialis), fasciculations
Joints	Effusions, rheumatoid arthritis nodules, psoriatic plaques
Alignment	Patellar alignment, tibial alignment
Position	Fixed flexion deformity of the knee (unable to straighten the knee)

✶ Feel

☐☐☐ **General**　　Palpate the knee with the patient still lying on the couch. Before palpating it ask if there is any pain. Feel the knee for warmth, effusions and position. State that you would like to perform the patella apprehension test to test for patella dislocation.

Skin　　Feel over the knee for warmth and temperature (infections, inflammation) comparing both knees.

☐☐☐ **Effusions**　　Perform the cross fluctuation, patella tap test and bulge test to assess the size of the effusion.

Cross Fluctuat.　　One hand empties the suprapatellar pouch while the other hand is placed just below the patella. A positive test is seen when an impulse is transmitted across the joint with alternate compressions. This test is used to detect large effusions.

Patella Tap　　Empty the suprapatellar pouch with one hand and then sharply tap the patella with the index finger.

A positive patella tap test will see the patella sink, striking the femur then bouncing back up again. This test elicits moderately sized effusions.

Patella
bounces up
and down

Patella Tap Test

Slide your hand down the patient's thigh emptying the suprapatellar pouch forcing the effusion below the patella. Next sharply tap the patella with the index finger of the other hand. Note if the patella bounces up

Bulge Test

After draining the medial compartment by massaging the medial aspect of the joint, swiftly stroke the lateral aspect of the knee, and observe for the appearance of a ripple on the medial surface. This test can detect the presence of small effusions in the joint.

Bulge Test

Empty the suprapatellar pouch before emptying the medial compartment by compressing it with your free hand. Lift the hand away and then quickly compress the lateral side. A positive test is noted if a 'bulge' is seen on the medial surface

▢▢▢ **Joints**

Have the knee flexed at 90° and feel along the joint line for tenderness. Feel for the ligaments and synovial thickening, as well as bony landmarks such as the tibial tuberosity and femoral condyles. Palpate in the popliteal fossa for a Baker's cyst.

Patella

Ask permission to perform the patella apprehension test. Flex the knee while pressing the patella laterally.

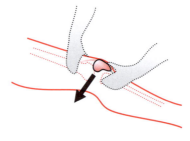

**Patella
Apprehension Test**

Flex the knee to approximately 30 degrees while pushing the patella firmly in the lateral direction. The patient will anticipate patella dislocation and discontinue the test

If the patella is unstable the patient will anticipate patella dislocation and discontinue the test.

✳ Move
☐☐☐ Active

Note any limited range of movement or the reporting of pain. Test for knee flexion by asking the patient to bend their leg backwards without providing assistance. Then ask them to straighten their leg as far as possible for knee extension.

Passive

Place one hand on the knee and the other on the ankle. Attempt to flex the patient's knee back as far as possible (140°). Then test for extension by straightening the leg while feeling for crepitus in the knee (−10°).

✳ Special Tests
☐☐☐ Collateral Lig.

The medial and lateral collateral ligaments can be assessed by applying a valgus or varus force at the knee. Have the patient's foot tucked under your armpit while holding the patient's knee with both hands. Apply a valgus force by steering the knee medially to test the medial ligament. Next apply a varus stress by pushing the knee laterally to test for the lateral ligament.

Alternatively, hold the ankle in one hand and the knee in the other. Test the medial ligament by abducting the ankle whilst pushing the knee medially. Test the lateral ligament by adducting the ankle whilst pushing the knee laterally. Apply the stresses

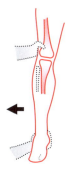

Test medial collaterals

Hold the patient's ankle in one hand and the knee in the other. Test for medial instability by applying a valgus stress to the knee while abducting the ankle

Excessive joint movement

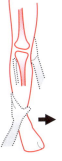

Test lateral collaterals

Hold the patient's ankle in one hand and the knee in the other. Test for lateral instability by applying a varus stress to the knee while adducting the ankle

Excessive joint movement

at 0° and repeat with the leg slight flexed at 20°. Excessive movement suggests a torn or stretched collateral ligament.

Cruciate Lig.   Look for the sag sign and perform the Drawer test and Lachman test to assess the cruciate ligaments.

Sag Sign   Have the knee flexed to 90° and observe for sagging of the upper end of the tibia compared to the patella. The sag sign indicates a posterior cruciate ligament tear.

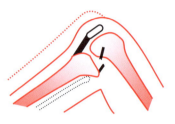

Sag Sign

Observe for the posterior tibial sag sign by having the patient's knee in 90 degrees of flexion. Note the sagging of the tibia suggesting the presence of a posterior cruciate ligament tear. Compare the knee to the opposite side

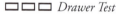 *Drawer Test*   Ask the patient if they have any pain in their feet. Have the knee flexed to 90° and then anchor the foot by sitting on it, requesting permission before doing so. Hold the knee with your thumbs on the tibial tuberosity and fingers in the popliteal fossa; rock it back and forth assessing for any give. An excessive anterior movement indicates anterior cruciate laxity while an excessive posterior movement suggest posterior cruciate laxity.

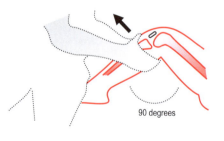

Drawer Test

Have the patient's knee flexed to 90 degrees before sitting on his foot. Grasp hold of the proximal tibia with both hands with thumbs on the tibial tuberosity and fingers in the popliteal fossa. Pull the tibia forward while noting degree of anterior tibial displacement

90 degrees

Lachman Test   Have the patient's knee flexed to 20°. Hold the lower thigh in one hand and place the other hand behind the proximal tibia. Gently glide the tibia forward by

272

pulling anteriorly. An intact anterior cruciate should prevent the forward gliding movement of the tibia on the femur. The Lachman test is a more sensitive test for anterior cruciate ligament laxity and is often carried out if the Drawer test cannot be performed due to foot pain, for example.

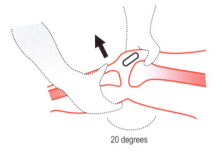

20 degrees

Lachman Test

Have the patient's knee flexed at 20 degrees. Stabilise the femur with one hand and place the other hand behind the proximal tibia with the thumb on the tibial tuberosity. Attempt to pull the tibia anteriorly checking for forward translational movement

Meniscus Tears

Perform the McMurray test and Apley's grinding test to assess for torn meniscal tags.

McMurray Test

Before undertaking this test, warn the patient that this test may cause pain. Flex the knee as far as possible while holding the knee joint. Externally rotate the leg and slowly extend it while stressing it into valgus. Repeat, but this time internally rotate the leg and extend it while stressing it into varus. A positive test is signalled by a painful click felt or heard. This indicates that a torn meniscal tag is caught between the articular surfaces of the femoral condyle and the tibial plateau.

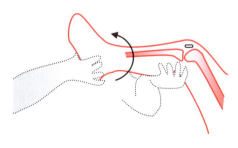

McMurray Test

Flex the patient's knee and have one hand stablising the knee with the other hand holding the sole of the foot. Test for a medial meniscus tag by externally rotating the leg and applying a valgus stress while slowly extending the knee. Test for lateral meniscal tags by repeating the test but internally rotating the knee while applying a varus stress.

Externally rotate the leg and extend while applying a valgus stress.

Grinding Test

Ask permission to perform Apley's grinding test. Have the patient lying prone with their knee flexed to 90° and the examiner resting their knee on the patient's thigh. Apply a grinding force by rotating and applying compression to the knee joint. Elicited pain suggests a torn meniscus. Repeat but instead rotate and pull the leg upwards simultaneously with patient's thigh anchored down with the examiner's knee. Pain indicates ligament damage.

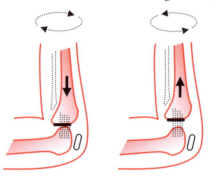

Apley's Grinding Test

Test for a meniscal tear by applying pressure and rotational force to the foot with the patient lying prone with his knee flexed 90 degrees. Test for ligament damage by reversing the direction of pressure and rotation. Elicit pain for a positive test

☐☐☐ **Neurovascular**   State that you would like to check for the presence of any distal neurovascular deficits. Check for presence of peripheral pulses (dorsalis pedis and posterior tibial arteries). Also test sensation and proprioception along both legs comparing both sides.

Request   State that you would also like to perform a hip and ankle examination.

☐☐☐ **Summarise**   Thank the patient and offer to assist them to put on their clothes. Acknowledge the patient's concerns and encourage questions. Summarise your findings to the examiner.

'This is Mark Hughes, a 20-year-old man who was playing football on the weekend. He is complaining of sharp pain in the medial aspect of the knee. He states that when he was playing football he twisted his knee. Shortly afterward he developed pain and swelling. Now he notes that his knee does not fully extend and can occasionally give way. On examination, he has a large fluctuant bulge on the medial aspect of the knee, and walks with an antalgic gait. The swelling had a positive bulge test. Of note he also had a positive McMurray test. In view of his history and examination findings I suspect he has a meniscal tear.'

0 1 2 3 4 5

☐ ☐ ☐ ☐ ☐ ☐ Overall assessment of knee examination

☐ ☐ ☐ ☐ ☐ ☐ Role player's score

Total mark out of 31

DIFFERENTIAL DIAGNOSIS

Osteoarthritis of the Knee

The knee represents the commonest site of presentation for osteoarthritis. It can be primary in nature or secondary due to injury, torn meniscus, recurrent patella dislocation or ligament instability. Patients are classically over 50 years of age, overweight, and may have a bow-leg deformity. They often complain of pain with stiffness. The pain originates in the knee and is severe in nature. It is made worse after the individual attempts to move after a period of inactivity. However, stiffness usually occurs after periods of rest. On examination, there may be limited movement with patellofemoral crepitus and flexion or varus deformities. The quadriceps muscle is often wasted and there is no effusion or warmth.

Meniscal Tears

The menisci are C-shaped cartilaginous tissues that are located above, and in addition to, the articular cartilage of the tibia. They act as shock absorbers and provide smooth movement and stability in the knee joint. Meniscal tears are common sport injuries in young athletes. They result from a twisting force applied to a bent knee that is also weight bearing, commonly seen in footballers as they strike a ball or when they are running and attempt to change direction. Tears vary in size and location and can be partial or full length. Longitudinal tears that extend along the length of the meniscus, with the cartilage still attached front and back, are known as a bucket handle tear. The 'handle' may flip over, displace and be caught between the femur and tibia, locking the knee and preventing full extension. Symptoms of meniscal tears include pain, swelling and loss of knee function. The pain often occurs when attempting to extend the leg and is felt within the knee joint. Swelling of the knee often develops several hours after the injury as a result of inflammation caused by the tear. The patient may describe that his knee occasionally gives way with pain and swelling developing afterwards. The locking of the knee is synonymous with bucket handle tears. Often patients are able to manually manipulate their leg and 'unlock' the knee so that it can be straightened once again. On examination, the knee is held partially flexed, there is localised tenderness in the joint line, an effusion is often present and there is limitation to knee extension. McMurray and Apley's grinding tests are positive.

Baker's Cyst

Baker's cyst is a collection of fluid in the synovial sac which protrudes out of the back of the knee below the joint line from the popliteal fossa. It is differentiated from a popliteal aneurysm by the absence of a palpable pulse. This type of Baker's cyst is commonly associated with a tear in the meniscal cartilage of the knee. In older adults, this condition is frequently associated with degenerative arthritis of the knee. It can present as a painless or painful swelling behind the knee. Occasionally, the cyst may rupture, causing pain, swelling and bruising on the back of the knee and calf. Transillumination of the cyst can demonstrate that the mass is fluid filled.

Bursitis

The semimembranosus bursa (Brodie's bursa) is found between the medial head of gastrocnemius and the semimembranosus tendon. Inflammation of the bursa presents as a painless fluctuant lump within the medial aspect of the popliteal fossa behind the knee. It is best examined whilst standing with the knee in extension. Prepatellar bursitis (housemaid's knee) is caused by repeated friction between the skin and the patella. It used to be synonymous with housemaids due to the time they spent washing the floors on their knees. However, it occurs more often in carpet fitters and miners. On examination, a swelling can be noted directly over the patella. The rest of the knee examination is unremarkable. Infrapatellar bursitis (clergyman's knees) similarly is caused by friction between the skin and patella. However, the swelling is found distal to the patella and superficial to the patellar ligament. This is caused by the kneeling posture taken up by a person in prayer as opposed to the one who cleans floors.

ORTHOPAEDICS: **Ankle and Foot Examination**

INSTRUCTIONS: Examine this patient, who is complaining of sudden onset of ankle pain. Report your findings to the examiner as you go along, and make an appropriate diagnosis.

HISTORY

0 1 2

☐☐☐ **Introduction** Introduce yourself. Elicit the patient's name, age and occupation. Establish rapport with the patient.

★ **History of Presenting Complaint**

☐☐☐ **Pain** Where is the pain located? Does the pain move anywhere? How severe is the pain graded out of ten? Can you describe the pain? What were you doing at the time it first started?

☐☐☐ **Stiffness** Do you have any stiffness in your ankle or foot?

Swelling Have you noticed any swelling (bunion, gout)?

EXAMINATION

Consent Explain the examination to the patient and seek consent.

☐☐☐ **Expose** Ask the patient to expose his lower limbs including his feet.

★ **Gait**

☐☐☐ **Walk** Observe the patient's gait. Ask the patient if they could walk to the end of the room and return. Note the presence of an antalgic gait.

Signs to Look for in Gait	
Use of a walking aid	Sticks, frames
Speed	Rhythm, presence of a limp
Phases of walking	Heel strike, stance, push off and swing
Stride length	Reduced, limited
Arm swing	Present, absent

★ **Look**

☐☐☐ **Inspect** Look at the patient's shoes for signs of abnormal wear. Inspect with the patient standing and then observe the ankles and feet from behind. Assess the patient's posture, alignment of the feet and joint deformity.

7.7

Ask the patient to lie down on the couch and continue your inspection.

Signs to Look for in the Ankle and Foot Examination

Skin	Colour, scars, sinus, corns, callosities, ulcers, fungal infections, in-growing toenails
Muscle	Wasting of the calf (gastrocnemius) and lower leg muscles
Alignment	Valgus deformity (foot deviated away from the midline)
	Varus deformity (foot deviated to the midline)
Deformity	Pes planus (flat foot), pes cavus (high-arched foot), talipes (club foot)
	Bunion (1st MTP joint), hallux valgus/rigidus, claw toe, mallet toe, hammer toe

✴ Feel
☐☐☐ **Palpate**

Ascertain if the foot is painful. Ask the patient to locate the pain before palpating it. Assess the skin temperature by running the back of your hands along both feet simultaneously comparing both sides. Palpate for presence of peripheral pulses. Palpate the joint margin, hindfoot, midfoot and forefoot noting any tenderness.

Signs to Palpate in the Ankle and Foot Examination

Skin	Temperature (infections, inflammation)
Pulses	Dorsalis pedis, posterior tibial
Joints	Effusions, oedema, lumps
Bones	Localise any tenderness (malleoli, MTP, IP, metatarsal head)

✴ Move
☐☐☐ **Movement**

Assess the range of movement at the ankle, subtalar, midtarsal joints and toes. Check active and passive movements for each joint.

Ankle

Grasp the heel in one hand and hold the midfoot in the other. Test ankle dorsiflexion (10°) and plantar-flexion (40°).

Subtalar

Maintain your grasp of the patient's foot. Using the ankle as a pivot, assess foot inversion (30°) by directing the sole towards the midline and foot eversion (30°) by turning the sole away from the midline.

Midtarsal	Hold the heel firmly in one hand and the forefoot in the other to stabilise the subtalar joint. Attempt to move the forefoot up and down and then from side to side.
Toe	Assess flexion and extension in each toe in turn.

★ Special Tests

☐☐☐ **Simmonds'** — Before performing this test, palpate the calf muscle and Achilles' tendon for wasting and tenderness. Note for depression in the lower calf signifying a tendon rupture. Perform Simmonds' test to confirm a ruptured Achilles' tendon. Have the patient lying prone with their feet hanging off the edge of the bed. Squeeze the calves simultaneously and note for reflex plantar flexion in both feet. Absence of plantarflexion of a foot suggests a ruptured tendon.

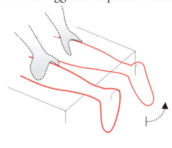

Simmonds' Test

Examine the patient lying flat on the couch with legs hanging off the edge. Squeeze both calves simultaneously and note plantarflexion in both feet. Absence of plantarflexion in a foot is a positive test and suggestive of a ruptured Achilles' tendon

☐☐☐ **Neurovascular** — State that you would like to check for the presence of any distal neurovascular deficits. Perform a full arterial examination to check for the presence of peripheral pulses. Test sensation and proprioception along both legs and feet comparing both sides.

Request — State that you would also like to perform a hip and knee examination.

☐☐☐ **Summarise** — Thank the patient and offer to assist them to put on their clothes. Acknowledge the patient's concerns. Summarise your findings to the examiner.

'Mr Peckham, a 15-year-old teenager, complains of sudden onset of pain in his right lower ankle. On examination, he was found to walk with an antalgic gait and unable to bear weight fully on his right side. A depression was noted in his right lower calf with weakness of plantar flexion of the ankle. Simmonds' test was positive. In view of the history and examination, I suspect Mr Peckham has a ruptured right Achillies' tendon.'

EXAMINER'S EVALUATION

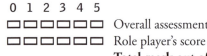

0 1 2 3 4 5

☐ ☐ ☐ ☐ ☐ ☐ Overall assessment of ankle and foot examination
☐ ☐ ☐ ☐ ☐ ☐ Role player's score

Total mark out of 25

DIFFERENTIAL DIAGNOSIS

Hallux Valgus

Hallux valgus is a valgus deformity of the hallux (1st MTP joint) with lateral deviation of the great toe exceeding 15°. Such angulation results in subluxation of MTP joint of the big toe which protrudes laterally and becomes prominent forming a bunion on the first metatarsal head. Friction with shoes may cause the bunion to be swollen and inflamed. It is associated with wide splaying of the forefoot, second digit hammer toe, metatarsalgia, flat feet and secondary osteoarthritis affecting the MTP joint of the big toe. It is commonly bilateral and often the result of inappropriate footwear, such as pointed shoes.

Pes Planus (Flat Foot)

Flat foot is the obliteration of the medial arch of the foot that persists through childhood and into adolescence. Commonly the condition is asymptomatic but a visible abnormality may be noticed by concerned parents. They may note that their child has an awkward gait and wears shoes poorly. Adults may complain of foot strain or aches in the feet after prolonged walking or standing. On examination, the medial arches of the feet are absent. The patient should be examined whilst sitting to observe for sites of tenderness and range of movement. Particular attention should be spent looking at the individual's shoes, which may reveal excessive wear along the medial border of the sole and outer side of the heel. A complete examination should include the knees, hips and spine to exclude an underlying disorder.

Pes Cavus (High-arched Foot)

Pes cavus describes a higher than normal medial arch. It is often associated with clawing of the toes and varus deformity of the heel. Pes cavus is normally idiopathic; however, neurological disorders such as Charcot-Marie-Tooth disease, Friedreich's ataxia and peroneal muscular atrophy should be excluded. The patient complains of pain in the metatarsal heads and callosities may form over the same sites.

Causes of Pes Cavus
Mnemonic: 'Disease Can Shorten The Foot'
Diabetes, Charcot-Marie-Tooth, Syringomyelia, Tabes Dorsalis, Friedreich's
Ataxia

Ruptured Achilles' Tendon

The Achilles tendon is a large fibrous cord that connects the calf muscles to the calcaneus. It typically ruptures during strenuous sports activities such as running, football or basketball, which require a forceful push off with the feet. The patient describes the sudden onset of pain at the back of the ankle, as if they had been struck above the heel. On occasion, a tearing snap can be heard at the time of the incident. On examination, there is tenderness and swelling around the affected tendon. A gap or defect can be seen and palpated 4–5 cm above the calcaneus. There is also associated weakness to plantar flexion of the affected foot with a positive Simmonds' test.

Emergency Medicine

Cannulation and I.V. Infusion

INSTRUCTIONS: Set up a normal saline drip into this model arm using the cannula provided. Explain to the examiner what you are doing as you go along.

INTRODUCTION

0 1 2

☐☐☐ **Introduction**   Introduce yourself. Check the patient's identity. Elicit the patient's name, age and occupation. Establish rapport with the patient.

☐☐☐ **Explain**   'I have been asked to set up a drip to give you some fluids. It is a simple procedure that involves inserting a thin, plastic tube into a vein in the back of your hand. The tube will then be connected to a bag of fluid. You may feel a sharp scratch as the needle is being inserted. Do you have any questions?'

Consent   Obtain consent before carrying out the procedure.

8.1

EQUIPMENT

– Correct fluid bag
– Drip stand
– Tray
– Alcohol swab
– Sharps bin
– Adhesive plaster

– Giving set
– Pair of non–sterile gloves
– Tourniquet
– Cannula (16G grey, 18G green, 20G pink)
– Sterile dressing/tape

PROCEDURE

☐☐☐ **Wash Hands**   Clean hands with appropriate disinfectant.

    ✷ **Fluid Bag**

☐☐☐ **Chart**   Inform examiner that you would refer to the drug chart to check fluid prescription.

☐☐☐ **Check**   Select correct fluid bag (fluid type, concentration, volume). Check integrity of fluid bag looking for any holes or contaminants. Check expiry date.

☐☐☐ **Prepare**   Remove fluid bag from its cover and place on drip stand. Remove the giving set from its cover as well, immediately closing its clamp by moving the roller down. Uncover the bag inlet and the giving set spike and then insert the spike into the fluid bag using aseptic technique.

□□□ **Run Through**   Squeeze the reservoir in the giving set until it is half filled with fluid. Remove cap at the end of the giving set. Slowly run fluid through the giving set by opening the clamp. Check for absence of air bubbles. Replace cap at the end of the giving set and then hang on the stand.

✴ Cannulation

Expose   Ensure that there is adequate exposure at the area of insertion.

□□□ **Tourniquet**   Apply tourniquet. Request patient to clench and unclench fist repeatedly. Identify vein. Put on gloves. Clean area with alcohol swab. Remove cannula from wrapping and take off cap.

□□□ **Sharp Scratch**   Retract skin. Warn patient of an impending 'sharp scratch'. Insert the cannula into vein at a shallow angle and look for flashback. Slowly advance the cannula whilst keeping the needle stationary. Remove the tourniquet.

□□□ **Sharps Bin**   Remove the needle and discard immediately into the sharps bin. Press over the vein at the tip of the cannula.

□□□ **Secure Cannula**   Cap the cannula and secure the cannula in place using the dressing or tape.

I.V. Cannulas and Fluid Composition
Infusion rates for cannulas and composition of i.v. fluids

Gauge	Colour	Diameter	Infusion rate	1 L saline stat
14 G	Orange	2.0 mm	270 mL/min	3 min 45 sec
16 G	Grey	1.7 mm	180 mL/min	5 min 33 sec
18 G	Green	1.2 mm	80 mL/min	12 min 30 sec
20 G	Pink	1.0 mm	54 mL/min	18 min 30 sec
22 G	Blue	0.8 mm	33 mL/min	30 min 20 sec
24 G	Yellow	0.7 mm	13 mL/min	76 min 55 sec

Fluids	Na^-	K^+	Cl^-	Ca^{2+}	HCO_3^-	Osmol	pH
0.9% N. saline	154	0	154	0	0	300	5.5
5% Dextrose	0	0	0	0	0	278	4.1
Hartmann's	131	5	112	4	29	281	6.5
Gelofusine	154	0.4	123	0.4	0	350	7.4

★ Drip

☐☐☐ **Open Clamp**

Attach the end of the giving set to cannula and open the giving set clamp. Ensure that the flow rate is appropriate.

Infusion Rates for Varying Volumes of I.V. fluids			
Infusion time	250 mL	500 mL	1L
4 hrs	62 mL/hr	125 mL/hr	250 mL/hr
6 hrs	41 mL/hr	83 mL/hr	166 mL/hr
8 hrs	31 mL/hr	62 mL/hr	125 mL/hr
12 hrs	20 mL/hr	41 mL/hr	83 mL/hr
24 hrs	10 mL/hr	21 mL/hr	42 mL/hr

☐☐☐ **Extravasation**

Ensure absence of swelling around the point of insertion of the cannula. Ensure the patient is comfortable.

☐☐☐ **Document**

Inform the examiner that you would sign the fluid chart and record the date and time when drip was commenced.

☐☐☐ **Waste**

Dispose of any remaining waste.

EXAMINER'S EVALUATION

0 1 2 3 4 5

☐☐☐☐☐☐ Overall assessment of cannulation and drip

Total mark out of 23

EMERGENCY MEDICINE: **Suturing a Wound**

INSTRUCTIONS: You are a foundation year House Officer in A&E. Mr Smith, a 20-year-old man, has presented to you following an assault. He has a 5 cm laceration to his forearm. You decide he requires three stitches. Demonstrate on the manikin provided what you would do to achieve wound closure.

INTRODUCTION

0 1 2

☐☐☐ **Introduction** — Introduce yourself. Elicit the patient's name, age and occupation. Establish rapport with the patient.

☐☐☐ **Explain** — 'I understand that you have an open wound following an assault. In order to help the healing process and prevent an unsightly scar, the wound needs to be stitched closed using a needle and special thread. You should not feel much pain since we will be using local anaesthetic.'

☐☐☐ **Consent** — Obtain the patient's consent before beginning the procedure.

EQUIPMENT

- Pair of sterile gloves
- 2 × needles (green and blue)
- Sharps box
- Lignocaine 1% local anaesthetic
- Alcohol swabs
- Suture pack
- Antiseptic solution and swabs
- Suture needle holder
- Forceps (one toothed, one normal)

PRE-PROCEDURE

☐☐☐ **Inspect** — Inspect the wound for any debris and dirt. Debris and dirt would require cleaning and debridement before continuing with the procedure.

☐☐☐ **X-ray** — Mention the need for an X-ray if there is potential of a foreign body.

☐☐☐ **Examine** — Examine the distal motor and sensory function. Check for the presence of peripheral pulses.

Position — Position the patient to ensure they are comfortable.

Equipment — Collect and set up the equipment on a trolley.

PROCEDURE
★ Preparation

☐☐☐ **Wash Hands** — Wash your hands before commencing the procedure.

8.2

☐☐☐ **Sterile Field**   Open the suture pack using sterile technique and drop a pair of sterile gloves, syringe, sutures and both needles into the field.

☐☐☐ **Sutures**   Select the correct type and thickness of suture for the wound (3/0).

Suture Size and Type and Time of Removal

Part of Body	Suture and Size	Time of Removal
Scalp	3/0, non-absorbable	7 days
Trunk	3/0, non-absorbable	10 days
Limbs	4/0, non-absorbable	10 days
Hands	5/0, non-absorbable	10 days
Face	6/0, non-absorbable	3–5 days

Wound	Employ appropriate sutures for deep and superficial wounds
Deep	Use absorbable sutures, e.g. Monocryl, Vicryl or Dexon
Superficial	Use monofilament non-absorbable sutures, e.g. nylon (Ethilon) or Prolene

☐☐☐ **Antiseptic**   Pour antiseptic solution into the receptacle and drop swabs into the bowl.

☐☐☐ **Gloves**   Put on the sterile gloves using a sterile technique.

☐☐☐ **Clean Wound**   Cleanse the surrounding skin by using antiseptic soaked swabs held with forceps. Clean the wound from the centre outwards on both sides.

☐☐☐ **Drape**   Cover the wound using a drape, leaving a hole over the region to be stitched.

★ Anaesthetic

☐☐☐ **Lignocaine**   Attach the 21 G (green) needle to the syringe. Seek assistance when drawing up 10 mL of 1% lignocaine. Dispose of the green needle and attach a 25 G (blue) needle.

Inject blebs of lignocaine anaesthetic into the skin encompassing the wound approximately 0.5–1 cm from its edge. Aspirate the needle on insertion to make sure a vessel has not been entered. Dispose of the needles into the sharps bin. Wait 5–10 minutes for the anaesthetic to work and then test by prodding around the wound.

☐☐☐ **Toxicity**   Ask the patient if they have noticed any signs of lignocaine toxicity such as tingling in mouth, a metallic taste, dizziness or light-headedness, ringing in ears or difficulty in focusing the eyes.

Lignocaine Toxicity

While administering the injection ensure that you talk to the patient and ask them how they feel. Any signs of drowsiness or confusion should make you suspect possible toxicity. You should immediately stop any further injections

Mild Toxicity	Light-headedness, dizziness, tinnitus, circumoral numbness, abnormal taste (metallic taste), confusion and drowsiness
Severe Toxicity	Tonic-clonic convulsion leading to progressive loss of consciousness, coma, respiratory depression and respiratory arrest

★ **Sutures**

Hold Needle

Grasp the curved needle with the needle holder properly (using the short, blunt forceps with a straight jaw) by holding the needle two-thirds along its shaft from its tip. Hold the needle holder between the thumb and middle finger using the index finger as a stabiliser.

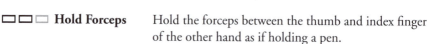

Suturing Technique

Hold the needle 2/3 along its shaft and pass it through the skin about 0.5 cm from the wound edge leaving 3 cm of suture behind. Pass the needle through the opposite skin edge using the forceps to hold the skin and then tie a knot

Needle holder

Hold Forceps

Hold the forceps between the thumb and index finger of the other hand as if holding a pen.

Suturing

Begin at the middle of the wound about 0.5 cm away from its edge. Pick up the skin with toothed forceps and pass the needle perpendicularly through. Pass the needle's full thickness through the skin and pull a length of suture through the needle's hole leaving about 3–5 cm of suture outside the wound.

Pick up the opposite skin edge and pass the needle through. Make sure the stitch is neither too tight nor too loose. Ensure that the needle emerges on the other side exactly opposite the site of insertion at an equal distance from the wound edge.

□□□ **Tie Knot**

Tie a knot by grabbing the needle end with the forceps and wind two loops of the long end of the suture in a clockwise motion around the needle holder. Pull the short end of the stitch through the loops using the mouth of the needle holder. Pull the knot gently down to the skin, apposing the two edges of the wound as you do so. Tighten the knot ensuring that the skin edges are apposed but held without tension.

To complete the knot, repeat the whole process but this time, wind once or twice anticlockwise and pull the end of the stitch through. The suture material may then be cut to complete the stitch. Ensure the knots created are everted and spaced 5–10 mm apart.

□□□ **Halves**

Offer to place the next suture (using the rule of halves) halfway between the present suture and the distal/medial end of the wound. Advise that you will repeat until satisfactory wound closure is achieved.

CLOSING

Dressing

Dress the wound appropriately.

□□□ **Immunisation**

Consider giving tetanus immunisation if the wound is contaminated or the patient had not received a booster within the last 10 years.

Tetanus Prophylaxis

Tetanus Vaccination	Last Dose	Type of Wound	Td	TIG
Uncertain or <3 doses	–	Clean, minor	√	X
	–	Contaminated, other	√	√
Immunised (≥3 doses)	<5 yrs	All types	X	X
	5–10 yrs	Clean, minor	X	X
	5–10 yrs	Contaminated, other	√	X
	>10 yrs	Contaminated, other	√	X

Consider tetanus toxoid vaccine if Td is contraindicated
Abbreviations: Td, tetanus-diphtheria vaccine; TIG, tetanus immunoglobulin

☐☐☐ **Document**	Make sure the details of the suture are documented in the patient's notes, including the strength of the lignocaine anaesthetic.
☐☐☐ **Waste**	Dispose of all sharps into the yellow sharps container. Dispose of gloves and other waste appropriately.
Questions	Thank the patient and ask if they have any questions.
☐☐☐ **Inform**	Inform the patient when the sutures can be removed (between 7 and 10 days).

EXAMINER'S EVALUATION

0 1 2 3 4 5

☐☐☐☐☐☐ Overall assessment for suturing a wound
Total mark out of 33

DIFFERENT SUTURING TECHNIQUES

Vertical Mattress Suture Technique

The vertical mattress suture technique represents a variation of the simple suture. It is especially useful in achieving wound eversion and reducing the tension across the wound. This is achieved by incorporating a larger amount of tissue within the passage of the suture loops. For this reason it is highly recommended for use in areas of the skin where there is a tendency for wound edges to invert, such the back of the neck or other concave surfaces. The vertical mattress suture applies the 'far–far, near–near' method. The first interrupted suture is placed far and deep across both sides of the wound edge. The second stitch is more superficial and closer to the wound edge and it is made in the opposite direction. Subsequently both ends of the threads are tied to form a knot that resides on the side where the suture was initiated.

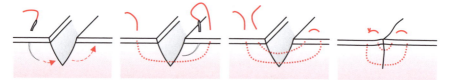

Modified Vertical Mattress Sutures

The modified vertical mattress suture adopts a far–near, near–far system that shares functionality with the pulley suture. The needle is passed into the skin approximately 5 mm from the wound edge before emerging on the contralateral side 2.5 mm from the

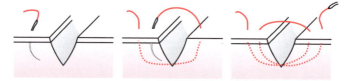

wound border. The suture is then inserted once again on the original side but instead introduced 2.5 mm from the wound edge before exiting once again on the opposite side to complete the loop, 5 mm away from the wound boundary. Once tied, this arrangement generates a pulley effect.

Horizontal Mattress Suture Technique

The horizontal mattress suture technique promotes wound eversion but also spreads the tension along the edge of the wound. The technique permits wound edges to be pulled together over large distances. They are effective in holding skins flaps in place as well as in holding fragile skin together. The horizontal mattress suture is initiated by entering the skin approximately 5 mm away from the wound edge, a small distance further away than normal sutures. The needle should then exit the skin at an equal distance from the wound edge. The needle is then reinserted into the skin on the ipsilateral side of the wound edge approximately 5 mm from the exit point, and passed through the wound to the opposite side, about 5 mm away from the wound edge. A knot is made on the same side as to where the suture began.

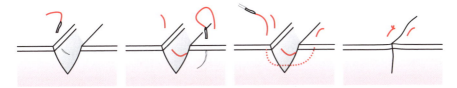

Corner Stitch Technique (Half-buried Horizontal Suture)

The modified or half-buried horizontal mattress suture (or corner stitch) is the best method for closing a flap. Apart from relieving tissue tension, it avoids compromising the blood supply to the tissue tip. It also securely fastens the tip of flaps into their primary positions without the need for a number of smaller sutures to hold both edges of the corner down. The suture is initiated on the side to which the flap is to be attached. It is passed though the bordering skin, across the wound space and through dermis of the flap, tip held up with the forceps. Finally, the suture is guided back into the skin to which the flap is to be attached, where the knot is made.

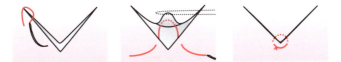

INSTRUCTIONS: A patient has collapsed in outpatients in front of you. Following your assessment, you have decided to stabilise their airway using a laryngeal mask. Demonstrate on the manikin how you would go about doing this.

NOTE: A laryngeal mask is commonly used in anaesthesia and in medical emergencies to secure the airway. It comprises a tube with an inflatable cuff that forms a seal around the laryngeal opening. Insertion requires the patient to be unconscious or have a depressed cough reflex.

PROCEDURE

0 1 2

☐☐☐ **Wash Hands**   Clean your hands with an appropriate disinfectant.

Gloves   Put on non-sterile gloves.

☐☐☐ **Equipment**   Assemble the equipment and choose the appropriate sized laryngeal mask. Sizes range from infant size (1) to adult size (5). A size 4 cuff is appropriate for an average-sized adult.

☐☐☐ **Ventilation**   Ensure that the patient is pre-oxygenated using a bag and mask before attempting the procedure.

EQUIPMENT

- Pair of non-sterile gloves
- Lubrication gel
- LMA of appropriate size
- Bite block
- Giving set
- 50 mL syringe
- Tape or bandage

★ Insertion

☐☐☐ **Deflate**   Deflate the cuff of the mask fully before inserting.

☐☐☐ **Lubricate**   Lubricate the laryngeal mask.

Position   Stand behind the patient and open the airway by head tilt and chin lift.

Stop Ventilate   Ask your colleague to stop ventilating the patient temporarily and count for 30 seconds while you attempt to insert the LMA. If the individual is being resuscitated continue with chest compressions.

8.3

☐☐☐ **Hold**	Hold the tube like a pen and allow your index finger to guide it into the mouth. Ensure the black line on the tube can be seen anteriorly.
☐☐☐ **Insert**	Have the apex of the mask pointing downwards to the tongue. Run the tip of the mask against the hard palate towards the uvula. Allow it to follow the natural bend of the oropharynx. Push the mask downwards until resistance is felt and then stop. Ensure that the procedure is completed within 30 seconds. If you are unable to do so, pre-oxygenate the patient again for 1 minute before reattempting.
☐☐☐ **Alignment**	Position is confirmed when the black line on the tube is in alignment with the nose.
☐☐☐ **Inflate**	Inflate the cuff with adequate volume of air to create a tight seal. Note that the laryngeal tube may slightly project outwards as the mask secures itself into position.

Laryngeal Mask Airway

Select the correctly sized airway before inserting it into the mouth. Hold it like a pen using your index finger to guide it. Run it against the palate until you reach the posterior wall of the pharynx. Inflate the cuff.

✶ **After Insertion**

☐☐☐ **Ventilation**	Attach a bag and mask that is connected to 100% oxygen and ventilate the patient. Watch for chest to rise bilaterally. Auscultate the lungs in the axilla to confirm placement. The absence of breath sounds or chest rise requires the removal of the airway adjunct and its reinsertion.
☐☐☐ **Secure**	Insert a bite block alongside the tube and secure the airway by tying it into place with tape.
Resuscitation	If the patient is being resuscitated ensure the airway is secure before commencing uninterrupted chest compressions. Continue to ventilate the patient at 10 breaths per minute.

✳ Removal

Instructions	*The patients shows signs of life with spontaneous respirations and finds the LMA uncomfortable.*
▭▭▭ **Remove**	Remove the laryngeal mask from the airway with the cuff still inflated. Consider suction of any collecting fluid in the mouth.
▭▭▭ **Oxygen**	Apply a face mask (a non-rebreathable bag) with 100% oxygen.
Waste	Dispose of any remaining waste.

EXAMINER'S EVALUATION

0 1 2 3 4 5
▭ ▭ ▭ ▭ ▭ ▭ Overall assessment of inserting a LMA
Total mark out of 20

EMERGENCY MEDICINE: **Adult Basic Life Support (BLS)**

INSTRUCTIONS: You are leaving a busy medical outpatient clinic when a man suddenly collapses in front of you. No one else is immediately available to help you. Assess the situation and commence resuscitation.

PROCEDURE

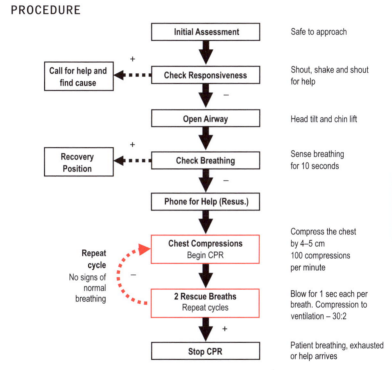

Initial Assessment	Safe to approach
Check Responsiveness → **Call for help and find cause** (+)	Shout, shake and shout for help
Open Airway	Head tilt and chin lift
Check Breathing → **Recovery Position** (+)	Sense breathing for 10 seconds
Phone for Help (Resus.)	
Chest Compressions Begin CPR	Compress the chest by 4–5 cm 100 compressions per minute
2 Rescue Breaths Repeat cycles	Blow for 1 sec each per breath. Compression to ventilation – 30:2
Stop CPR	Patient breathing, exhausted or help arrives

Repeat cycle — No signs of normal breathing

8.4

★ Assessment (*Mnemonic* – SSSS)

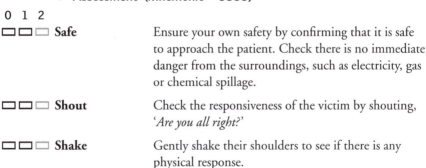

0 1 2

☐☐☐ **Safe**   Ensure your own safety by confirming that it is safe to approach the patient. Check there is no immediate danger from the surroundings, such as electricity, gas or chemical spillage.

☐☐☐ **Shout**   Check the responsiveness of the victim by shouting, '*Are you all right?*'

☐☐☐ **Shake**   Gently shake their shoulders to see if there is any physical response.

295

☐☐☐ **Shout for Help**   If there is no response from the patient, shout for help.

Responsive   If the patient is responsive, leave them in the position you found them ensuring that the surrounding environment poses no danger to them. Establish cause of current state and attempt to obtain assistance. Reassess the patient regularly in case of deterioration.

∗ Airway
☐☐☐ **Open Airway**   If necessary turn the patient onto their back and then open their airway by gently tilting their head back and lifting their chin. If you suspect a cervical spine injury then open the airway by jaw thrust only.

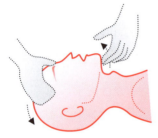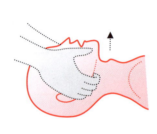

Airway Management

Open the patient's airway by placing your hand on his forehead and tilting his head backwards. Lift his chin by using your fingertips beneath his chin. In a suspected cervical spine injury perform a jaw thrust only

∗ Breathing
☐☐☐ **Sense**   Keeping the airway open, bring your ear to the victim's mouth and sense for signs of breathing. Look for chest movements, listen for breath sounds and feel for breathing against your cheeks for no more than 10 seconds. Simultaneously place two fingers on the carotid to assess the presence of a pulse.

Assessing Breathing

Assess the patient's breathing by bringing your head to the patient's mouth and feeling for a breath against your cheek. Look for chest movements and listen for breath sounds for no more than 10 seconds. If in any doubt treat as if the patient's breathing is abnormal

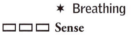

☐☐☐ *Not Breathing*   If the victim is not breathing, ask an individual to call the resuscitation team. If you are alone, leave the side

of the victim and seek assistance by telephoning the emergency number. Dial 2222 or equivalent.

'I am a foundation year House Officer in the medical outpatients department. A person has collapsed in front of me and has no cardiac output. Please call the resuscitation team immediately.'

Agonal Gasps

Agonal gasps are infrequent, noisy breaths and should not be assumed to be evidence of normal breathing. This occurs in the proceeding minutes after a cardiac arrest and should be treated as abnormal breathing.

Breathing

If the victim is breathing, reposition him into the recovery position and check for signs of continued breathing. Send for help or, if alone, seek assistance.

★ Circulation

NOTE: Following the vital few minutes after a cardiac arrest, the circulating blood oxygen concentration levels remain elevated. For this reason, chest compressions are more important than ventilation so that the residual oxygen in the blood is distributed to the vital organs.

☐☐☐ **Compressions**

Start chest compressions immediately. Go down to the level of the patient. Superimpose one hand over the other and interlock your fingers. Place the heel of your hand over the centre of the patient's chest (approximately the middle section of the lower half of the sternum) and apply compressions. Avoid the patient's ribs, upper abdomen or base of the sternum.

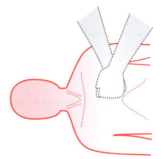

Chest Compressions

Interlock your fingers and place the heel of your hands over the centre of the chest. Avoid the ribs and upper abdomen. Begin chest compressions at 100 per minute and at a rate of 30 per 2 rescue breaths. Depress the chest by 4–5 cm

☐☐☐ *Technique*

Ensure that you are positioned vertically above the victim with your arms straightened and with your shoulders above your wrists. Press down, depressing the chest by a depth of 4–5 cm with the same duration taken for compression and release.

☐☐☐ **Rescue Breaths** After completing 30 compressions, give the patient two effective rescue breaths. Maintain the airway by ensuring that the head is tilted and chin is lifted. Pinch the patient's nose and place your lips around his mouth, forming a good seal. Blow steadily for 1 second making sure each breath causes the chest to rise and fall. If a face mask is made available apply it over the patient's mouth before providing rescue breaths. After providing two rescue breaths, continue with chest compressions.

Unwilling If you are unable or are reluctant to give rescue breaths (e.g. if a face mask is unavailable), continue to give chest compressions only, at the same rate of 100 per minute, stopping only if the patient breathes normally again.

☐☐☐ *Obstruction* If after giving two rescue breaths you fail to see the chest rise, inspect the mouth for any obstructions. Remove any visible obstructions (using finger sweep method) such as dislodged dentures, vomit or foreign bodies. Leave in place any well-fitting dentures.

☐☐☐ **Rate & Ratio** Employ a chest compression to ventilation ratio of 30:2, delivering two effective breaths for every 30 compressions. Maintain compressions at a rate of 100 per minute (just under two compressions per second). If assistance is available alternate chest compressors every 2 minutes to prevent exhaustion. Ensure the duration of the transitions is kept to a minimum.

☐☐☐ **Stop CPR** Continue resuscitating the patient until help arrives, the victim shows signs of life or you feel exhausted.

EXAMINER'S EVALUATION

0 1 2 3 4 5
☐☐☐☐☐☐ Overall assessment of BLS
Total mark out of 23

EMERGENCY MEDICINE: Adult Advanced Life Support (ALS)

INSTRUCTIONS: You are leaving the hospital grounds when suddenly a man in the car park collapses in front of you. Nobody else is available for help. Assess the situation and commence resuscitation.

PROCEDURE

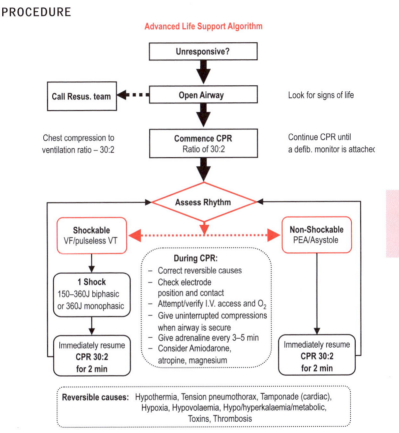

Advanced Life Support Algorithm

Unresponsive?

Call Resus. team ◄···· Open Airway — Look for signs of life

Chest compression to ventilation ratio – 30:2 — Commence CPR Ratio of 30:2 — Continue CPR until a defib. monitor is attached

Assess Rhythm

8.5

Shockable
VF/pulseless VT

Non-Shockable
PEA/Asystole

During CPR:
– Correct reversible causes
– Check electrode position and contact
– Attempt/verify I.V. access and O_2
– Give uninterrupted compressions when airway is secure
– Give adrenaline every 3–5 min
– Consider Amiodarone, atropine, magnesium

1 Shock
150–360J biphasic
or 360J monophasic

Immediately resume
CPR 30:2
for 2 min

Immediately resume
CPR 30:2
for 2 min

Reversible causes: Hypothermia, Tension pneumothorax, Tamponade (cardiac), Hypoxia, Hypovolaemia, Hypo/hyperkalaemia/metabolic, Toxins, Thrombosis

★ Responsiveness

0 1 2

☐☐☐ **Unresponsive**   Ensure that it is safe to approach and there are no immediate dangers. Check the responsiveness by shouting at the patient, '*Are you all right?*' Shake their shoulders to see if there is a physical response. If there is no response, shout for help.

✳ Airway and Breathing

□□□ **Position**

Open the patient's airway by gently tilting their head back and lifting their chin. If you suspect a cervical spine injury then open the airway by jaw thrust only.

□□□ **Sense Breath**

Bring your ear to the victim's mouth. Look for chest movements, listen for breath sounds and feel for breathing for no more than 10 seconds. Simultaneously place two fingers on the carotid to assess the presence of a pulse.

□□□ *Not Breathing*

If the victim is not breathing normally, ask an individual to call the resuscitation team. If you are alone, leave the side of the victim and seek assistance by telephoning the emergency number. Dial 2222 or equivalent.

✳ Circulation

□□□ **Compressions**

Start chest compressions immediately. Superimpose one hand over the other and interlock your fingers. Place the heel of your hand over the centre of the patient's chest. Press down, depressing the chest by a depth of 4–5 cm.

□□□ **Rescue Breaths**

After completing 30 compressions, give the patient two effective rescue breaths. Blow steadily for 1 second making sure each breath causes the chest to rise and fall. If a face mask is made available apply it over the patient's mouth before providing rescue breaths. After providing two rescue breaths, continue with chest compressions.

□□□ **Rate and Ratio**

Employ a chest compression to ventilation ratio of 30:2. Maintain compressions at a rate of 100 per minute.

ASSESS RHYTHM

Instructions

The resuscitation team arrives with a defibrillator. Since you were the first on the scene you take charge of the team.

□□□ **Defibrillator**

Attach the salmon pink pads to the correct location on the patient. Place the pads on the right lung apex just below the right clavicle and over the cardiac apex. Switch on the monitor and connect the monitor leads to the pads. Ensure you are reading lead II.

□□□ **Interpret**   Correctly interpret the rhythm strip and identify
whether it is a shockable (VF/pulseless VT) or non-
shockable (PEA/asystole) rhythm. If there is any
uncertainty or ambiguity as to whether the rhythm is
asystole or fine VF, treat as a non-shockable rhythm
and do not administer a shock.

✳ Shockable (VT/pulseless VT)

Shockable   Shockable rhythms include ventricular fibrillations
(VF) and pulseless ventricular tachycardias (pulseless
VT). They should be defibrillated.

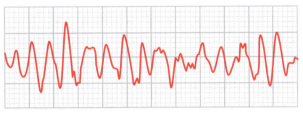

Ventricular fibrillation (VF)

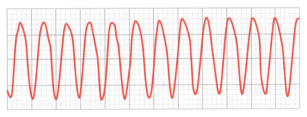

Pulseless ventricular tachycardia (VT)

□□□ **First shock**   Choose an appropriate charge for defibrillation
(150–200 J biphasic or 360 J monophasic). Take
shock pads and place them onto the chest. Warn all
around you to stand back, remove the oxygen and
perform a visual check of the surrounding trolley

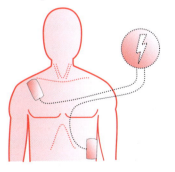

Defibrillation

Place one electrode pad over the
cardiac apex with the other over the
right lung apex just below the clavicle.
Attach it to the defibrillator. Identify
the shockable rhythm (VF, pulseless
VT) before performing a visual sweep,
charging and delivering 1 shock.
Perform CPR for 2 min before
reassessing the rhythm strip for
shockable rhythms

area. Shout: '*Top clear, middle clear, bottom clear, self clear. Oxygen away. Charging!*' Charge pads and dispense.

☐☐☐ **CPR**

After one shock, immediately resume compressions at a rate of 30 chest compressions per two effective breaths. However, give uninterrupted chest compressions when the airway is secure. Do not assess the rhythm strip or assess carotid pulse until 2 complete minutes of CPR have elapsed.

☐☐☐ **Second Shock**

Recheck the rhythm strip and if the shockable rhythm persists give a second shock of equal amplitude (150–200 J biphasic or 360 J monophasic). Continue CPR for 2 minutes and then recheck monitor for rhythm change.

☐☐☐ **Third Shock**

Inspect the rhythm and note if VF or VT persists before giving adrenaline 1 mg i.v. Administer a third shock of equal amplitude and restart CPR for 2 minutes. Recheck the monitor for rhythm change.

☐☐☐ **Fourth Shock**

Re-examine the monitor and note if VF or VT persists. Give a bolus amiodarone 300 mg i.v. before dispensing a fourth shock of equal amplitude. Resume CPR for 2 minutes. Recheck monitor for rhythm change.

☐☐☐ **Repeat**

Repeat shock cycles as stated above for persistent VF or VT. Administer adrenaline 1 mg i.v. on alternate cycles (every 3–5 minutes) immediately before shocks. Consider a further dose of 150 mg of amiodarone for recurrent or refractory VF/VT, followed by an infusion of 900 mg over 24 hours. Only consider lidocaine (1 mg per kg) if amiodarone is not available.

Praecordial Thump in Advance Life Support

A praecordial thump is a medical procedure used in a witnessed and confirmed cardiac arrest when a defibrillator is not immediately available. It should be considered only by a trained provider and attempted only once.

Form a tight clenched fist with one hand and apply a sharp impact blow to the lower sternum from a distance of 20 cm. Make contact with only the ulnar edge of your fist retracting immediately after dispensing to create an impulse like stimulus.

Praecordial thumps are most successful at converting ventricular tachycardia (VT) to a sinus rhythm. It is believed to produce an electrical depolarisation of 2–5 J

Rhythm Change If there is a change in the rhythm strip to an organised electrical activity at the end of 2 minutes of CPR when the monitor is reassessed, check for a viable pulse. An absent pulse will require the application of the non-shockable algorithm, while if the pulse is present, post-resuscitation care should be commenced.

□ □ □ **Reversible** During the course of CPR the healthcare professional should consider reversible causes:

Reversible Causes of a Cardiac Arrest

Reversible Cause	Management
Hypoxia	Signs of cyanosis, low oxygen levels on ABG. Give 100% oxygen
Hypovolaemia	Signs of active bleeding, pale skin, dehydrated. Give rapid i.v. fluids, group O negative blood and consider urgent surgery
$\uparrow\downarrow$ K$^+$, $\downarrow$ Ca^{2+}, acidaemia	Take bloods, ABG and ECGs. Consider calcium (10 mL 10% calcium chloride) in hyperkalaemia, hypocalcaemia
Hypothermia	History of drowning. Patient feels cold with low core temperature. Give warm fluids, remove wet clothing and consider blanket
Tension pneumothorax	History of penetrating injury, signs of absent breath sounds and tracheal deviation. Needle thoracocentesis before chest drain
Tamponade	History of chest trauma and signs of distended neck veins ($\uparrow$ JVP) and low BP. Needle pericardiocentesis
Toxic substances	History of drug abuse or suicide. Consider antidotes for specific agents. Treatment is supportive
Thromboembolism	History of PE/DVT, leg stockings, warfarin. Consider thrombolysis

✷ Non-Shockable (PEA/Asystole)

Non-shockable Non-shockable rhythms include pulseless electrical activity (PEA) and asystole. They should not be defibrillated.

PEA Identify pulseless electrical activity (PEA) on the cardiac monitor.

Pulseless Electrical Activity (PEA)

Pulseless electrical activity (PEA) is a clinical condition that is regarded as the loss of a palpable pulse in the presence of recordable cardiac electrical activity. It was previously known as electromechanical dissociation or non-perfusing rhythm. Unless the underlying condition is identified and corrected, the patient is unlikely to be resuscitated. The most common cause is hypovolaemia

☐☐☐ **CPR**

Resume compressions at a rate of 30 chest compressions per two effective breaths. However, give uninterrupted chest compressions when airway is secure. Reassess the rhythm strip after 2 minutes of CPR has elapsed.

☐☐☐ **Adrenaline**

Give adrenaline 1 mg i.v. as soon as i.v. access is obtained.

Recheck

Assess the rhythm strip and check for an ECG change from a non-shockable rhythm.

No ECG Change

If there are no ECG changes noted, recommence CPR for 2 minutes giving adrenaline 1 mg i.v. on alternative cycles (every 3–5 minutes).

ECG Changes

If the ECG changes to organised electrical activity, check if a pulse is palpable. If a pulse is palpable, start post-resuscitation care and consider transferring to ITU. If a pulse is not palpable, treat as a PEA and continue CPR for 2 minutes rechecking the rhythm strip. Give adrenaline, as before, only on alternative cycles.

Asystole

Identify asystole on the cardiac monitor. Consider increasing the gain to rule out low voltage VF.

Asystole (absence of cardiac electrical activity)

☐☐☐ **CPR**

Resume compressions at a rate of 30 chest compressions per two effective breaths. However, give uninterrupted chest compressions when airway is secure.

	Leads	Ensure that the chest leads are attached correctly to the patient and that incorrect placement is not causing the perceived asystole.
☐☐☐	**Adrenaline**	Give adrenaline 1 mg i.v. as soon as i.v. access is obtained.
☐☐☐	**Atropine**	Provide atropine 3 mg i.v. once only.
	Recheck	Reassess the rhythm strip after 2 minutes of CPR has elapsed. Check for an ECG change from a non-shockable rhythm.

EXAMINER'S EVALUATION

0 1 2 3 4 5

☐☐☐☐☐☐ Overall assessment of advanced life support

Total mark out of 30

PROCEDURE

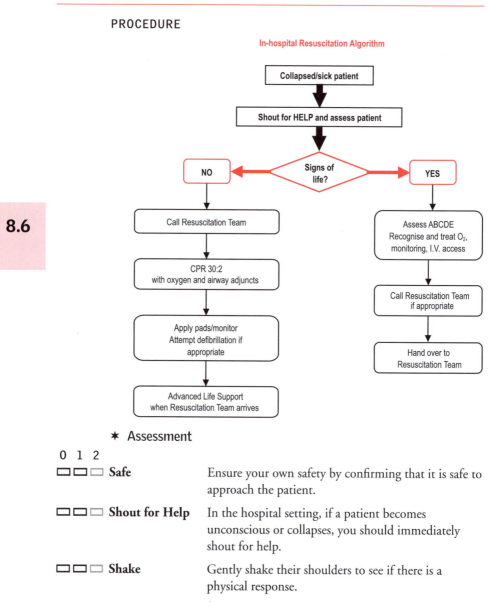

8.6

✱ Assessment

0 1 2

☐☐☐ **Safe**   Ensure your own safety by confirming that it is safe to approach the patient.

☐☐☐ **Shout for Help**   In the hospital setting, if a patient becomes unconscious or collapses, you should immediately shout for help.

☐☐☐ **Shake**   Gently shake their shoulders to see if there is a physical response.

□□□ **Shout**   Check the responsiveness of the victim by shouting, '*Are you all right?*' If the patient is unresponsive, open patient's airway and assess breathing.

Responsive   If the patient is responsive, obtain urgent medical assessment to review the patient. Assess the patient using the ABCDE approach and attempt to establish the cause of the current state. Give oxygen, attach monitor leads and acquire i.v. access.

✳ Airway

□□□ **Open Airway**   If you have not already done so, shout for help. If necessary turn the patient onto their back and then open their airway by gently tilting their head back and lifting their chin. If you suspect a cervical spine injury then open the airway by jaw thrust only. If a life-threatening obstruction persists consider tentative head tilt. A patent airway is more important than a potential cervical spine injury.

□□□ **Obstruction**   Inspect the mouth and remove any visible obstructions (by suction or forceps if available) such as dislodged dentures, vomit or foreign bodies, but leave in place any well-fitting dentures.

✳ Breathing and Circulation

□□□ **Sense**   Keeping the airway open, bring your ear to the patient's mouth and sense for signs of breathing. Look for chest movements, listen for breath sounds and feel for breathing against your cheek for no more than 10 seconds. Simultaneously assess the presence of a carotid pulse.

□□□ *No Signs of Life*   If the patient lacks signs of life or does not have a pulse, ask an individual to call the resuscitation team (dial 2222 or equivalent) and collect essential resuscitation equipment. If you are alone you may have to leave the side of the patient to perform this. Prepare to perform urgent CPR.

'I am a foundation year House Officer on AMU. A person has collapsed in front of me and has no cardiac output. Please call the resuscitation team immediately.'

Signs of Life   If the patient shows signs of life or has a palpable pulse obtain urgent medical assessment. Assess the patient using the ABCDE approach and attempt to establish the cause of the current state. Give oxygen, attach monitor leads and acquire i.v. access.

Resp. Arrest   If the patient has a palpable pulse but is not breathing (respiratory arrest), ventilate the patient's lungs at 10 ventilations per minute and check the pulse every minute.

✴ Cardiopulmonary Resuscitation (CPR)

Chest Thump   Consider giving a single praecordial thump if a VT or VF cardiac arrest is confirmed but a defibrillator is not immediately available.

⬜⬜⬜ **Compressions**   Start chest compressions immediately. Give 30 chest compressions before giving two effective breaths. Superimpose one hand over the other and interlock your fingers. Place the heel of your hand over the lower half of the sternum and apply compressions depressing the chest by 4–5 cm. Compress at a rate of 100 compressions per minute.

Breaths   If a pocket mask or other ventilation equipment is unavailable commence mouth to mouth resuscitation. If you are unable or unwilling to perform mouth to mouth contact, continue uninterrupted chest compressions until the necessary equipment is available.

Instructions   *A nurse arrives on the scene and provides you with airway adjuncts as well as with a bag valve mask.*

Ventilate   In the hospital setting a number of airway adjuncts are readily available to maintain the airway. Consider a pocket mask or bag and mask to ventilate the lung and oropharyngeal, nasopharyngeal or laryngeal mask airway (LMA) to maintain the airway. Use an inspiratory time of 1 second when delivering oxygen and ensure that the chest elevates as in normal breathing. Add supplemental oxygen as soon as possible. Tracheal intubation is the gold standard but should be attempted only by a trained and skilled individual.

⬜⬜⬜ *Oropharyngeal*   Consider an oropharyngeal airway if the patient remains semiconscious or unconscious. A patient who is not unconscious will not tolerate the device due to presence of his gag reflex.

Choose an appropriate-sized Guedel airway by selecting one that is equivalent in length to the distance from the corner of the mouth to the angle of the mandible. Insert the airway upside down into the patient's mouth. Once contact is made with the back of the throat, rotate the airway through 180°, assuring that the tongue is secured. To remove the device, pull the airway out without rotating it, following the curvature of the tongue.

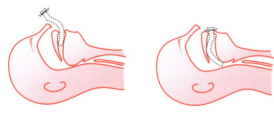

Oropharyngeal Airway

Select the correctly sized airway by measuring from the corner of the mouth to the angle of the jaw. Insert it upside down and then rotate it 180 degrees in order to secure the tongue in place

Nasopharyngeal

A nasopharyngeal airway is tolerated better in an alert patient. It is contraindicated in patients with severe head or facial injuries, or a basal skull fracture (Battle's sign) due to the possibility of introducing the device into brain tissue.

Establish the correct size of airway by measuring the device on the patient. The airway adjunct should reach from the patient's nostril to their earlobe or the angle of the jaw. Pass the device into the nasal passage and along the floor of the nose with the tip pointing downwards until the flange end or safety pin rests against the nostril.

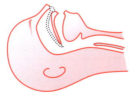

Nasopharyngeal Airway

Measure the nasopharyngeal airway against the patient from the nostril to the earlobe. Insert the device with the tip pointing downwards until the safety pin lies against the nostril

Laryngeal Mask

Consider a laryngeal mask if the patient is unconscious and has a depressed gag reflex.

Hold the mask like a pen. Run the tip of the mask against the palate until you reach the posterior wall of the pharynx and meet resistance. Inflate the cuff and check position. Auscultate the chest and check for chest rise.

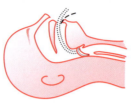

Laryngeal Mask Airway

Select the correctly sized airway. Insert the mask with the tip running against the palate until resistance is noted. Inflate the cuff and note the tube lift out slightly. Confirm position by auscultation

☐☐☐ *Pocket Mask*

Establish a good seal with the patient's mouth by making a C shape on the pocket face mask with your thumbs and index fingers. Use the rest of your fingers to clutch the patient's jaw.

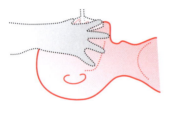

Portable Face Mask

The face mask contains a one-way valve and filter that permits gases passing through but prevents contaminants returning. Make a good seal with the patient's mouth by using your thumbs and index fingers to form a 'C' shape on the mask. Use your remaining fingers to clutch onto the patient's jaw

☐☐☐ *Bag and Mask*

Attach the valve end of the mask to an oxygen supply, if one is available, before adjusting the flow to 15 L/minute to deliver 100% oxygen. Hold the mask over the patient's face and make a tight seal by securing it over their nose and jaw with your thumb and fingers. Use your free hand to compress the bag while looking for a rise in their chest. If you have assistance, hold the mask with both your hands and get your assistant to squeeze the bag.

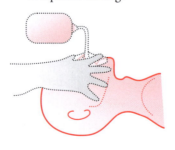

Bag Valve Mask (Ambu bag)

Hold the mask over the patient's face making a tight seal with your thumb and fingers. Use your other hand to compress the bag. If you have help, get them to squeeze the bag while you form a tight seal with your hands

□□□ **Airway Secure**   Give uninterrupted chest compressions at a rate of 100 per minute when the airway is secure. Ventilate the patient at a rate of 10 breaths per minute (or every 6 seconds).

Instructions   *The resuscitation team arrives with a defibrillator. Since you were the first on the scene you take charge of the team.*

□□□ **Defibrillator**   Attach the salmon pink pads to the correct location on the patient. Place the pads on the right lung apex just below the right clavicle and over the cardiac apex. Switch on monitor and connect the monitor leads to the pads. Ensure you are reading lead II. If you are using an automated external defibrillator (AED), follow the voice commands, otherwise implement the advanced life support (ALS) algorithm.

□□□ **Rhythm**   Interpret the rhythm strip and determine if it is a shockable or non-shockable rhythm. If a shockable rhythm is noted administer a single shock (150–200 J biphasic or 360 J monophasic).

□□□ **Compressions**   Restart compressions immediately. Do not assess the rhythm strip or assess carotid pulse until 2 complete minutes of CPR have elapsed. Rotate with the person performing chest compressions every 2 minutes to prevent exhaustion.

EXAMINER'S EVALUATION

0 1 2 3 4 5

□□□□□□   Overall assessment of in-hospital resuscitation
Total mark out of 26

INSTRUCTIONS: You are in the hospital canteen having your lunch when you hear a person struggling to breathe and pointing to his throat. Assess the situation and manage appropriately.

NOTE: Choking is the mechanical obstruction of the airway by a foreign body which prevents the victim from breathing. It can cause mild or severe airway obstruction. Partial obstruction can cause inadequate flow of air into the lungs, while severe airway obstruction results in asphyxiation causing hypoxia, unconsciousness or cardiopulmonary arrest. Choking must not be confused with a myocardial infarction, faint, collapse or seizure.

PROCEDURE

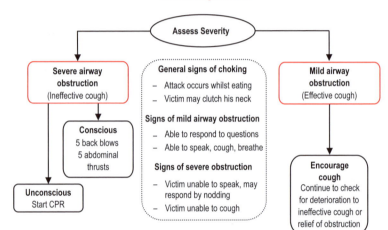

8.7

★ Assessment

0 1 2
☐ ☐ ☐ **Severity**

Ascertain the severity of the choke. Ask the patient: '*Are you choking?*' Differentiate between mild and severe forms of obstruction. If the victim is able to answer coherently, this is suggestive of mild airway obstruction. Inability to respond or ineffective coughing indicates severe obstruction.

Signs and Symptoms of Choking

General signs	Attacks mostly occur when the patient eats
	The victim desperately grabs at their throat
Mild obstruction	Patient is able to speak and respond replying 'yes'
	Signs of cough and breathing
Severe obstruction	Patient is unable to speak but may respond by nodding

Signs include an inability to breathe, wheezy
breath sounds, attempts to cough are silent,
cyanosis, unconsciousness

✳ **Mild Airway Obstruction**

☐☐☐ **Cough**

Encourage the victim to continue coughing in the presence of mild airway obstruction. Monitor for signs of relief or deterioration.

✳ **Severe Airway Obstruction**

☐☐☐ **Position**

Note signs of severe airway obstruction. Stand obliquely behind the patient. Have the patient leaning forward with one of your hands supporting his chest.

☐☐☐ **Back Blows**

Administer five sharp back slaps to the patient between the shoulder blades striking with the heel of your hand. With each blow observe if the offending article has been dislodged and coughed out. Attempt to relieve the obstruction with each slap rather than giving all five.

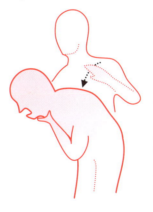

Back Blows

A blow to the back creates a percussion impulse that generates pressure beneath the blockage dislodging the foreign body. With the victim leaning forwards, the offending object is encouraged to exit through the mouth rather than to descend further down the airway and worsen the obstruction. The physical vibration of the back slap alone can cause movement of the obstructing object and permit clearance of the airway

☐☐☐ **Abdo. Thrusts**

If the offending object fails to dislodge and clear the airway after five back blows, attempt five abdominal thrusts. Stand directly behind the patient and wrap your arms around his upper abdomen. Lean the patient forwards to enable any dislodged articles to escape through their mouth. Form a fist with one hand and place it in the epigastric area (between the umbilicus and lower edge of sternum). Put your other hand over the fist and pull sharply inwards and upwards. Give up to five abdominal thrusts.

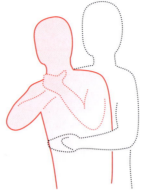

Abdominal thrust (Heimlich manoeuvre)

An abdominal thrust involves exerting a pressure at the bottom of the diaphragm. This increases the intrathoracic pressure creating effective energy to expel the foreign body through the mouth. This manoeuvre can cause injury including fracture of the xyphoid process or ribs. Patients should be assessed by a doctor for injury

☐☐☐ **Repeat Cycle**   If the airway fails to clear with five abdominal thrusts, repeat the cycle and administer five back blows with five abdominal thrusts.

☐☐☐ **Unconscious**   If the patient deteriorates and becomes unconscious, immediately call for help (dial 2222 or equivalent). Begin CPR with chest compressions without delay even in the presence of a palpable carotid pulse.

☐☐☐ **Recovery**   If the patient recovers ask for an urgent medical review to assess if the respiratory tract is clear of any obstructions and if the patient has sustained any injury from abdominal thrusts. Persistent coughing, difficulty swallowing and a sensation of an obstruction at a particular level should warrant further investigation.

EXAMINER'S EVALUATION

0   1   2   3   4   5
☐☐☐☐☐☐   Overall assessment of managing choking
Total mark out of 15

INSTRUCTIONS: You are a foundation year House Officer in casualty. Mr Hamond is a 29-year-old motorcyclist who has been brought in after a road-traffic accident. Manage the patient, explaining your steps to the examiner as you go along.

PRIMARY SURVEY

0 1 2

☐ ☐ ☐ **Emergency**

Declare your intention to follow an ABC approach and state that this is an acute emergency.

<hr>

Systematic Approach to Primary Survey

Mnemonic: 'ABCDE': **A**irway, **B**reathing, **C**irculation, **D**isability, **E**xposure

<hr>

✶ **Airway**

☐ ☐ ☐ **Patency**

Ascertain if the airway is patent, obstructed or partially obstructed (snoring, gurgling, stridor). Determine whether the airway needs to be secured.

Responsive

Introduce yourself to the patient and establish his identity. Enquire as to whether he knows where he is. Verbal communication is always a good sign and confirms the airway is patent with adequate breathing and circulation taking place.

Unresponsive

Failure to respond may suggest reduced levels of consciousness and may require action to maintain and secure the airway. Follow the BLS guidelines, check and remove any obstructions (blood, vomit or foreign bodies), perform a jaw thrust and chin lift manoeuvre (in the absence of a spinal injury) and consider artificial airways (oropharyngeal, nasopharyngeal, endotracheal tube).

Look, feel and listen for signs of breathing. Absence of breathing may suggest a foreign body obstruction or apnoea. Partial obstructions present with snoring, drooling, gurgling, hoarseness of voice and stridor.

☐ ☐ ☐ **C-Spine**

Consider the possibility of a cervical spine injury (c-spine). Immobilise the neck by placing sandbags either side of his head and taping across his forehead or by using a well-fitting hard collar. Determine the collar size by measuring the vertical distance between the top of the shoulder (trapezius) and the tip of the

8.8

315

chin, when the head is in the desired alignment, using your finger width (average: three or four finger-widths wide).

Suspicion of Cervical Spine Injury

Cervical spine immobilisation is vital in patients with suspected cervical spine injuries and involves applying a single-piece, rigid cervical collar with three-point fixation to the patient's neck. Cervical spine immobilisation should be left in place until significant trauma to the spine can be excluded clinically (with a neurological examination) or radiologically (AP, lateral, odontoid views)

Indications for cervical spine immobilisation
- Unresponsive/unconscious patient
- History of multiple trauma (polytrauma)
- History of neck trauma (or mechanism)
- Unexplained neck pain or tenderness to C-spine
- Poor range of movements
- Neurological deficit (pain, paraesthesia)

'Mr Hamond is alert, conscious and replying to my questions. He states that he was involved in a motorcycle accident and collided with a moving vehicle. I am not immediately concerned about his airway at this moment in time but want to immobilise his neck with a rigid collar.'

★ Breathing

☐☐☐ **Oxygen**

Attach a pulse oximeter and determine the patient's oxygen saturation. Administer high flow oxygen if the oxygen saturation is less than 95%.

☐☐☐ **Chest**

Observe his chest movements and look for any evidence of chest injuries. Determine the respiratory rate (fast, slow – respiratory arrest, narcotics). Examine the chest checking for tracheal shift and displaced apex beat, reduced chest expansion, hyper-resonance or dullness to percussion and unequal or abnormal breaths sounds on auscultation. Exclude a tension pneumothorax. Check for any paradoxical chest movements (flail chest).

☐☐☐ **ABG**

Ask for an ABG and interpret the result.

★ Circulation

☐☐☐ **Injury**

Look for signs of external haemorrhage. Control any bleeding by direct pressure.

☐☐☐ **Examine**

Observe skin colour, temperature and capillary refill. Feel the pulse, assess peripheral pulses and check JVP.

Ask the examiner for the blood pressure. Auscultate the heart for heart sounds. Observe for signs of shock and exclude a cardiac tamponade (low BP, raised JVP, absent HS).

☐☐☐ **ECG** Attach an ECG monitor and interpret the waveform.

☐☐☐ **I.V. Access** Establish venous access by inserting two large i.v. cannulas (orange or grey coloured).

☐☐☐ **Bloods** Group and cross-match 10 units of blood. Take 20 mL of blood and check full blood count, coagulation profile, urea and electrolytes, amylase, liver function test, glucose and toxicology screen.

☐☐☐ **Fluid Resus.** Commence fluid resuscitation, normal saline and colloid. Consider group O negative blood in cases of severe haemorrhage.

★ **Disability**

☐☐☐ **AVPU** Assess the patient's level of consciousness using **AVPU** (**A**lert, responds to **V**ocal stimuli, responds to **P**ain, **U**nresponsive) or the Glasgow coma score.

Glasgow Coma Score (GCS) to Assess Consciousness

The Glasgow coma score is a sensitive tool to assess the level of consciousness of a patient. Three types of responses are assessed with an overall score of 15. The minimum GCS score is three, a comatosed patient scores eight or less and a normal responsive person scores 15.

Best motor response	Score	Best verbal response	Score
Obeys commands	6	Orientated	5
Localises pain	5	Confused	4
Withdraws from pain	4	Inappropriate words	3
Abnormal flexion	3	Incomprehensible speech	2
Extension to pain	2	None	1
No response	1		

Eye opening	Score
Opens spontaneously	4
Opens to speech	3
Opens to pain	2
No response	1

☐☐☐ **Pupils** Check pupil size, equality of pupils and pupillary reaction to light and accommodation (constricted, unresponsive pupils – opioids, unilateral dilated pupil – brain disease).

□□□ **Motor**   Ask patient to wiggle their fingers and toes. Note any abnormal postures or limb movements.

Importance of Glucose in Primary Survey
Mnemonic: 'DEFG ': Don't Ever Forget Glucose

★ Exposure

□□□ **Clothes**   Expose the whole body for examination. Recheck the body for signs of missed injuries or sources of haemorrhages. Remove any wet clothes and consider warm intravenous fluids in hypothermia.

SECONDARY SURVEY

□□□ **History**   Take an **AMPLE** history. Ask about: **A**llergies, **M**edications (anticoagulants, insulin, cardiovascular medications), **P**ast medical history, **L**ast food and drink, **E**vents/**E**nvironment surrounding the injury

□□□ **Examine**   State that you would like to perform a head to toe examination. Mention that you will need assistance to examine the back as the patient will have to be log-rolled. Examine the thoraco-lumbar spine and listen to the lung fields. Perform a PR examination to assess anal tone.

Monitor   State that you would like to monitor the heart with a cardiac monitor, blood pressure, oxygen saturation and core temperature.

□□□ **Catheter**   State you would insert a urinary catheter after excluding a high riding prostate by a digital rectal examination.

□□□ **NG Tube**   State you would consider using an NG tube (if there is vomiting, the patient is unconscious or if there is no gag reflex).

□□□ **Investigations**   State you would order X-rays of the lateral cervical spine, chest and pelvis.

□□□ **Seniors**   State that you would request a senior review.

EXAMINER'S EVALUATION

0 1 2 3 4 5
□□□□□□ Overall assessment of motorcycle accident
Total mark out of 33

Abdominal Aortic Aneurysm

You are a foundation year House Officer in casualty. Mr Benard is a 75-year-old man with known atherosclerotic heart disease. He is complaining of a sudden onset of tearing intra-abdominal pain radiating to the back. Manage the patient, explaining your steps to the examiner as you go along.

ABC APPROACH

0 1 2

☐ ☐ ☐ **Emergency** | Declare your intention to follow an ABC approach and state that this is an acute emergency. State your intention to call for help.

✶ Airway

☐ ☐ ☐ **Patency** | Ascertain if the airway is patent, obstructed or partially obstructed. Determine whether the airway needs to be secured.

Responsive | Introduce yourself to the patient and establish his identity. Enquire as to whether he knows where he is. Verbal communication is always a good sign and confirms the airway is patient with adequate breathing and circulation taking place.

8.9

'Mr Benard is alert, conscious and replying to my questions. He states that he has a history of atherosclerotic heart disease and suddenly experienced a bout of severe abdominal pain that radiates to the back. I suspect he has a ruptured aortic aneurysm. I am not immediately concerned about his airway at this moment in time but advised him to keep his neck and head as still as possible.'

✶ Breathing

☐ ☐ ☐ **Oxygen** | Attach a pulse oximeter and determine the patient's oxygen saturation. Administer high flow oxygen if oxygen saturation is less than 95%.

☐ ☐ ☐ **Chest** | Observe chest movements and look for any evidence of chest injuries. Determine the respiratory rate. Examine the chest checking for tracheal shift and displaced apex beat, reduced chest expansion, hyper-resonance or dullness to percussion and unequal or abnormal breath sounds on auscultation.

☐☐☐ **ABG**   Request an ABG and interpret the result.

✳ Circulation

☐☐☐ **Injury**   Look for signs of external haemorrhage. Control any
                               bleeding by direct pressure.

☐☐☐ **Examine**   Observe skin colour (pallor), temperature (coolness)
                               and capillary refill (>2 seconds). Feel the pulse
                               (tachycardia), assess peripheral pulses (absent) and
                               check JVP. Ask examiner for the blood pressure.
                               Auscultate the heart for heart sounds. Observe for
                               signs of shock.

Signs of Hypovolaemic/haemorrhagic Shock

Hypovolaemic shock can be caused by external blood loss (laceration),
internal blood loss (pelvic fracture or leaking AAA) or through severe
dehydration (poor fluid intake, fluid loss – diarrhoea, sweating, third
space loss – pancreatitis)
- Tachycardia
- Low blood pressure
- Delayed capillary refill time (>2 sec)
- Altered conscious levels
- Pale, cool skin and extremities
- Poor urine output

                               Examine the abdomen for tenderness, expansile
                               palpable mass and signs of peritoneal irritation.

☐☐☐ **Seniors**   State that this is a surgical emergency and you
                               suspect a leaking abdominal aortic aneurysm. Inform
                               theatres and fast bleep a senior vascular surgeon and
                               anaesthetist urgently.

☐☐☐ **I.V. Access**   Establish venous access by inserting two large i.v.
                               cannulas (orange or grey coloured).

☐☐☐ **Bloods**   Group and cross-match eight units of blood.
                               Take 20 mL of blood and check full blood count,
                               coagulation profile, urea and electrolytes, amylase,
                               liver function test and glucose.

☐☐☐ **Fluid Resus.**   Commence fast fluid infusion (Gelofusine 500 mL
                               stat) while monitoring the patient's blood pressure.
                               Lay the patient flat and elevate his legs if BP
                               <100 mmHg (if C-spine injury is not suspected). Aim
                               for systolic BP between 90–100 mmHg. If clinical
                               signs of severe shock are present give group O Rh-ve
                               blood as soon as possible.

Classification of Haemorrhagic Shock
Mnemonic: Blood loss based on tennis scores: 15, 30, 40, 45

Classification	I	II	III	IV
Blood loss (%)	<15	15–30	30–40	>45
Blood loss (mL)	750	750–1500	1500–2000	>2000
Systolic BP	No change	Normal	Reduced	Very low
Pulse (bpm)	Elevated	100–120	>120	>140
Capillary refill (sec)	<2	slow >2	slow >2	Undetectable
Urine output	>30	20–30	10–20	0–10
Consciousness	Alert	Anxious	Drowsy	Very drowsy

☐☐☐ **Theatre** Take patient immediately to the theatre.

☐☐☐ **Monitor** Monitor the patient with an ECG and pulse oximeter.

☐☐☐ **Catheterise** Perform bladder catheterisation and ensure fluid balance is closely monitored.

Antibiotics Administer prophylactic antibiotics prior to surgery.

EXAMINER'S EVALUATION

0 1 2 3 4 5
☐☐☐☐☐☐ Overall assessment of AAA
Total mark out of 23

EMERGENCY MEDICINE: **Severe Asthma**

INSTRUCTIONS: You are a foundation year House Officer in casualty. Mr McScholes is a 34-year-old man who is a known asthmatic and has been brought in with sudden onset of breathlessness. He is unable to complete his sentences. Manage the patient, explaining your steps to the examiner as you go along.

ABC APPROACH

0 1 2

□ □ □ **Emergency** — Declare your intention to follow an ABC approach and state that this is an acute emergency.

★ Airway

□ □ □ **Patency** — Ascertain if the airway is patent, obstructed or partially obstructed. Determine whether the airway needs to be secured.

Responsive — Introduce yourself to the patient, sit the patient upright and establish his identity. Enquire whether he knows where he is. Verbal communication is always a good sign and confirms the airway is patent with adequate breathing and circulation taking place. Note that the patient may not be able to complete his sentences.

'Mr McScholes is alert, conscious and replying to my questions despite having difficulty in completing his sentences. He states that he has a history of asthma and suddenly experienced a bout of severe shortness of breath. I suspect he is suffering from an asthma attack. I am not immediately concerned about his airway at this moment in time but I advised him to stay still as possible.'

History — Take a more focused history from the patient about his asthma. Ask about the current episode, previous episodes, treatment, best peak flow, previous hospital or ITU admissions and known precipitants.

★ Breathing

□ □ □ **Oximeter** — Attach a pulse oximeter and determine the patient's oxygen saturation.

□ □ □ **ABG** — Ask for an ABG and interpret the result. A low PaO_2 and low $PaCO_2$ suggest hyperventilation. Normal or elevating $PaCO_2$ suggests respiratory muscle fatigue and possible imminent respiratory failure.

8.10

☐☐☐ **Oxygen**   Start the patient on 100% oxygen using a non-rebreather mask.

☐☐☐ **Rate**   Measure the heart rate (tachycardia, bradycardia) and respiratory rate (tachypnoea or feeble respiratory effort).

☐☐☐ **Peak Flow**   State that you would like to measure the patient's peak flow. Greater than 75% of predicted PEFR indicates mild asthma, less than 75% is suggestive of a moderate, severe or life threatening asthma.

☐☐☐ **Examine**   Observe chest movements (accessory muscles) and look for any evidence of chest injuries (fractured ribs). Examine the chest, checking for tracheal deviation, reduced chest expansion, hyper-resonance or dullness to percussion, abnormal or absent breath sounds (life threatening if silent) and added sounds (wheezes) on auscultation.

✷ Circulation

☐☐☐ **Examine**   Observe skin colour (pallor, cyanosis), temperature and capillary refill. Feel the pulse (tachycardia, bradycardia), assess peripheral pulses and check JVP. Ask examiner for the blood pressure (hypotension). Auscultate the heart for heart sounds.

☐☐☐ **I.V. Access** Establish venous access by inserting two large i.v. cannulas (orange or grey coloured).

☐☐☐ **Bloods**   Take 20 mL of blood and check full blood count, CRP, coagulation profile, urea and electrolytes, liver function test and theophylline levels.

☐☐☐ **Assess**   Make an initial assessment of severity.

Assessing Asthma Severity

Moderate Exacerbation:	Increasing symptoms
	PEFR >50-75% best or predicted
	No features of acute severe asthma
Acute Severe Attack: (any one of)	Unable to complete sentences in one breath
	PEFR 33-50% best or predicted
	Respiratory rate ≥25/min
	Heart rate ≥110/min
Life Threatening: (any one of)	PEFR <33% predicted
	SpO_2 <92% or PaO_2 <8 kPa
	$PaCO_2$ normal or high

Silent chest or feeble respiratory
effort
Cyanosis, bradycardia, dysrhythmia
or hypotension
Exhaustion, confusion or coma

TREATMENT
★ General

□□□ **Oxygen**   Deliver high flow oxygen via non-rebreather bag
(100%).

□□□ **Nebuliser**   Start oxygen-driven nebulised bronchodilators:
salbutamol 5 mg with ipratropium bromide 0.5 mg.

□□□ **Steroids**   Hydrocortisone 100 mg i.v. or prednisolone 40 mg
PO

Antibiotics   Antibiotics are not routinely given unless evidence of
infection.

Low BP   If hypotensive, state intention to start i.v. fluids.

Treatment of Asthma
Mnemonic: 'O SHIT'
Oxygen at 40–60%, 100% if not improving
Sit the patient up, Salbutamol nebulised 5 mg every 4 hr
Hydrocortisone 100 mg i.v. or prednisolone 40 mg PO
Ipratropium bromide 0.5 mg qds, nebulised, inform ITU (life threatening)
Theophylline (aminophylline), CXR to exclude pneumoThorax

★ Life Threatening

□□□ **Critical**   If life threatening features are present or if there is
a poor initial response to bronchodilator therapy,
inform ITU and your seniors before considering
magnesium sulphate 1.2–2 g i.v. over 20 minutes.
Also consider repeating salbutamol nebulisers every
15 min or 5–10 mg continuously per hour.

Improving   Continue high flow oxygen (40–60%). Administer
prednisolone 40 mg PO every 24 hours and nebulised
salbutamol every 4 hours. Monitor peak flow and
oxygen saturation.

Not Improving   After 15 minutes, continue 100% oxygen. Give
salbutamol nebulisers every 15 minutes or 10 mg
continuously every hour. Give ipratropium nebulised
0.5 mg every 4–6 hours.

No Improve.			Inform ITU and discuss with seniors. Repeat salbutamol nebuliser every 15 min. Give 1.2–2 g magnesium sulphate i.v. over 20 min. if not already given. Consider aminophylline: discuss this with a senior colleague. If the patient is still not improving intubation may be required.

* General Points

☐☐☐ **PEFR**

Repeat PEFR 15–30 minutes after first treatment dose (peak flow should be recorded before and after bronchodilator therapy) and maintain oxygen saturation >92%.

☐☐☐ **ABG**

Check arterial blood gases within 2 hours of deterioration, if patient was initially hypoxic (low PaO_2) or if patient initially had a normal or raised $PaCO_2$. Otherwise check after 4 hours.

☐☐☐ **Chest X-ray**

Request chest X-ray to exclude pneumothorax, infection or inhaled foreign body, once stable.

EXAMINER'S EVALUATION

1 2 3 4 5
☐☐☐☐☐ Overall assessment of managing severe asthma
Total mark out of 28

Anaesthetics

ANAESTHETICS: **Pre-operative Assessment**

INSTRUCTIONS: You are a foundation year House Officer in a pre-operative assessment clinic. Carry out a pre-operative assessment in order to ascertain the patient's fitness for surgery and address any concerns they may have regarding the procedure.

INTRODUCTION

0 1 2

☐ ☐ ☐ **Introduction**   Introduce yourself. Elicit the patient's name, age and occupation. Establish rapport with the patient.

☐ ☐ ☐ **Ideas**   Find out what the patient knows about his operation and why he has attended today.

'You are here today for an assessment as to whether you are medically fit to proceed for an operation. Can you please tell me what operation you will be having and what you understand by it?'

☐ ☐ ☐ **Concerns**   Elicit the patient's concerns about having the operation.

'Is there anything that is concerning you about your operation at the moment?'

Explain   Explain to the patient that you will need to ask some questions regarding his health and perform an examination before he can proceed with the operation.

9.1

HISTORY

☐ ☐ ☐ **Type**   Determine the type of surgery planned (elective, emergency).

☐ ☐ ☐ **General Health**   Ask the patient about his general health. Establish whether he has had a cough, shortness of breath, pain (chest, abdomen), fever, weakness, loss of consciousness, weight loss, diarrhoea, constipation and urinary frequency.

☐ ☐ ☐ **Medical History**   Ask about the patient's previous medical problems including cardiac (IHD, HTN, HF, AF), respiratory (asthma, COPD, TB), neurological (stroke, TIA, epilepsy), gastroenterological (liver disease, jaundice) and haematological (sickle cell, thalassaemia) problems. Also ask the patient if they are pregnant if relevant.

☐☐☐ **Prev. Surgery** Ask about any previous operations and post-op. complications. Enquire about previous types of anaesthesia received (local, general) and enquire about any anaesthetic complications (malignant hyperpyrexia).

☐☐☐ **Drug History** Ask about any prescribed medications the patient is taking including insulin or hypoglycaemics, anticoagulants (warfarin, aspirin), β-blockers, steroids, ACE inhibitors, diuretics and inhalers. Enquire about any over-the-counter medication, contraception (COCP) and HRT.

Indications for Pre-op. Medications (Elective)

Medication	Pre-operative Advice
Antihypertensives	Continue taking including morning of surgery (excludes diuretics)
Digoxin	Continue taking including morning of surgery
NSAIDs	Stop 7 days before surgery
Aspirin, clopidogrel	Stop 7 days before surgery
Warfarin	Stop 3–5 days before surgery. INR should be <1.5 pre-op. (lower in spinal or epidural). Prosthetic heart valves require I.V. heparin when warfarin stopped
Metformin	Stop 2 days before surgery. Put patient first on list
Insulin	Patient should be started on insulin infusion pump
Bronchodilators	Take prior to surgery
Contraception	COCP stopped 4 weeks before operation. Patient should consider alternatives (barrier methods). HRT can continue (with DVT prophylaxis)
Steroids	Continue throughout surgery, may require extra cover during operation

Please consult the anaesthetist on call or follow hospital guidelines for further guidance

☐☐☐ **Allergies** Enquire about allergies to antibiotics, plasters, latex, eggs and antiseptic solutions.

☐☐☐ **Family History** Check for family history of any illnesses including myotonic dystrophy, malignant hyperpyrexia, porphyria, cholinesterase disorders and sickle cell disease. Enquire about any other anaesthetic complications and allergic reactions in the family.

Dental Ask about any history of dental problems, false teeth, caps, bridges and dentures.

Social History Elicit the patient's alcohol history noting the number of units consumed in a week. Determine if the patient is a smoker and how many cigarettes he smokes per day.

EXAMINATION

□□□ **BMI** Measure the patient's height and weight and calculate his body mass index. Ideal BMI is between 18.5 and 24.9.

□□□ **Observations** Document the patient's blood pressure, oxygen saturation on air, pulse, respiratory rate and temperature.

□□□ **Systems** Perform a brief chest, abdomen, cardiovascular and neurological examination.

Joint Mobility Ask the patient to flex and extend his neck and to open and close his mouth.

Teeth Inspect the teeth and see if there are any obvious abnormalities.

Mallampati If appropriate, assess ease of intubation by performing a Mallampati assessment. This is done by asking the patient to open his mouth as wide as possible and sticking his tongue out. Grade according to what is visible.

Mallampati Pharyngeal Assessment

Class	Parts Visible	Intubation Difficulty
I	Soft palate, uvula, fauces, pharyngeal pillars	No difficulty
II	Soft palate, uvula, fauces	No difficulty
III	Soft palate, base of uvula	Moderate difficulty
IV	Hard palate only	Severe difficulty

Class I   Class II   Class III   Class IV

Note: Class III/IV represents difficult intubation, relative contraindication to surgery

ASA Score   Grade the patient for pre-operative fitness based upon the American Society of Anesthesiologists (ASA) score.

ASA Scores

Score	Mortality	Physical status	Example
I	0.07%	Healthy patient	Fit with inguinal hernia
II	0.24%	Mild systemic disease, no incapacitation	Essential hypertension
III	1.4%	Severe systemic disease, some incapacitation	Unstable angina
IV	7.5%	Life threatening disease, incapacitating	CCF
V	8.1%	Moribund patient, death expected ≤24 hrs	Ruptured AAA
E	Double	Emergency case	

Mortality rates are for 48 hours post-op. Emergency case rates are double the risk of any class

Investigations   State that you would order investigations (bloods, chest X-ray, ECG, further imaging) if clinically appropriate.

Indications for Pre-op. Investigations

Investigation	Indication
FBC	Exclude infection, anaemia
SS screen	Sickle cell disease (African, Mediterranean, FH)
U&E	Diabetic (creatinine), vomiting and diarrhoea, renal disease (failure), >60 yr, cardiovascular disease, drugs (steroids, diuretics, ACE inhibitors)
LFT	Alcoholic, liver disease, malnutrition, metastatic disease
Coag. screen	Warfarin, liver disease, jaundice
Calcium	Malignancy, chronic renal impairment
Glucose	Diabetes (type 1 and 2), PVD, steroids
TFT	Hypo- or hyperthyroidism or suspicion
Urine β-HCG	Women of child bearing age to exclude pregnancy
ECG	Hypertension, heart disease, arrhythmia, >50 years old, DM
CXR	Respiratory (asthma, COPD) or cardiac disease (heart failure), malignancy, thoracic surgery, respiratory symptoms (cough, SOB, sputum), previous TB
C-spine	Rheumatoid arthritis, previous neck surgery, major trauma
Echo	Undiagnosed systolic murmur (AS), unexplained SOB, poor exercise tolerance, impaired ventricular function

CLOSING

NBM Advise the patient that they should not eat 6 hours pre-operatively or drink clear fluids 2 hours before the operation.

☐☐☐ **Conclude** Ask the patient if he has any further questions or concerns. Offer the patient an information leaflet. Thank the patient.

☐☐☐ **Drug Chart** Write up a drug chart documenting the date of admission (operation), patient's name, date of birth, hospital number, drug allergies and regular medications. Write up prophylactic anticoagulation (Clexane 20 mg SC or Tinzaparin 4500 U SC), analgesia and antiemetic (as required) and TED stockings. Consider pre-operative antibiotics or bowel preparation depending on the type of operation.

☐☐☐ **Anaesthetist** State to the examiner that if there were any concerns raised from the pre-op. assessment, you would contact the anaesthetist on call or more preferably the anaesthetist performing the list.

EXAMINER'S EVALUATION

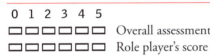

0 1 2 3 4 5

☐☐☐☐☐☐ Overall assessment of pre-op. assessment
☐☐☐☐☐☐ Role player's score
Total mark out of 34

ANAESTHETICS: **Pain Relief Management**

INSTRUCTIONS: You are a foundation year House Officer in general surgery. Mr Jones is scheduled to have major abdominal surgery in 2 weeks time. He has asked to speak to a member of the surgical team about pain relief following the operation. Elicit his concerns and explain the pain relief options that can be used.

INTRODUCTION

0 1 2

☐☐☐ **Introduction**   Introduce yourself. Confirm the patient's name, age and occupation. Establish rapport with him.

☐☐☐ **Ideas**   Confirm the reason for attendance and elicit the patient's understanding and ideas of post-operation pain relief.

'I understand that you are going to have an operation soon and would like to know more about pain relief. Can I ask you what you have already been told?'

☐☐☐ **Concerns**   Elicit the patient's concerns, i.e. post-op. pain and side effects of pain killers.

'Do you have any particular concerns, about the operation or receiving pain relief? Are there any matters you wish me to clarify?'

9.2

☐☐☐ **Expectations**   Clarify what the patient would like to know.

'I'm going to explain to you some things about pain relief after your operation. Is that OK? If you have any questions or queries along the way, please stop me and ask'.

EXPLANATION

☐☐☐ **Pain Relief**   Reassure the patient that post-operative pain can be controlled with drugs. Explain that good pain relief reduces recovery time as patients are able to become mobile sooner.

☐☐☐ **Epidural**   Explain epidural pain relief to the patient.

'There are a number of ways to control your pain after the operation. This includes an epidural, PCA device and oral medications. I will explain to you each one of these in turn.

'An epidural is a fine tube that is passed between the bones in your back. This fine tube allows small amounts of painkillers to be given directly and continuously to the nerves that relay pain. This tube is taped to your back and connected to a pump which delivers an accurate dose of medication and can be adjusted by the doctor to meet your requirements.'

☐ ☐ ☐ **Advantages**   Explain to the patient the advantages of epidural pain relief.

'Because the painkiller acts directly on the nerves that relay pain, smaller amounts of analgesia can be used, so you will receive good pain relief and be less likely to feel drowsy or sick than with other methods. You should also be able to move about in bed more easily and get out of bed sooner than with most other kinds of pain killers. Patients with good pain control progress more quickly and go home earlier. Epidurals are known to be extremely safe and have been used for many years.'

☐ ☐ ☐ **Side Effects**   Explain the side effects of epidurals.

'Although epidurals are performed routinely, there is a small chance of suffering from some side effects. The most common of these are relatively minor. You may experience headaches, backaches and problems passing urine. However, you may also experience weakness and numbness of your legs. If you suffer from any of these symptoms and you are worried, please let a doctor or nurse know.

'Although very uncommon, I must inform you that there is a slight possibility that the epidural tube may become infected or bleed around the insertion site. At all times during your stay in hospital you will be regularly checked and monitored so that any potential problems can be treated promptly.'

☐ ☐ ☐ **PCA**   Explain to the patient what the PCA is.

'PCA stands for patient-controlled analgesia. This means that you are in direct control of how much pain relief you require for your pain as and when you need it. A special pump that contains the pain relief medication is connected to you by a small tube. This tube may be attached to your i.v. line or your epidural. You control your pain relief mainly by pushing a button that makes the pump deliver you a small safe dose of analgesia. The total amount of the drug is fixed so that there is no risk of overdosing.'

☐ ☐ ☐ **Advantages**   Explain the advantages of PCA pain relief.

'Because the drug enters your body through your veins, it works much faster than tablets. You should feel better within 10 minutes of delivering a dose. This means that you should be able to move about in bed and get out of bed sooner than with tablets alone and this will help your recovery. PCA is known to be extremely safe and has been used for many years.'

☐☐☐ **Side Effects** Explain the side effects of PCAs.

'Pain-relieving drugs often cause mild sleepiness, nausea and vomiting. Some symptoms are fairly common but can easily be treated. Although the medication should not hurt you as it goes into your vein, you may feel a slight burning or warm feeling. Let a nurse or doctor know if this bothers you.'

☐☐☐ **Alternatives** Explain that there are other forms of pain relief including tablets and suppositories once pain becomes milder.

'The epidural/PCA will stop when your pain becomes mild and can be treated in other ways. Eventually, you will be able to take oral medications to control your pain. This will usually be a few days after your operation and may be as tablets, taken orally, or suppositories, through your back passage.'

CLOSING

☐☐☐ **Understanding** Confirm that the patient has understood what you have explained to them.

☐☐☐ **Questions** Respond appropriately to the patient's questions.

Leaflet Offer to give him more information in the form of a handout. Advise that the leaflet contains much of the information you have mentioned.

COMMUNICATION SKILLS

☐☐☐ **Rapport** Attempt to establish rapport with the patient through the use of appropriate eye contact. Maintain appropriate body language and open posture throughout.

☐☐☐ **Listening** Demonstrate interest and concern in what the patient says. Show active listening and listen empathetically.

☐☐☐ **Fluency** Deliver information in a fluent manner. Avoid jargon and repetition.

☐☐☐ **Summary** Provide an appropriate summary to the patient.

EXAMINER'S EVALUATION

0 1 2 3 4 5
☐☐☐☐☐☐ Overall assessment of explaining post-op. analgesia
☐☐☐☐☐☐ Role player's score
Total mark out of 32

ANAESTHETICS: **Post-herpetic Neuralgia Pain Relief**

INSTRUCTIONS: You are a foundation year House Officer in neurology outpatients. Mr Edward Smith has previously been prescribed amitriptyline for post-herpetic neuralgia. He now presents to the clinic refusing to take the drug as his neighbour has been prescribed the same medication for depression. Deal with this problem appropriately.

INTRODUCTION

0 1 2

☐ ☐ ☐ **Introduction** — Introduce yourself. Confirm the patient's name, age and occupation. Establish rapport with him.

☐ ☐ ☐ **Ideas** — Confirm the reason for attendance and elicit the patient's understanding and ideas about his medication. Identify the patient's current medication and ascertain the dosage.

'I understand that you have been prescribed some pain relief medication recently. Can you tell me more about it and how much you are taking?'

☐ ☐ ☐ **Concerns** — Elicit the patient's concerns about being prescribed antidepressants.

'Do you have any particular concerns about the medication you have been prescribed?'

9.3

☐ ☐ ☐ **Expectations** — Clarify what the patient would like to know.

HISTORY

☐ ☐ ☐ **Pain History** — Take a focused pain history including site, onset, character, radiation, associated symptoms, timing, exacerbating and relieving factors.

☐ ☐ ☐ **Drug History** — Ask the patient if any other medications have been tried in the past to control the pain.

EXPLAIN

☐ ☐ ☐ **Reassure** — Reassure the patient that he is not being treated for depression.

'As you may be aware, your pain symptoms are consistent with a condition called post-herpetic neuralgia. One of the recommended medications is a drug called amitriptyline which is effective in controlling this type of pain. However, this drug is also used to treat people suffering from depression. The dose of amitriptyline used for your condition is much lower than that required to treat depression. Taking amitriptyline tablets does not mean that you are depressed.'

☐☐☐ **Mechanism**   Explain the mechanism of action of amitriptyline and why it is used for pain relief.

'Whenever you hurt or injure yourself, the body senses this through the nerves and interprets it as pain. Amitriptyline is believed to alter the way the body responds to these pain signals and therefore reduces the pain you feel.'

☐☐☐ **Advantages**   Explain the advantages of the medication.

'Amitriptyline is able to effectively control the pain of post-herpetic neuralgia where other oral medications have failed. It is extremely effective and safe with very few side effects when taken in the low dose form.'

☐☐☐ **Disadvantages**   Explain the disadvantages of the medication.

'However, with all medications there are risks of side effects. These include having a dry mouth, feeling nauseous and slightly drowsy. If you experience any of these please contact your GP.'

CLOSING

☐☐☐ **Understanding**   Confirm that the patient has understood what you have explained to them.

☐☐☐ **Questions**   Respond appropriately to patient's questions.

Leaflet   Offer to give him more information in the form of a handout. Advise that the leaflet contains much of the information you have mentioned.

COMMUNICATION SKILLS

☐☐☐ **Rapport**   Attempt to establish rapport with the patient through the use of appropriate eye contact. Maintain appropriate body language and open posture throughout.

☐☐☐ **Listening**   Demonstrate interest and concern in what the patient says. Show active listening and listen empathetically.

☐☐☐ **Fluency**   Deliver information in a fluent manner. Avoid jargon and repetition.

☐☐☐ **Summary**   Provide an appropriate summary to the patient.

0 1 2 3 4 5

☐☐☐☐☐☐ Overall assessment of explaining amitriptyline use

☐☐☐☐☐☐ Role player's score

Total mark out of 29

ANAESTHETICS: Trigeminal Neuralgia Pain Relief

INSTRUCTIONS: You are a foundation year House Officer in neurology outpatients. Mr Petite has previously been prescribed carbamazepine medication for trigeminal neuralgia. He now presents to the clinic refusing to take the drug as his relative has been prescribed the same medication for epilepsy. Deal with this problem appropriately.

INTRODUCTION

0 1 2

☐☐☐ **Introduction**   Introduce yourself. Confirm the patient's name, age and occupation. Establish rapport with the patient.

☐☐☐ **Ideas**   Confirm the reason for his attendance and elicit the patient's understanding and ideas about his medication. Identify the patient's current medication and ascertain the dosage.

'I understand that you have been prescribed some pain relief medication recently. Can you tell me more about it and how much you take?'

☐☐☐ **Concerns**   Elicit the patient's concerns about being prescribed antiepileptic medication.

9.4

'Do you have any particular concerns about the medication you have been prescribed?'

☐☐☐ **Expectations**   Clarify what the patient would like to know.

FOCUSED HISTORY

☐☐☐ **Pain History**   Take a focused pain history including the site, onset and character of the pain, radiation, associated symptoms, timing, exacerbating and relieving factors.

☐☐☐ **Drug History**   Ask the patient if any other medications have been tried in the past to control the pain.

EXPLAIN

☐☐☐ **Reassure**   Reassure the patient that he is not being treated for epilepsy.

'As you may be aware, your pain symptoms are consistent with a condition known as trigeminal neuralgia. Patients experience sharp nerve pain over areas of the face. Because of the type of pain we recommend carbamazepine, which is the first step in treating this condition. However, this drug is more commonly known for treating epilepsy. The dose of carbamazepine used for your condition is much lower than that required to treat epilepsy. Taking carbamazepine tablets does not mean that you suffer from epilepsy.'

☐☐☐ **Mechanism** Explain the mechanism of action of antiepileptics and why they are used for pain relief.

'In trigeminal neuralgia, the nerve that supplies the area of your face becomes overactive. Thus, when you touch those areas you may feel a sharp nerve-like pain. In epilepsy, it is believed that a similar mechanism takes place by the over-stimulation of the brain cells. Carbamazepine works by dulling nerve hyperactivity, which is why it is effective in both conditions.'

☐☐☐ **Advantages** Explain the advantages of the medication.

'You may have noticed that normal pain-relieving medications are ineffective against this pain. Carbamazepine is able to effectively control the pain of trigeminal neuralgia where other oral medications have failed. It is extremely effective against the pain of trigeminal neuralgia, safe and fast acting, with very few side effects when taken in a low dose. Your GP will perform blood tests now and again to check everything is OK (such as no agranulocytosis or liver dysfunction). If you do notice any side effects, such as feeling sleepy or confused, then let your GP know.'

☐☐☐ **Disadvantages** Explain the disadvantages of the medication.

'However, as with all medications there is a risk of side effects. These include feeling sick and vomiting, headaches, blurred vision and numbness of the hands or legs.

'This medication very rarely can weaken your immune system. This may present as a persistent sore throat (agranulocytosis). If you experience this please contact your GP as soon as possible. They will arrange a blood test. I would like to reassure you that this side effect is very rare and unlikely to occur since you are on the low dose form.'

CLOSING
☐☐☐ **Understanding** Confirm that the patient has understood what you have explained to them.

☐☐☐ **Questions** Respond appropriately to the patient's questions.

Leaflet Offer to give him more information in the form of a handout. Advise that the leaflet contains much of the information you have mentioned.

COMMUNICATION SKILLS

☐☐☐ **Rapport**   Attempt to establish rapport with the patient through the use of appropriate eye contact. Maintain appropriate body language and an open posture throughout.

☐☐☐ **Listening**   Demonstrate an interest and concern in what the patient says. Show active listening and listen empathetically.

☐☐☐ **Fluency**   Deliver information in a fluent manner. Avoid jargon and repetition.

☐☐☐ **Summary**   Provide an appropriate summary to the patient.

EXAMINER'S EVALUATION

0 1 2 3 4 5

☐☐☐☐☐☐ Overall assessment of explaining carbamazepine use

☐☐☐☐☐☐ Role player's score

Total mark out of 30

Geriatrics

INSTRUCTIONS: You are a foundation year House Officer in care-of-the-elderly outpatients' clinic. You have been asked to see Mr Parkinson, a 77-year-old retired war veteran who is being followed up after a recent admission to hospital. You will be marked on your communication skills and your ability to take the history from the patient.

INTRODUCTION

0 1 2

☐ ☐ ☐ **Introduction**   Introduce yourself appropriately and establish rapport with the patient.

Name & Age   Elicit the patient's name and age.

☐ ☐ ☐ **Occupation**   Enquire about the patient's occupation or previous occupation if retired.

HISTORY

☐ ☐ ☐ **Admission**   Elicit the reason why the patient was recently admitted into hospital, how long he was hospitalised for and the date of his discharge.

☐ ☐ ☐ **History**   Elicit the patient's acute and chronic symptoms. For each complaint ascertain the time of onset, presenting features and associated symptoms. Explore systematically each complaint (e.g. chest pain) by asking about individual aspects and symptoms (e.g. site, onset, character, radiation, associations, exacerbating/alleviating factors and severity).

10.1

☐ ☐ ☐ **Impact on Life**   Ask the patient about how this current problem is affecting his life.

'How has this affected your life? How is it preventing you from doing things that you could do before?'

ASSOCIATED HISTORY

☐ ☐ ☐ **Medical History**   Has he had any previous hospital admission or operations? Does he suffer from any medical problems including hypertension, diabetes, epilepsy, stroke, angina, MI, cholesterol, cancer or COPD?

☐ ☐ ☐ **Drug History**   Is he taking any regular medications, prescribed or over the counter? Does the patient use a dossett box and take his own medication or does someone else administer it to him? Does the patient have any known allergies?

□□□ **Family History** Ask about inherited family disorders and major illnesses (e.g. heart disease, diabetes, stroke, Alzheimer's, cancer).

Social History Does he smoke? How many cigarettes a day and for how long has he smoked? Does he drink alcohol? How many units a week does he drink?

□□□ *Accommodation* What type of accommodation does he live in (flat, house, rented, owned, residential home, nursing home, warden-controlled) and does it have stairs? Are the toilet, bedroom, bathroom and kitchen all on the same level?

Nutrition Ask the patient how often he eats and what types of food he eats (if less than two meals a day he is at risk of under-nutrition)? Does he prepare his own meals or does he receive Meals on Wheels?

□□□ *Social Support* Does the patient live alone or does he live with anyone? How much support does he receive from friends or family? Does he have any carers or social services input? Does he attend day centres? Does he receive a pension?

FUNCTIONAL STATUS

□□□ **Normal Day** Enquire about the patient's normal daily routine, including activities such as reading, work, hobbies and interaction with others (friends, family). If appropriate, systematically enquire about his daily activities to assess his physical function.

□□□ **Adaptations** Has he had any adaptations installed in the accommodation (hand rails, toilet bars, hoist)?

SYSTEMIC ENQUIRY

□□□ **Vision** Has the patient experienced any problems with his vision which have led to any accidents or caused difficulties in taking medication?

□□□ **Balance** Has the patient had any problems with balance or falling? Has he experienced any dizziness, unsteadiness or fainting?

Mnemonic: 'SPLATT'

Symptoms before fall	LOC, leg weakness, coughing, urination – frequency, palpitations, angina, dizziness, giddiness
Previous falls	Note history of previous falls and frequency
Location of the fall	Ask the patient where and when the fall took place (toilet, stairs, bedroom, pavement). Establish the time of the fall and how long the patient remained on the floor unaided
Associated symptoms	Note any symptoms associated with the fall
Trauma of the fall	Elicit any bone or muscle tenderness, bruising or reduced range of movement of joints. Consider X-rays (pelvis, hip, knee, wrist, elbow), to exclude trauma or fractures
Tablets, i.e. medications	Take a thorough drug history noting anti-hypertensive drugs, diuretics, sedatives, hypoglycaemic drugs

▭▭▭ Memory

Has the patient or a family member noticed any long-term or short-term memory loss? Enquire about any memory loss and cognitive problems and carry out a cognitive assessment if appropriate.

Psychiatric

Has the patient experienced any mood changes recently? Has he recently had disturbed sleep or a low mood?

GI Symptoms

Has the patient experienced any dyspepsia or gastrointestinal symptoms? Has he experienced any appetite changes or weight loss?

Mnemonic for Causes of Recurrent Falls

Mnemonic: 'CATASTROPHE'

Carer and housing (housebound, living alone), **C**ognition impaired (confusion, impaired judgement)

Alcohol excess or withdrawal

Treatment (>3 diuretics, antihypertensives, hypnotics, antidepressants, hypoglycaemics)

Affect (low mood), **A**ids (stick, frame, wheelchair, crutches)

Syncope, **S**hoes (poor footwear)

Teetering (dizziness)

Recent illness (hospitalisation)

Old (elderly >75-years old), **O**cular problems

Previous falls, **P**ain on mobility, **P**MH (vertigo, arthritis, OA, DM, CVA, epilepsy, IHD, neuro)

Hearing problems

Environmental hazards (poor lighting, loose carpets)

COMMUNICATION SKILLS

☐☐☐ **Rapport**   Establish and maintain rapport and demonstrate listening skills.

☐☐☐ **Response**   React positively to and acknowledge the patient's emotions.

☐☐☐ **Fluency**   Speak fluently and do not use jargon.

☐☐☐ **Summarise**   Check that the patient has no further concerns and deliver an appropriate summary.

'This is Mr Parkinson, a 77-year-old man, who was admitted 2 months ago after having a fall at home. He states that he woke up in the early hours of the morning and fell down two stairs trying to get to the bathroom. Later he was diagnosed with a fractured neck of femur and had a dynamic hip screw inserted. Following the operation he was mobilising well and was discharged home a month later. Today he is complaining of pain over the operation site for which he is taking only prn paracetamol. He is a known type 2 diabetic on metformin. He lives alone in a first-floor split-level flat in which his bathroom and kitchen are downstairs. He has no social service input or adaptations to the house. On systematic enquiry he says he is generally well and his previous hip fracture was due to a mechanical fall. Taking into account his history and social circumstances, I would like to perform a thorough examination (dislocation, infection) before considering increasing his analgesia.'

EXAMINER'S EVALUATION

0 1 2 3 4 5

☐☐☐☐☐☐ Overall assessment of geriatric history

☐☐☐☐☐☐ Role player's score

Total mark out of 35

INSTRUCTIONS: You are a foundation year House Officer in General Practice. Mr Brown is an elderly man who has come to the practice as he has been feeling very low. Assess his problem and psychiatric state. You will be marked on your ability to elicit an appropriate psychiatric history and to reach a diagnosis, and on your communication skills.

INTRODUCTION

0 1 2

☐ ☐ ☐ **Introduction**   Introduce yourself. Establish rapport with the patient.

Patient Details   Elicit the patient's name, age, and former occupation (if he is retired).

HISTORY

☐ ☐ ☐ **Complaint**   Elicit all the patient's presenting complaints.

☐ ☐ ☐ **History**   When did it first start? What has been happening recently? How long has it been going on for? What do you think caused it? How has this affected you?

DEPRESSIVE SYMPTOMS

✴ Core Symptoms

☐ ☐ ☐ **Low Mood**   Have you been feeling depressed or feeling low in spirits recently?

☐ ☐ ☐ **Anhedonia**   Do you still enjoy the activities that you used to enjoy?

☐ ☐ ☐ **Fatigue**   Do you feel that you don't have the same amount of energy as before? Do you find that you tire easily?

☐ ☐ ☐ **Cause**   What do you think caused you to feel this way? Are there any particular stresses in your life or has something happened recently which may have contributed (such as bereavement, chronic illness, abuse)?

✴ Cognitive Symptoms

☐ ☐ ☐ **Concentration**   Are you finding it hard to concentrate? How easy do you find it to read a newspaper or follow a television programme?

☐ ☐ ☐ **Hopelessness**   How do you feel about the future? Do you see things getting any better?

10.2

☐☐☐ **Helpless**	Do you feel helpless about your current situation?
Worthless	How do you feel about yourself? Do you feel you are of any value?
Self-esteem	Would you say you have low self-esteem?
Guilt	Do you feel that you are to blame for the situation you are in?

✴ Biological Symptoms

☐☐☐ **Sleep**	How well have been you sleeping? Do you find yourself waking early in the morning?
☐☐☐ **Diurnal**	At what the time of the day do you feel the worst? Does the day improve as it progresses?
☐☐☐ **Appetite**	How is your appetite? Is your weight steady?
☐☐☐ **Bowels**	Have you been feeling constipated recently?
Libido	How has your libido been recently? Have you recently lost interest in sex?

✴ Systemic Review

☐☐☐ **Symptoms**	Enquire about non-specific symptoms including headache, palpitations, abdominal or back pain, weakness, lethargy and shortness of breath.

✴ Differential

☐☐☐ **Dementia**	How has your memory been recently? Do you mind if I ask you a few questions? (Perform an AMTS if appropriate.)
Bipolar	I know you feel low now, but have you recently felt so high and energetic that others have said that you seem elated?
Psychosis	Have you ever heard voices when no one was there? Have you seen something that you did not expect to see or that others could not see?

✴ Suicidal Ideation

☐☐☐ **Thoughts**	Do you find it difficult to face the next day? Have you ever thought of ending it all by taking your own life? How often do you get these thoughts? Do you try and resist them?
Method	Have you thought about ways of doing it? Have you gained the means to do this at home (gun, pills, etc.)?

Attempt   Have you actually tried to kill or harm yourself? What stopped you from doing this?

☐☐☐ **Impact**   Do you have any particular concerns or worries about the symptoms you are experiencing? How have these symptoms affected your life and your family?

ASSOCIATED HISTORY

☐☐☐ **Psych. History**   Have you ever harmed yourself in the past? Have you suffered from depression in the past? Do you suffer from any illnesses that have affected you for a long time (chronic)? Have you ever had any previous treatments for depression (counselling, psychotherapy, ECT)?

☐☐☐ **Drug History**   Are you taking any medication? Do you have any drug allergies?

Family History   Has anyone in your family suffered from depression or psychiatric illness? Has anyone in your family ever harmed themselves or taken their own life?

☐☐☐ **Social History**   Do you smoke? How many cigarettes do you smoke a day and for how long have you smoked? Do you drink alcohol? How many units a week do you drink? Enquire about previous or current substance abuse.

Accommodation   What type of accommodation do you live in (flat, house, rented, owned, residential home, nursing home, warden-controlled) and does it have stairs? Are the toilet, bedroom, bathroom and kitchen all on the same level?

Nutrition   Ask the patient how often he eats and what types of food he eats (if less than two meals a day he is at risk of under-nutrition)? Does he prepare his own meals or does he receive Meals on Wheels?

Social Support   Does the patient live alone or does he live with anyone? How much support does he receive from friends or family? Does he have any carers or social services input? Does he attend day centres? Does he receive a pension?

Risk Factors for Depression
- Female gender
- Living in sheltered accommodation
- Chronic disease (MS, arthritis)

- Past history of depression
- Poor social support (living alone)
- Neurotic personality
- Carer (e.g. for disabled/ill spouse)
- Adverse life events (bereavement)

□□□ **Insight** Do you think you are depressed? How would you feel about taking medication for your problem? Do you think you can be helped?

COMMUNICATION SKILLS

□□□ **Rapport** Establish and maintain rapport and demonstrate listening skills.

□□□ **Response** React positively to and acknowledge the patient's emotions.

□□□ **Fluency** Speak fluently and do not use jargon.

□□□ **Summarise** Check with the patient and deliver an appropriate summary.

'This is Mr Brown, a 77-year-old retired banker, who has been complaining of a low mood for the last 3 months. He mentions that he is still grieving from the loss of his wife from cancer. He is complaining of low mood, insomnia, lack of appetite, poor concentration and fatigue. There is no current suicidal ideation or evidence of psychosis. Previously he suffered from depression after being made redundant in the early 1990s for which he took a short course of antidepressants. He also suffers from diabetes and hypertension for which he takes regular medication. He currently lives alone in a two-bedroom bungalow and his children visit frequently. In view of his history, I suspect that Mr Brown is experiencing a bereavement reaction. However, I would also like to exclude severe depression.'

EXAMINER'S EVALUATION

0 1 2 3 4 5

□□□□□□ Overall assessment of elderly depression
□□□□□□ Role player's score
Total mark out of 41

DIFFERENTIAL DIAGNOSIS
Depression

Depression is common in the elderly, with an overall prevalence of between 5 and 10%. It is estimated that two-thirds of adults will suffer from depression at some point in their life. Depression is more common in women. Risk factors for depression include previous depression, significant past medical illnesses and other psychiatric illnesses. It is defined by the presence of at least two of three core symptoms (low mood, anhedonia and fatigue) for at least 2 weeks. In elderly people, a new onset of neurotic symptoms such as phobias, anxiety, obsessive–compulsive behaviour and hypochondria are likely to be secondary to depressive illness rather than primary diagnoses on their own. In the elderly, unusual presentations of common symptoms may be the only presentation of depression.

Signs and Symptoms of Depression
Mnemonic: 'SAD FACES'

Sleep Changes	**A**gitation (psychomotor)
Anhedonia	**C**oncentration (poor)
Dysphoria (low mood)	**E**steem (poor)
Fatigue (lack of energy)	**S**uicide

Dementia

Dementia is an irreversible, progressively deteriorating illness that is characterised by global impairment of cognitive function and personality without impairment to consciousness. Diagnosis is reached when symptoms persist for more than 6 months. Pseudodementia is the term given to severe depression in which the cognitive changes mimic those of dementia. Although differentiation between the two can initially be challenging, there are distinguishing features that can point towards a correct diagnosis. Whereas in dementia onset is usually insidious, severely depressed patients usually develop pseudodementia rapidly in comparison, and symptoms are typically of short duration only. Dementia sufferers will frequently try and hide their poor memory whereas those with pseudodementia will draw attention to it. Characteristically, when asked questions about memory and time–space orientation, those with dementia will give answers that are slightly incorrect whereas those with pseudodementia will give apathetic replies (e.g. 'don't know'). An important differentiating feature between the two conditions is the presence in dementia and absence in pseudodementia of cortical dysfunction (apraxia, aphasia, agnosia, etc.).

Organic Mood Disorder

Organic mood disorders caused by medical illness and/or drugs need to be excluded in an elderly patient presenting with mood change. A full history, examination and investigations will need to be carried out as appropriate in order to consider and exclude metabolic, infective and neoplastic causes as well as organic brain disease. Blood tests to investigate the first presentation of a depressive episode in the elderly include a full blood count, urea and electrolytes, thyroid function, liver function, calcium, B12 and folate. In an atypical presentation, syphilis serology should also be considered. A computed tomography scan of the brain should be performed if appropriate in light of the clinical picture and if other tests have been negative. Electro-encephalography (EEG) is used in specific cases to distinguish between depression and organic brain syndromes. Drugs that can contribute to causing organic mood syndromes include antihypertensives, steroids, antiparkinsonian drugs, analgesics and sedatives.

Bipolar Disorder

Bipolar disorder consists of episodes of mania/hypomania and depression. Men and women have the same incidence of bipolar disorder, with the age of onset usually being in the 20s. For a diagnosis to be considered it is necessary for two episodes of mood disturbance to occur. Manic phases are characterised by behaviour that is overactive and irritable. Patients will often spend extravagantly and incur debts, feel extremely energetic and embark on unrealistic activities that are left unfinished. The libido may also be increased as part of a general disinhibition and this is particularly important in elderly people where the partner may have noticed the patient suddenly wishing to engage in sexual activity. Speech and thought patterns may seem erratic and when severe, the patient may exhibit a flight of ideas. Persecutory and grandiose delusions are common, and insight is usually extremely limited. Diagnostic difficulty can occur during depressive phases, and some patients will experience mainly depression with only occasional manic episodes.

Signs and Symptoms of Mania
Mnemonic: 'MANIC'
Mood (irritable), **M**outh (pressure of speech)
Activity increased, **A**ttention (distractability)
Naughty (disinhibition)
Insomnia, **I**deas (flight of)
Confidence (grandiose ideas)

Dysthymia

Dysthymia is part of the spectrum of depressive disorders. It is less severe than major depression and is characterised by a mood that is mildly depressed or irritable which has been present for most of the day for at least 2 years with no more than a 2-month period free of symptoms. For diagnosis, at least two of six symptoms (poor appetite or overeating, sleep disturbance, fatigue/low energy, poor self-esteem, poor concentration/difficulty in decision-making and feelings of hopelessness) should be present. Although dysthymia has been considered to be mainly a condition of the young, onset can be in later life.

Bereavement Reaction

A bereavement reaction is a natural reaction that occurs after the loss of a close individual (a friend or relative). It can also include other forms of losses, such as the loss of health (mental or physical), status or a family pet. The stages of normal bereavement include alarm (a highly stressed state with physiological arousal), numbness (emotionally disconnected), pining (preoccupation with the deceased, bouts of intense anxiety), depression and recovery (acceptance of loss, return to normal daily activities). These phases do not represent a rigid sequence and people fluctuate between these phases. The duration of symptoms varies from person to person but tends to last longer if the death occurred suddenly and unexpectedly. If symptoms last for more than 6 months then an adjustment disorder should be considered.

GERIATRICS: **Assessing Suicide Risk**

INSTRUCTIONS: You are a foundation year House Officer in A&E. Miss Carey is a 76-year-old song writer who has been brought in after an overdose of paracetamol tablets. Her blood tests show that her paracetamol levels are below the levels needed to commence treatment. Take a history from the patient and establish her current suicide risk.

INTRODUCTION

0 1 2

☐ ☐ ☐ **Introduction** Introduce yourself. Establish rapport with the patient.

Patient's Details Elicit the patient's name, age and former occupation (if retired).

HISTORY

☐ ☐ ☐ **Complaint** Elicit all the patient's presenting complaints.

☐ ☐ ☐ **History** How are you feeling today? What made you feel that you had to do this? What exactly happened?

Deliberate Self-harm and Suicide in the Elderly

Although the incidence of deliberate self-harm decreases with age, there is a higher rate of suicidal intent associated with deliberate self-harm in the elderly. Risk factors in the elderly include being diagnosed with a psychiatric illness, the death of a spouse, separation from a cohabitee (one of the two partners going to a nursing home), threat of transfer to a nursing home, divorce, loneliness, social isolation and cognitive impairment. The rate of suicide in the elderly is higher compared to the overall rate for the general population. Elderly men have a preponderance of up to 2:1 for completed suicide compared with elderly women. The risk factors for suicide in the elderly are largely the same as those for the general population except that widowhood and physical illness is more common in the elderly. An important aspect of self-harm or suicide in the elderly is that in many cases where an overdose has taken place, the choice of drug and dose used are not indicators of suicidal intent. Elderly people attempting suicide will frequently consume a drug of a certain dose and believe the choice to be fatal whereas it is not. In addition, an elderly patient's perception of the severity of an illness and its suitability for warranting a suicide attempt (e.g. mild arthritis) may be at odds with what most people may believe, and a dismissive approach to a patient's grievances regarding mild illnesses should be avoided. Generally elderly men adopt more violent methods than women. In the UK, the most common method of male suicide is hanging, whereas a drug overdose or self poisoning is more common in women

10.3

PSYCHIATRIC SYMPTOMS

✳ Before the Attempt

☐☐☐ **Before** — What happened just before you tried ending your life? Have you been feeling low or depressed? How long have you felt like this?

☐☐☐ **Planning** — Did you plan this to happen or was it spontaneous? Did you go out and buy the tablets for this purpose?

Seeking Help — Did you tell anyone about the attempt? Did you try to get help?

Precautions — Did you take any precautions against getting caught or discovered?

Final Actions — Did you make a will? Or leave a note? Did you close your bank accounts or make any changes to your finances?

✳ The Attempt

☐☐☐ **Incident** — What did you do? How did you do it? When did you do it? Where were you at the time?

☐☐☐ **Meaning** — Did you really want to die and escape your problems?

☐☐☐ **Fatality** — Did you think the amount of tablets you took would be sufficient to end your life?

Discovery — How were you discovered?

Alcohol — Did you drink any alcohol before the attempt? Were you drunk?

✳ After the Attempt

☐☐☐ **Feeling** — How do you feel know? Do you feel angry that it was not successful? Do you feel relieved that you failed?

☐☐☐ **Thoughts** — Do you still have any lingering thoughts about taking your life?

☐☐☐ **Mood** — Do you feel depressed? How do you see the future?

✳ Risk Factors

☐☐☐ **Home** — Do you live alone? Were you to be transferred to sheltered accommodation?

☐☐☐ **Family** — Are you in a relationship? Do you have a partner? Do you have any family?

☐☐☐ **Bereavement** — Did you experience a recent bereavement?

354

□□□ **Chronic Illness**   Do you suffer with any chronic illnesses (HF, COPD, epilepsy, MS, arthritis, cancer)?

Risk Factors for Suicide
Mnemonic: 'SAD PERSONS'

Sex (male)
Age (elderly or young)
Depression
Previous attempts/Plan to do it again
Ethanol abuse or other drugs

Rational thinking lost (psychosis)
Social support lacking (single)
Organised suicide plan
No job (retired) or No spouse
Sickness (chronic)

ASSOCIATED HISTORY

Psych. History   Have you ever tried to end your life before? Have you ever harmed yourself in the past? Do you suffer from any psychiatric illnesses such as depression, schizophrenia or mania?

Medical History   Do you suffer from any illness that has affected you for a long time (e.g. cancer, multiple sclerosis, chronic back pain, renal failure, heart failure, diabetes)?

□□□ **Drug History**   Are you taking any medications? Do you have any drug allergies?

□□□ **Family History**   Has anyone in your family suffered from depression or psychiatric illness? Has anyone in your family ever harmed themselves or taken their own life?

□□□ **Social History**   Do you drink alcohol? How much and how often? Do you smoke? Have you tried any recreational drugs? Who do you live with? Have you got a partner? Do you have support from family or friends?

□□□ **Insight**   Do you feel you need help? Would you accept any help if it was offered to you?

Follow up   Provide appropriate patient risk assessment and advise on management, i.e. need for inpatient admission or outpatient follow up.

COMMUNICATION SKILLS

□□□ **Rapport**   Establish and maintain rapport with the patient and demonstrate listening skills.

□□□ **Response**   React positively to and acknowledge the patient's emotions.

□□□ **Fluency**   Speak fluently and do not use jargon.

☐☐☐ **Summarise**   Check with the patient and deliver an appropriate summary.

'This is Miss Carey, a 76-year-old song writer. She was admitted to hospital last night following a suicide attempt by taking 10 paracetamol tablets with alcohol. She states that she has been suffering from a number of chronic illnesses, including COPD and epilepsy, which have severely restricted her quality of life. She mentions that her family are finding it difficult to cope with her needs and are considering transferring her to a residential home. She states that this was the final straw and last night wanted to 'end it all'. She believed that the 10 tablets of paracetamol with alcohol would kill her and left a suicide note by her side. She was surprised when her son found her in the early hours of the morning. She continues to describe suicidal intent and is unhappy that this attempt was unsuccessful. In view of her history and current mental state, I believe that Miss Carey is still at high risk of suicide and I would recommend her to be admitted and observed in hospital by a psychiatrist.'

EXAMINER'S EVALUATION

0 1 2 3 4 5

☐☐☐☐☐☐ Overall assessment of elderly suicide risk
☐☐☐☐☐☐ Role player's score
Total mark out of 37

GERIATRICS: Abbreviated Mental Test Score (AMTS)

INSTRUCTIONS: You are a foundation year doctor in care-of-the-elderly. Mr Dawkins has attended today as his family members have been telling him that he is becoming a little forgetful. Perform an abbreviated mental test score (AMTS) screen and provide an interpretation of your findings.

INTRODUCTION

0 1 2

☐☐☐ **Introduction**   Introduce yourself to the patient as appropriate and establish rapport with him.

Name & Occ.   Elicit the patient's name and former occupation.

HISTORY

☐☐☐ **Problems**   Elicit the patient's awareness of his forgetfulness and memory loss. Elicit the patient's concerns regarding this problem.

☐☐☐ **Explain**   'I am going to ask you a series of questions and ask you to carry out a number of commands to assess your mental state. The commands may appear a little silly but we routinely ask all our patients these.'

ABBREVIATED MENTAL TEST SCORE

NOTE: One point is scored for each correct answer with a maximum of 10 points awarded. A score of six or less suggests the possibility of dementia or, in an acute setting, delirium. Further investigations and more formal tests are needed for a reliable diagnosis. More detailed screening tests include the 30-point mini mental state examination (MMSE). Other factors which can lead to low scores include poor cooperation from the patient, poor understanding of the English language, hearing difficulties, depression and receptive or expressive dysphasia.

10.4

☐☐☐ **Age**   Could you tell me how old you are? (Score 1)

☐☐☐ **Time**   Could you tell me what time it is without looking at a clock? (Score 1)

The time should be stated to the nearest hour to be awarded a point.

☐☐☐ **Address**   I am going to tell you an address. Could you repeat it back to me? 42 West Street.

Ask the patient to repeat the address at the end of the test. A point can only be given if the patient successfully recalls the address at the end of the test. A point is not awarded for repetition.

☐☐☐ **Year**   Could you tell me what year it is? (Score 1)

☐☐☐ **Location**   Could you tell me the name of the building (hospital/surgery/clinic) we are currently in? (Score 1)

☐☐☐ **Recognition**   Could you tell me what my job is? Next gesture to a nurse and ask, 'Could you tell me what that person's job is?' (Score 1)

Only one point can be awarded for correctly recognising two peoples' roles.

☐☐☐ **Date of Birth**   Could you tell me your date of birth? (Score 1)

☐☐☐ **WWII Date**   Could you tell me when the Second World War started? (Score 1)

☐☐☐ **Monarch**   What is the name of the current monarch (or current PM)? (Score 1)

☐☐☐ **Counting**   Ask the patient to count backwards from 20 to 1. (Score 1)

☐☐☐ **Recall**   Ask the patient to recall the address stated to the patient earlier. (Score 1)

☐☐☐ **Total**   Calculate the patient's AMTS score. (Total out of 10)

☐☐☐ **Closing**   Thank the patient for their time and state that you would like take a collateral history and perform a 30-point MMSE if indicated.

COMMUNICATION SKILLS

☐☐☐ **Rapport**   Establish and maintain rapport with the patient and demonstrate listening skills.

☐☐☐ **Response**   React positively to and acknowledge the patient's emotions.

☐☐☐ **Fluency**   Speak fluently and do not use jargon.

☐☐☐ **Summary**   Check with the patient and deliver an appropriate summary.

EXAMINER'S EVALUATION

0 1 2 3 4 5

☐☐☐☐☐☐ Overall assessment of performing AMTS

☐☐☐☐☐☐ Role player's score

Total mark out of 31

GERIATRICS: **Activities of Daily Living (ADL)**

INSTRUCTIONS: You are a foundation year House Officer. Mrs Sharone has been in hospital for a month following a stroke that has caused weakness to her right arm and leg. She has been performing well with OT and physiotherapy and may be discharged in the coming weeks. Assess the patient in order to prepare a discharge plan. You will be marked on your ability to perform the assessment and your communication skills.

INTRODUCTION

0 1 2

☐☐☐ **Introduction**   Introduce yourself to the patient and confirm their name and age.

☐☐☐ **Purpose**   Explain the purpose of the consultation.

'I understand that you have been in hospital for 1 month now. The consultant in charge of your care is considering planning for your discharge soon. I am here to ask you a few questions regarding what treatments you received in hospital and what you understand by your condition. I am also going to ask you what issues you think there might be surrounding your discharge home and whether you think any changes may need to be made there. Is it OK for me to proceed?'

HISTORY

✷ Elicit the Patient's understanding of their situation

☐☐☐ **Ideas**   Establish the patient's understanding of their planned discharge. What have they already been told?

☐☐☐ **Concerns**   Does the patient have any particular concerns with her illness or with going home? Find out if the patient has home help or a social network.

☐☐☐ **Home**   Establish the patient's type of accommodation, and whether she will have to use stairs or a stair lift. Is there anyone else at her home and in what ways do they help her? Was the patient receiving any social services before admission that need to be restarted?

☐☐☐ **Treatment**   Establish from patient what treatments she has been given.

'You have had a stroke that has left you with a degree of disability. Unfortunately, you will not be at the same level of function as you were prior to the stroke. However, I wish to assess how well you have been functioning in a number of areas whilst you have been in hospital as we can offer some services that may be able to assist you to live

10.5

359

as independently as possible. Is it all right for me to ask you a few questions regarding how you have been coping on the ward?'

✴ Assessment of ADLs

☐☐☐ **Washing**   Have you managed to wash yourself on the ward? Do you require help?

☐☐☐ **Dressing**   Have you been able to dress yourself? Do you have any difficulty with grooming such as combing and shaving? Do you need assistance?

☐☐☐ **Mobility**   Are you able to walk independently? Do you require a frame, stick or wheelchair?

☐☐☐ **Transferring** Are you able to stand from sitting and get out of bed on your own?

☐☐☐ **Stairs**   Are you able to manage the stairs?

☐☐☐ **Cooking**   Are you able to cook a meal? What can you do by yourself?

☐☐☐ **Feeding**   Have you been managing to eat and drink yourself? Do you have any difficulty cutting your food or with chewing and swallowing? Do you require any special food thickeners?

☐☐☐ **Continence**   Have you had any accidents with passing stools or urine? Does this happen all the time or only on occasions?

✴ Patient's Discharge Needs

☐☐☐ **Carers**   Identify any need for carers to help with washing and dressing.

☐☐☐ **Single Level** Identify whether the patient is unable to walk up stairs and advise her to seek single floor accommodation.

☐☐☐ **Shopping**   Identify the need to organise shopping delivery for the patient.

☐☐☐ **Meal Prep.**   Identify if the patient is unable to cook and suggest 'Meals on Wheels'.

☐☐☐ **Continence**   Explain need for a commode next to bed and the use of continence pads.

When assessing a patient's discharge needs, it is important to know the services each department can offer. The **mnemonic SPOTS** is a useful tool for remembering which services are involved in discharging elderly patients.

Social services	This service can help in a number of areas, from establishing entitlement for financial benefits, arranging carers and services that provide freshly cooked meals, and deal with issues regarding suitable accommodation needs. They can also arrange respite care and can deal with the financial issues pertaining to home modification and care homes
Physiotherapist	Movement specialists who can help to identify the root mechanical cause of a disability and can improve function through exercise or compensation
OT	Occupational therapists are able to provide aids and adaptations but also have an important role by working with physiotherapists to improve function, in their case using occupation or functional skills to improve balance, strength and sequencing to ultimately improve rehabilitation
Other	Other services that can assist include the continence nursing, speech and language (also deal with swallowing issues), district nurses (providing wound care and support at home) and dieticians (assessing patients' nutritional needs)

CLOSING

☐ ☐ ☐ **Follow-up**　　Offer the patient an outpatient appointment.

☐ ☐ ☐ **Understanding**　　Check that the patient has understood the information provided.

☐ ☐ ☐ **Questions**　　Encourage patient's questions and respond to them.

The Barthel Index

The Barthel Index (BI) or score has been recommended for the functional assessment of elderly patients. It consists of 10 categories that assess a patient's activities of daily living such as mobility, self-grooming and eating. The score is ranked out of 20 with higher scores suggestive of a more 'independent' person. It is a useful tool to assess whether extra services or needs are required for a patient on discharge and whether it is safe for them to go home

Bowels	Control bowels with no accidents	Bladder control	Urinary control day and night
0	Incontinent	0	Incontinent (or catheterised)
1	Occasional accident	1	Occasional accident
2	Continent	2	Continent (manages catheter alone)
Grooming	Brush teeth, shaving and washing	Bathing	Getting in and out of the bath and wash
0	Needs help	0	Dependent
1	Independent	1	Independent
Mobility	Ability to mobilise in house	Transfer	Ability to get up from a bed or chair
0	Immobile or <50 metres	0	Unable
1	Wheel chair independent	1	Major help
2	Walks with help	2	Minor help
3	Independent	3	Independent
Eating	Ability to eat food independently	Un/dressing	Ability to put clothes on and off
0	Unable to eat unassisted	0	Dependent
1	Needs help	1	Needs help
2	Independent	2	Independent
Toilet use	Ability to independently use the toilet	Stairs	Ability to negotiate stairs
0	Dependent	0	Unable
1	Needs help	1	Needs help
2	Independent	2	Independent
Total	Total score out of 20. Scores 0–9: high dependency, 10–19: moderate dependency, 20: independent		

COMMUNICATION SKILLS

☐☐☐ **Rapport** — Establish rapport with the patient and maintain it throughout the interview.

☐☐☐ **Listening** — Demonstrate interest and concern in what the patient says. Show active listening and listen empathically.

☐☐☐ **Summary** — Give a brief summary to the patient about what has been discussed. Jointly agree on an action plan and conclude the interview.

'I am happy to hear that despite your illness you are able to provide help for yourself in a number of areas and you have demonstrated this whilst on the ward. However, there are a few areas in which you need some assistance and I feel we can offer some help. Regarding your problems with washing and dressing, we are able to provide carers who will come to visit you at regular intervals during the day to help you wake up, dress and wash you. As you are no longer able to use the stairs, we recommend you should live on a single level downstairs so that your bed, toilet or commode and kitchen are on the ground floor. As you are finding it difficult to cook for yourself, we can offer a service where we provide ready cooked hot meals for you to eat. We can also organise someone to do your shopping. Regarding issues with continence, we can provide you with pads which should help avoid any messy accidents. We also suggest you place a commode next to your bed in case you need to go in the night. Are you happy with these arrangements?'

EXAMINER'S EVALUATION

0 1 2 3 4 5

☐ ☐ ☐ ☐ ☐ ☐ Overall assessment of assessing ADL

☐ ☐ ☐ ☐ ☐ ☐ Role player's score

Total mark out of 37

Palliative Care

PALLIATIVE CARE: **Pain Management**

INSTRUCTIONS: You are a foundation year House Officer in outpatients. You are asked to see Mrs Kalie, a 45-year-old woman with advanced metastatic breast cancer who is complaining of increasing back pain. You will be marked on the information you provide and your communication skills.

INTRODUCTION

0 1 2

☐☐☐ **Introduction** — Introduce yourself appropriately to the patient and establish rapport with her.

☐☐☐ **Ideas** — Explore the patient's ideas of what she believes may be causing her symptoms.

☐☐☐ **Concerns** — Explore any concerns the patient may have regarding her symptoms.

Expectations — Explore the patient's expectations of what she hopes to achieve during this consultation.

FOCUSED HISTORY

☐☐☐ **Pain** — Ask about where the pain is (site), its severity, time of its onset and character (dull/sharp/colicky or cramp-like). Elicit where the pain radiates and any exacerbating or relieving factors (posture, straining, eating, coughing).

Carcinomas that Metastasise to the Bone
Mnemonic: 'Kinds Of Tumours Leaping Promptly To Bone'
Kidney, Ovary, Testis, Lung, Prostate, Thyroid, Breast

11.1

☐☐☐ **Assoc. Symp.** — Enquire about fever, nausea and vomiting and pain (in the chest or abdomen). Enquire about fatigue, weight loss, changes in appetite and neurological symptoms (urinary and faecal incontinence, leg numbness and weakness – metastases).

☐☐☐ **Impact on Life** — Enquire how this symptom has impacted on her life.

Experience of Pain

Type	Features
Pleural/peritoneal	Well-localised pain exacerbated by inspiration
Visceral Pain	Pain is poorly localised and may refer to other sites (pain is experienced in epigastrium and can radiate to upper lumbar spine)

	Retroperitoneal structures (e.g. pancreas except tail), finds pain worse on lying down and is relieved by sitting forward flexed
Biliary/ureteric/bowel	Episodic colicky/cramp-like pain
Bone/somatic	Often aching, dull and localised over the involved bone. Worse when stressed, e.g. weight bearing. It is typically worse at night
Neuropathic	Pain can be continuous or intermittent, and experienced in the distribution of a peripheral nerve or nerve root. Pain is often described as stabbing, burning or cold. Numbness, paraesthesia and allodynia are common

ASSOCIATED HISTORY

☐☐☐ **Medical History**   Enquire about any past medical history. Has the patient received any chemotherapy or radiotherapy and if so, how many cycles of treatment? Enquire about the prognosis of cancer and whether there are any metastases. Ask about a history of back pain, sciatica, falls, osteoporosis and disc prolapse. Ask about history of ulcers, asthma, heart and renal failure.

☐☐☐ **Drug History**   Establish current medications, including analgesia (NSAIDs – aspirin, opiate – fentanyl patch, morphine sulphate tablets, tramadol, co-codamol, co-dydramol). Enquire about how analgesia is administered (patches, PR, oral, syringe driver). Check patient sensitivities and allergies.

Variable Strengths of Analgesia		
Opioid	**Dose**	**Relative (Oramorph)**
Codeine	60 mg/qds, PO	0.1
Dihydrocodeine	60 mg/qds, PO	0.1
Pethidine	100 mg/qds, PO	0.175
Tramadol	50 mg/qds, PO	0.2
Pethidine	100 mg/qds, i.m.	0.375
Oramorph/MST	10 mg/4 hrly, PO	1
Oxycodone	5 mg/4 hrly, PO	2
Morphine	5 mg/1–4 hrly, sc, i.v., im	2
Diamorphine	2.5 mg/1–4 hrly, sc	3
Fentanyl	25 mcg/hour	150

☐☐☐ **Mental State**   Enquire about how their current symptom has affected their mood. Note that a psychosocial assessment is important, as depression and anxiety are associated with intractable pain.

☐☐☐ **Social History** Establish her home situation – does she live alone, does she receive help from friends, family or carers? Is she able to get out of the house much? Does she have any contact with a palliative care specialist or a Macmillan nurse?

SYMPTOM MANAGEMENT

Treatment Discuss with the patient the different options available for the treatment of her symptoms (pharmacological and non-pharmacological) and arrive at an agreed management plan.

☐☐☐ *Non-pharm.* Recommend rest, massages and acupuncture for the pain, and the avoidance of heavy lifting. Consider non-opioid analgesia (TENS, nerve blocks).

☐☐☐ *Pharmacological* After ascertaining the patient's current analgesic regime, consider optimising pain management by stepping up the WHO analgesic ladder or different routes (intranasal, PR, transdermal, SC).

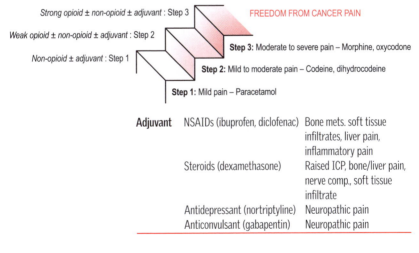

The Analgesic Ladder for Control of Pain
The WHO Three-Step Ladder for Cancer Pain Relief

Strong opioid ± non-opioid ± adjuvant : Step 3

Weak opioid ± non-opioid ± adjuvant : Step 2

Non-opioid ± adjuvant : Step 1

FREEDOM FROM CANCER PAIN

Step 3: Moderate to severe pain – Morphine, oxycodone

Step 2: Mild to moderate pain – Codeine, dihydrocodeine

Step 1: Mild pain – Paracetamol

Adjuvant		
	NSAIDs (ibuprofen, diclofenac)	Bone mets. soft tissue infiltrates, liver pain, inflammatory pain
	Steroids (dexamethasone)	Raised ICP, bone/liver pain, nerve comp., soft tissue infiltrate
	Antidepressant (nortriptyline)	Neuropathic pain
	Anticonvulsant (gabapentin)	Neuropathic pain

CLOSING

☐☐☐ **Follow-up** Offer the patient an outpatient appointment to review her response to treatment.

☐☐☐ **Understanding**　　Check that the patient understands the information provided.

Questions　　Encourage patient's questions and respond to them.

The Liverpool Care of the Dying Pathway

Approximately 16% of cancer-related deaths and less than 5% of non-cancer deaths occur in a hospice. The Liverpool Care of the Dying Pathway attempts to transfer best practice in the dying phase from the hospice model to the hospital setting. This is a framework that guides the multidisciplinary team in making decisions on the continuation or discontinuation of treatment and comfort measures during the last few hours of life. It emphasises the need to combine physical treatment with psychological support for both the patient and carer while taking into account the religious and spiritual desires of the individual. The patient and carer should be made aware that the focus of care has now changed from active treatment to more a palliative approach as the patient nears the end of their life

---

COMMUNICATION SKILLS

☐☐☐ **Rapport**　　Establish and maintain rapport with the patient throughout the interview.

☐☐☐ **Listening**　　Demonstrate an interest and concern in what the patient says. Show active listening and listen empathetically.

☐☐☐ **Verbal Cues**　　Use non-verbal and verbal cues, i.e. tone and pace of voice, and nodding head where appropriate.

☐☐☐ **Summarise**　　Give a brief summary to the patient about what has been discussed. Jointly agree on an action plan.

'This is Mrs Kalie, a 45-year-old woman suffering from advanced breast cancer that is now being treated palliatively. She had a right-sided mastectomy a number of years ago for her breast cancer. Unfortunately a CT scan of her back revealed significant metastases. Today she has been complaining of continuous pain in her back for the last month that has not been controlled by her slow-release morphine sulphate tablets. She states that the pain is severe and often disturbs her sleep. Her concern is that she will be living out her last remaining days in significant pain. It appears that Mrs Kalie's pain is not adequately controlled by her morphine sulphate tablets. In view of her discomfort I would recommend commencing a morphine syringe driver infusion according to the Liverpool Care Pathway and have her reviewed in the community by a palliative care nurse to ensure she is comfortable and pain free.'

0 1 2 3 4 5

☐ ☐ ☐ ☐ ☐ ☐ Overall assessment of pain management

☐ ☐ ☐ ☐ ☐ ☐ Role player's score

Total mark out of 32

PALLIATIVE CARE: Nausea and Vomiting Management

INSTRUCTIONS: You are a foundation year House Officer in outpatients. You are asked to see Mr Duke, who is an 83-year-old man with advanced colorectal cancer and is complaining of vomiting and feeling nauseous. Take a history and summarise your findings to the examiner.

INTRODUCTION

0 1 2

☐☐☐ **Introduction** Introduce yourself appropriately to the patient and establish rapport with him.

☐☐☐ **Ideas** Explore the patient's ideas of what he believes may be causing his symptoms.

☐☐☐ **Concerns** Explore any concerns the patient may have regarding his symptoms.

Expectations Explore the patient's expectations of what he hopes to achieve during this consultation.

FOCUSED HISTORY

☐☐☐ **N & V** Ask about when the nausea and vomiting first started (onset), how often it is (frequency) and how much is vomited (volume)? Enquire about the colour of the vomit and its content (bilious, faecal, coffee-ground, blood).

☐☐☐ *Timing* Note when the vomiting occurs. Is it after meals (gastric stasis), or on moving (vestibular disease) or does it wake the patient up (meningeal irritation/ raised ICP)? Establish if the nausea dissipates after prolonged periods of vomiting or if it persists. Note that nausea tends to predominate in chemical causes such as hypercalcaemia and renal failure.

☐☐☐ **Assoc. Symp.** Ask about abdominal pain and distension, time of last bowel motion (constipation – hypercalcaemia) and his ability to pass flatus (bowel obstruction), the passage of urine (obstructive renal failure), indigestion, headaches (ICP), vertigo and tinnitus (vestibular disease). Enquire about weight loss, change in appetite and neurological symptoms (mets).

11.2

☐☐☐ **Impact on Life**   Enquire about how these symptoms have impacted on his life.

Causes and Features of Vomiting

Causes	Features
Anxiety related	Nausea occurring in waves or spasms
Motion sickness	Nausea and vomiting on simple movement
Bowel obstruction	Abdominal pain (colicky), distension, worsening nausea and vomiting (vomiting is a late sign in large bowel)
Gastric stasis	Infrequent large volume vomiting followed by relief of symptom. Associated with hiccups, reflux, early epigastric fullness
Gastric outflow obst.	Associated with projectile vomiting
Oesophageal obst.	Sensation of food sticking in the oesophagus. Vomiting of unaltered food after ingestion
Chemical induced	Constant nausea with varying amounts of vomiting
Raised ICP	Early morning headaches with nausea and vomiting (can wake patient). Photophobia and papilloedema

---

ASSOCIATED HISTORY

☐☐☐ **Medical History**   Enquire about any past medical history. Has the patient received any chemotherapy or radiotherapy and how many cycles have they been given? Enquire about the prognosis of cancer and whether there are any metastases. Ask about motion sickness, endocrine conditions (DM, Addison's), previous reflux, ulcers (*Helicobacter pylori* test), surgery and adhesions.

☐☐☐ **Drug History**   Establish current medications including analgesia (NSAIDs – aspirin, opiate – morphine sulphate tablets, tramadol, co-codamol, co-dydramol), iron tablets, digoxin and antibiotics (erythromycin, gentamicin, cephalosporin). Check the patient's sensitivities and allergies.

Mental State   Enquire how his current symptom has affected his mood.

☐☐☐ **Social History**   Establish home situation – does he live alone, is he receiving help from friends, family or carers? Is he able to get out of the house much? Does he have any contact with a palliative care specialist or Macmillan nurse?

SYMPTOM MANAGEMENT

Treatment   Discuss with the patient the different options available for the treatment of his symptoms (pharmacological and non-pharmacological) and arrive at an agreed management plan.

☐☐☐ *Non-pharm.*   Recommend small palatable meals. If possible suggest he avoids exposure to foods or cooking that may precipitate the nausea. Ask him to consider requesting somebody else to cook for him or purchase prepared foods (to avoid contact with precipitants such as smells). Review his drugs and reduce or stop any identifiable offending medication.

☐☐☐ *Pharmacological*   Consider prescribing an antiemetic and describe to the patient the different forms available. Consider oral medication in mild nausea and vomiting (≤1/day) and subcutaneous or rectal routes for moderate forms of nausea. Severe or continuous symptoms may require a syringe driver.

Choice of Antiemetic

Causes	Antiemetic
Raised intracranial pressure	Cyclizine
Drug induced/chemical/metabolic	Haloperidol
Unknown or GI obstruction without colic	Metoclopramide
GI obstruction with colic	Hyoscine butylbromide
Gastric irritation	Stop the NSAIDs and PPI
Radiotherapy or chemotherapy	Granisetron
Multiple causes	Levomepromazine (broad spectrum)

CLOSING

☐☐☐ **Follow-up**   Offer the patient an outpatient appointment to review treatment response.

☐☐☐ **Understanding**   Check that the patient understands information provided.

Questions   Encourage the patient to ask questions and respond to them.

COMMUNICATION SKILLS

☐☐☐ **Rapport**   Establish rapport with the patient and maintain it throughout interview.

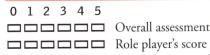 **Listening**   Demonstrate interest and concern in what the patient says. Show active listening and listen empathetically.

Verbal Cues   Use non-verbal and verbal cues, i.e. an appropriate tone and pace of voice, nodding head where appropriate.

Summarise   Give a brief summary to the patient of what has been discussed. Jointly agree on an action plan.

'This is Mr Duke, an 83-year-old man suffering from advanced colorectal cancer. He has failed to respond to a course of chemotherapy 3 months ago and is now being treated palliatively. A recent CT scan for his back pain has revealed secondary metastases for which he was commenced on morphine sulphate tablets 10 mg qds and metoclopramide. For the last two weeks he has been suffering from increased nausea and vomiting. The vomiting occurs at any time of the day and bears no relationship to meal times. There is no constipation or haematemesis. His main concern is that he is unable to keep food down and is feeling more fatigued. I suspect that Mr Duke's symptoms are a result of inadequate antiemetic cover for his analgesia and are unlikely to be a result of his failed chemotherapy. I would recommend changing his antiemetic to cyclizine and review the patient's analgesia (start long-acting morphine with low-dose morphine for break-through pain)'.

EXAMINER'S EVALUATION

0 1 2 3 4 5

☐ ☐ ☐ ☐ ☐ ☐ Overall assessment of nausea & vomiting management

☐ ☐ ☐ ☐ ☐ ☐ Role player's score

Total mark out of 35

PALLIATIVE CARE: **Dyspnoea Management**

INSTRUCTIONS: You are a foundation year House Officer in outpatients. You are asked to see Mrs Hamlet, a 63-year-old woman with a non-small cell carcinoma. You are here to review this woman as she has been referred from the community health centre because the district nurse is concerned about her increasing shortness of breath. Take a history and summarise your findings to the examiner.

INTRODUCTION

0 1 2

☐☐☐ **Introduction**   Introduce yourself appropriately and establish rapport with the patient.

☐☐☐ **Ideas**   Explore the patient's ideas of what she believes may be causing her symptoms.

☐☐☐ **Concerns**   Explore any concerns the patient may have regarding her symptoms.

Expectations   Explore the patient's expectations of what she hopes to achieve during this consultation.

FOCUSED HISTORY

☐☐☐ **Dyspnoea**   Ask about when the breathlessness started (onset acute or gradual), its nature (intermittent, continuous or exercise-induced), exacerbation and relieving factors (exertion, posture, environmental and stress). Establish whether the dyspnoea affects her sleep (are pillows required, orthopnoea, paroxysmal nocturnal dyspnoea).

☐☐☐ **Assoc. Symp.**   Do not assume that the patient's breathlessness is directly caused by her cancer. Enquire about wheezing, hoarseness of voice, stridor (airway obstruction), fever, cough, sputum (pneumonia), pleuritic chest pain, calf tenderness, haemoptysis (PE), lethargy (anaemia), chest pain, sweating (angina/MI) or palpitations (arrhythmia). Also enquire about weight loss, change in appetite and neurological symptoms (mets).

☐☐☐ **Impact on Life**   Enquire about how this symptom has impacted on her life.

11.3

☐☐☐ **Medical History** Enquire about any past medical history. Has the patient received any chemotherapy or radiotherapy and how many cycles has she been given? Enquire about the prognosis of cancer and whether there are any metastases. Ask about heart failure, asthma, COPD, previous PE and DVTs.

☐☐☐ **Drug History** Establish her current medications including analgesia (NSAIDs – aspirin, opiate – morphine sulphate tablets, tramadol, co-codamol, co-dydramol), digoxin and antibiotics (erythromycin, gentamicin, cephalosporin). Check the patient's sensitivities and allergies.

Mental State Enquire about how her current symptoms have affected her mood.

Social History Establish her home situation – does she live alone, is she receiving help from friends, family or carers? Is she able to get out of the house much? Does she have any contact with a palliative care specialist or Macmillan nurse?

SYMPTOM MANAGEMENT

Treatment Discuss with the patient the different options available for the treatment of her symptoms (pharmacological and non-pharmacological) and arrive at an agreed management plan.

☐☐☐ *Non-pharm.* Recommend breathing and relaxation techniques (positioning, breathing exercises) that can be helpful in controlling her dyspnoea. Encourage the patient to exercise to increase her exercise tolerance. Directing a stream of air (fan) over her face may reduced the sensation of breathlessness. Suggest she keeps the room cool and improves the air ventilation (fan, window). Establish a good position that is comfortable for the patient (sitting upright or forwards eases chest muscles and diaphragm).

☐☐☐ *Pharmacological* Treatment depends on the suspected cause.

Symptomatic Treatment of Dysnopea in Palliative Care

Treatment	Indication
Corticosteroids	Emergency airway obstruction (from tumour or superior vena cava obstruction)
Bronchodilators	Interim measure in partial airway obstruction or as a trial when definitive treatment is not appropriate. Also where reversible airway obstruction is present (asthma/COPD)
Opioids	Symptomatic relief of dyspnoea towards end of life
Benzodiazepines	Dyspnoea associated with anxiety
Oxygen	Dyspnoeic patients with oxygen saturations of ≤90%

Treatment of Specific Causes

Pneumonia	Antibiotics
Anaemia	Blood transfusions, iron tablets, erythropoietin
Pleural effusion	Pleural tap and pleurodesis (recurrent effusions)
Heart failure	Diuretics/ACE inhibitor
Ascites	Ascitic tap
Airway obstruction	Radiotherapy, stent, corticosteroids
Pulmonary embolism	Anticoagulation therapy (LMWH, warfarin)

CLOSING

☐☐☐ **Follow-up** Offer the patient an outpatient appointment to review treatment response.

☐☐☐ **Understanding** Check that the patient understands the information provided.

Questions Encourage the patient to ask questions and respond to them.

COMMUNICATION SKILLS

☐☐☐ **Rapport** Establish rapport with the patient and maintain it throughout interview.

☐☐☐ **Listening** Demonstrate an interest and concern in what the patient says. Show active listening and listen empathetically.

☐☐☐ **Verbal Cues** Use non-verbal and verbal cues, i.e. an appropriate tone and pace of voice, nodding head where appropriate.

☐☐☐ **Summarise** Give a brief summary to the patient about what has been discussed. Jointly agree on an action plan.

'This is Mrs Hamlet, a 63-year-old woman suffering from advanced lung cancer which is now being treated palliatively. She has been complaining of a gradual onset of shortness of breath over the last 2 weeks. Over this time she has had a swinging temperature, productive cough with green sputum and some pleuritic chest pain. The patient is concerned that her breathlessness is affecting her day-to-day activities. She has been gasping for air on exertion and is now struggling to climb the flight of stairs to her apartment. I suspect that Mrs Hamlet's symptoms are caused by a chest infection for which I would like to start a course of antibiotics. However, I would like to carry out a full examination and request for a chest X-ray and a set of blood tests to rule out other potential causes (pleural effusion, pulmonary embolism).'

EXAMINER'S EVALUATION

0 1 2 3 4 5

☐ ☐ ☐ ☐ ☐ ☐ Overall assessment of dyspnoea treatment

☐ ☐ ☐ ☐ ☐ ☐ Role player's score

Total mark out of 32

PALLIATIVE CARE: **Constipation Management**

INSTRUCTIONS: You are a foundation year House Officer in outpatients. You are asked to see Mr Bowell, who is 65-year-old man with advanced prostate cancer, and is complaining of constipation and excessive flatulence. Take a history and summarise your findings to the examiner.

INTRODUCTION

0 1 2

☐☐☐ **Introduction**   Introduce yourself appropriately to the patient and establish rapport with him.

☐☐☐ **Ideas**   Explore the patient's ideas of what he believes may be causing his symptoms.

☐☐☐ **Concerns**   Explore any concerns the patient may have regarding his symptoms.

Expectations   Explore the patient's expectations of what he hopes to achieve during this consultation.

FOCUSED HISTORY

☐☐☐ **Constipation**   Ask the patient what he means by 'constipation'. Ask when it started (onset), how often he passes stools (frequency), its quality (soft, hard) and quantity (large, small)? Enquire whether the stools are painful to pass. Ask if the patient has been immobile over the past few weeks.

11.4

Constipation

There is often a disparity in the understanding of the word 'constipation' between doctors and patients. It is often used by patients to describe painful hard stools or the sensation of incomplete emptying rather than the medical definition of an infrequent passage of stools (<3/week). It is always important to clarify the patient's own understanding of the word 'constipation' before going down the path of misdiagnosing and mistreating. Treatment is important in order to avoid complications (pain, bowel obstruction, overflow diarrhoea, urinary retention)

Causes of Constipation

Dietary	Dehydration, lack of fluid intake, poor diet (low fibre)
Drugs	Opioids, diuretics, aluminium antacids, iron and calcium supplements, anticholinergics (TCAs), calcium channel blocker
Bowel	Bowel obstruction (abdominal pain, distension, vomiting, tinkling bowel sounds), colon carcinoma (abdominal pain, weight loss, PR blood, mass),

	diverticular disease, stricture, irritable bowel syndrome
Anal	Anal fissure (perianal tags), haemorrhoids (fresh PR blood on toilet paper, pain)
Endocrine	Hypothyroidism, hypokalaemia, hypercalcaemia
Neuro.	Spinal cord injury, autonomic neuropathy

☐☐☐ **Bowel Habits**   Establish the patient's normal bowel habits, including their frequency, quality and quantity. Identify the presence of altered bowel habits. Ask about episodes of loose stools in between periods of constipation (overflow diarrhoea).

☐☐☐ **Assoc. Symp.**   Ask about abdominal pain and distension, nausea and vomiting, PR bleeding (fresh, melaena) and ability to pass flatus. Enquire about back pain (constant, even at night), weight loss, change in appetite and neurological symptoms (mets).

☐☐☐ **Impact on Life**   Enquire about how this symptom has impacted on their life. Note depression in its own right can cause constipation.

ASSOCIATED HISTORY

☐☐☐ **Medical History**   Enquire about any past medical history. Has the patient received any chemotherapy or radiotherapy and how many cycles has he been given? Enquire about the prognosis of cancer and whether there are any metastases.

☐☐☐ **Drug History**   Establish current medications including analgesia (opiate – morphine sulphate tablets, tramadol, co-codamol, co-dydramol), anticholinergics (TCA – amitriptyline), iron supplements and aluminium salts. Check the patient's sensitivities and allergies.

☐☐☐ **Mental State**   Enquire about how his current symptom has affected his mood.

☐☐☐ **Social History**   Establish his home situation – does he live alone, is he receiving help from friends, family or carers? Is he able to get out of the house much? Does he have any contact with a palliative care specialist or a Macmillan nurse?

SYMPTOM MANAGEMENT

Treatment Discuss with the patient the different options available for the treatment of his symptoms (pharmacological and non-pharmacological) and arrive at an agreed management plan.

□□□ *Non-pharm.* Advise the patient to drink at least 2 litres of fluid a day and ensure adequate fibre intake. Encourage the patient to mobilise. Also discuss opioid rationalisation – drop down pain ladder or stop offending medication.

Effects and Side Effects of Morphine
Mnemonic: 'MORPHINE'

Miosis	**H**ypotension
Out of it (sedation)	**I**nfrequency (constipation, urinary retention)
Respiratory depression	**N**ausea
Pain relief	**E**mesis, Euphoria

□□□ *Pharmacological* Consider prescribing a laxative and describe the different forms available (stimulant, softeners, osmotic laxatives).

Choices of Laxative for Constipation

Types	Laxative
Faecal impaction	Arachis oil enema (night), phosphate enema (morning)
Stimulant	(Senna, bisacodyl, co-danthramer) increase intestinal peristalsis but can cause diarrhoea, abdominal cramps and hypokalaemia. Avoid in intestinal obstruction, consider for opioid induced constipation
Softeners	(Docusate, co-danthramer) promote defaecation through softening or lubricating the faeces. Safer in resolving intestinal obstruction
Osmotic	(Movicol, lactulose) increase the amount of water in the bowel by drawing it in or retaining fluid administered with it. Avoid in palliative care (requires 2 L of water to function). Lactulose can cause flatus and bloating

Constipation	Laxative
Mild	Senna or bisacodyl, docusate, lactulose or movicol
Moderate to severe	Co-danthramer (dual stimulant and softener), glycerine suppositories

EVALUATION

☐☐☐ **Follow-up**   Offer the patient an outpatient appointment to review treatment response.

☐☐☐ **Understanding**   Check that the patient understands the information provided.

Questions   Encourage the patient to ask questions and respond to them.

COMMUNICATION SKILLS

☐☐☐ **Rapport**   Establish rapport with the patient and maintain it throughout the interview.

☐☐☐ **Listening**   Demonstrate an interest and concern in what the patient says. Show active listening and listen empathetically.

☐☐☐ **Verbal Cues**   Use non-verbal and verbal cues, i.e. an appropriate tone and pace of voice, nodding head where appropriate.

☐☐☐ **Summarise**   Give a brief summary to the patient about what has been discussed. Jointly agree on an action plan.

'This is Mr Bowell, a 65-year-old man suffering from advanced prostate cancer which is being treated palliatively. He is complaining for the last 2 weeks of abdominal bloating, pain and less frequent bowel motions. He is not vomiting and is passing flatus. He normally goes daily but recently has been opening his bowels every 2 to 3 days. Recently he has had his analgesia changed from co-dydramol to tramadol. He is concerned that he may suffer a recurrence of his painful haemorrhoids. Taking into consideration his medication, I suspect that Mr Bowell's constipation is secondary to opioids. I would recommend starting a laxative (docusate) and review the patient's analgesia (change to Tramacet). I also recommend that the patient drinks plenty of fluid and mobilises.'

EXAMINER'S EVALUATION

0 1 2 3 4 5

☐☐☐☐☐☐ Overall assessment of constipation treatment

☐☐☐☐☐☐ Role player's score

Total mark out of 36

Communication Skills

COMMUNICATION SKILLS: **Breaking Bad News**

INSTRUCTIONS: You are a foundation year House Officer in A&E. Mr Wallis' wife has been admitted for observation after falling off a ladder at home. She was unconscious for 5 minutes and is rather groggy. There is no skull fracture but she has a large scalp laceration and is awaiting an urgent CT scan. Inform Mr Wallis about the injury and the need for admission. You will be marked on communication skills, dealing with Mr Wallis' anxiety and the delivery of the information.

INTRODUCTION

0 1 2

☐☐☐ **Introduction** Introduce yourself to the relative. Confirm his name and relationship to the patient. Establish rapport with him.

☐☐☐ **Ideas** Elicit the relative's understanding of what is going on.

☐☐☐ **Concerns** Encourage the relative to express his concerns and deal with them appropriately.

☐☐☐ **Acknowledge** Acknowledge the relative's emotional state (recognise that he is fearful, anxious and angry).

'I understand that you have come to hospital to find out how your wife is doing. Can you tell me what have you been told so far? Has anything been explained to you already? Do you have any particular concerns you would like to raise?'

BREAKING THE NEWS

Breaking News Break the bad news empathetically, using pauses where appropriate. Pace the information provided using appropriate body language when necessary. Inform the relative about the details of the injury, the need for an urgent CT scan and possible hospital admission.

12.1

☐☐☐ *Injury* 'I'm afraid that I have some difficult news for you. Unfortunately, earlier on today your wife suffered an injury whilst at home. She was adjusting the TV aerial when she fell off her ladder and cut her forehead. She remained unconscious for a few minutes and at the moment appears a little confused. Thankfully, an X-ray has shown that there are no fractures to her skull. However, she has got quite a large wound on her head that needs stitches.'

☐☐☐ *CT Scan* 'I must inform you that because of the mechanism of the injury and the fact that she was unconscious we will be performing an urgent CT scan of her head to make sure that no serious internal harm has been done.'

□□□ *Admission*　　'We will be transferring her to one of the wards for close observation after the CT scan to make sure that she does not deteriorate overnight. In the morning we will reassess the situation and in light of the results decide if she is fit to go home.'

CLOSING

□□□ **Questions**　　Encourage the relative to ask questions.

'I appreciate that this has come as quite a shock to you and you are obviously concerned. Do you have any questions about what I have told you? Is there anything that still concerns you? Would you like any more information?'

□□□ **Understanding**　　Check the relative understands what has been explained.

'I know that I have given you a lot of information already. Is there anything you would like me to repeat or clarify?'

□□□ **Summarise**　　Summarise back to the relative what has been discussed.

'I am sorry to have had to break the news to you. It must be quite a shock to you. I would like to recap what has been already discussed to check that you are clear as to what has happened . . .'

COMMUNICATION SKILLS

□□□ **Rapport**　　Attempt to establish rapport with the relative through the use of appropriate eye contact. Maintain appropriate body language and an open posture throughout.

□□□ **Behaviour**　　Avoid dismissing the relative's fears and concerns. Avoid offering inappropriate reassurance.

□□□ **Manner**　　Remain calm and clear (use an appropriate tone and pace of voice, use simple sentences). If the relative becomes agitated and tries to get up and leave, gently ask him to sit down.

□□□ **Listening**　　Demonstrate interest and concern in what the relative says. Show active listening and listen empathetically.

□□□ **Pauses**　　Pace the information and use appropriate pauses. Allow the relative to speak his feelings freely and without interruptions.

□□□ **Empathy**　　Demonstrate an empathetic response (offer emotional support and validate his concerns).

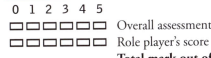 **Verbal Cues**   Use non-verbal and verbal cues, i.e. tone and pace of voice, nodding your head where appropriate.

EXAMINER'S EVALUATION

0 1 2 3 4 5

☐ ☐ ☐ ☐ ☐ ☐ Overall assessment of breaking bad news

☐ ☐ ☐ ☐ ☐ ☐ Role player's score

Total mark out of 29

COMMUNICATION SKILLS: **Angry Relatives**

INSTRUCTIONS: You are a foundation year House Officer in care-of-the-elderly. You have been looking after Mrs Gibbs, a frail old lady who was admitted 4 days previously with lower lobe pneumonia and had been started on broad-spectrum antibiotics. She is now is being transferred into a side room because she has developed diarrhoea. Her stool specimen is Clostridium difficile-toxin positive. You have been asked to see Mrs Gibbs's relatives who wish to complain about her treatment. Mrs Gibbs has already given you her consent to discuss the case with her relatives. You will be marked on your communication skills, your knowledge and your ability to deal with the issues surrounding their complaints.

INTRODUCTION

0 1 2

☐☐☐ **Introduction**   Introduce yourself. Confirm the relationship between the relatives and the patient.

☐☐☐ **Ideas**   Elicit the relatives' ideas and understanding of what is going on.

'I understand that you have asked to speak to a doctor about your relative Mrs Gibbs. I am one of the doctors involved in her care. Is there anything I can help you with?'

☐☐☐ **Concerns**   Encourage the relatives to express their concerns and deal with them appropriately. Their concerns include their relative being moved into a side room with delay in treatment and worries related to *C. difficile* and 'superbug' drug resistance.

☐☐☐ **Expectations**   Elicit the relatives' expectation as to what can be achieved in this consultation.

☐☐☐ **Acknowledge**   Acknowledge the relatives' emotional state (angry and demanding).

ADVICE

☐☐☐ *C. difficile*   Explain how the patient became infected with *Clostridium difficile* and how it will be treated.

'As you may be aware, Mrs Gibbs suffered from a severe chest infection which required antibiotic treatment. These antibiotics are necessary for killing the bugs that cause the chest infection, but they unfortunately also kill many of the useful bugs in the gut. The bowel contains many bugs and *Clostridium difficile* is one that can be found in healthy individuals. When some of the other healthy bugs are killed by antibiotics, *Clostridium difficile* can increase and produce toxins that

12.2

can cause diarrhoea and abdominal pain. These antibiotics have now been stopped and a new treatment for *Clostridium difficile* has been commenced. Hopefully her symptoms will improve over the coming days and we will monitor her closely.'

☐☐☐ **Respond**

Respond to the relatives' concerns about her side room isolation.

'I appreciate that you are upset that this has happened to your relative. I understand that you are unhappy she has been moved to a side room. I would like to explain why she has been moved and reassure you that she is receiving the correct treatment.'

☐☐☐ **Side room**

Explain why the patient has been moved.

'Your relative has been moved into a side room to prevent the spread of this bug. When a patient suffers from *Clostridium difficile* there is an increased chance of this infection being passed to other people (in the surrounding environment). To minimise the risk of it spreading, we move the patient to a side room and advise anyone who has contact with her to wear an apron and wash their hands before and after visiting her. These measures are in place to protect you, the staff and other patients from getting infected.'

☐☐☐ **Reassure**

Reassure the relatives that the patient's *Clostridium difficile* is unlikely to be related to poor hospital infection control.

'I appreciate your concerns about hospital hygiene and whether this may have contributed to Mrs Gibbs' infection. I would like to assure you that we are extremely conscious about hospital hygiene and this is why we insist on strict hand washing, which applies to staff as well as visitors. I would like to point out that it is unlikely that your relative's development of *Clostridium difficile* is the result of poor hospital hygiene. Her symptoms started soon after she was started on antibiotics for her chest infection. It is therefore highly likely that these antibiotics were the cause of her current illness. Those antibiotics have now been stopped.'

CLOSING

☐☐☐ **Understanding**

Check the relatives understand what you have said.

☐☐☐ **Questions**

Encourage the relatives to ask questions and respond to them.

Leaflet

Offer the relatives a leaflet for reference.

☐☐☐ **Summarise**

Summarise the situation to the relatives to confirm they understand it.

'I would like to reassure you again that although your relative has been affected by *Clostridium difficile*, we have removed the likely cause and are managing her in the best possible way. We will continue to treat and monitor her closely so that the quality of care she receives is not compromised. Hospital hygiene is one of our biggest priorities and guidelines are strictly adhered to. I would also like to reassure you that as healthy visitors you are at very little risk of being affected by the illness and there is very little evidence of it spreading outside the hospital. I appreciate that you are upset at what has happened but I assure you we are doing everything we can to ensure the best possible outcome.'

COMMUNICATION SKILLS

☐☐☐ **Rapport**

Attempt to establish rapport through the use of appropriate eye contact. Maintain appropriate body language and an open posture throughout the meeting.

☐☐☐ **Listening**

Demonstrate an interest and concern in what the relatives say. Listen empathetically.

☐☐☐ **Behaviour**

Avoid dismissing the relatives' fears and concerns. Avoid offering them inappropriate reassurance.

☐☐☐ **Manner**

Remain calm and clear (use an appropriate tone and pace of voice, use simple sentences). If the relatives become agitated and try to get up and leave, gently ask them to sit down.

☐☐☐ **Verbal Cues**

Use non-verbal and verbal cues, i.e. tone and pace of voice, nodding your head where appropriate.

EXAMINER'S EVALUATION

0 1 2 3 4 5

☐☐☐☐☐☐ Overall assessment in dealing angry relatives
☐☐☐☐☐☐ Role player's score
Total mark out of 31

INSTRUCTIONS: You are providing ward cover on-call as a foundation year House Officer in surgery. You have written up i.v. fluids for a patient who is pre-op. nil-by-mouth and handed this to the nurse to give them. When you return to the ward 5 hours later you notice the fluids have not yet been given. The nurse is sitting in the nurses' station.

INTRODUCTION

0 1 2

☐☐☐ **Introduction**   Use an appropriate introduction. Establish rapport with the nurse.

'Hi, I'm the on-call House Officer for surgery. I think I saw you earlier on. How have things been on the ward today?'

☐☐☐ **Purpose**   State the purpose as to why you would like to speak to her.

'I'm sorry to hear you have had such a busy day. There is something troubling me that I need to talk to you about. Could we go somewhere private and discuss this?'

MENTION PROBLEM

☐☐☐ **Verify**   Show empathy and highlight the problems encountered by the nurse, e.g. busy wards and understaffing. Now that rapport has been established, verify whether the i.v. fluids have been administered to the patient.

'I understand that there has been a shortage of staff on the ward today and it has been very busy for you. However, do you remember that earlier I handed you a drug chart for a patient who was due i.v. fluids? Can I just check that this has been given?'

12.3

☐☐☐ **Concerns**   Once the nurse has responded to you after you have mentioned the problem, explain your personal concerns that the request has not been carried out.

'Although I appreciate the problems you have been having, I am sure you will understand that the patient concerned required these fluids, particularly because they were nil-by-mouth and awaiting an operation. It is likely he is more dehydrated now and this may affect the decision to let him go for the operation.'

□□□ **Response**   Deal with the nurse's responses appropriately and empathetically.

'I understand that you had to deal with an emergency soon after I left you with the fluid prescription and that it was easy to forget about it afterwards. I agree that it has been a busy day for all of us. However the patient is now more dehydrated than before and needs his treatment right away.'

□□□ **Offer Advice**   Demonstrate an understanding of the situation and offer possible solutions.

'I appreciate that you have experienced significant difficulties today due to lack of staffing and you have been very busy coping with the additional workload. I suggest that a possible way in which the patients' care is not compromised would be to create a sheet of jobs for both doctors and nurses. These lists could be taped to the front desk so they are never missed and would remind any doctor or nurse on the ward of jobs that had not been done. This would avoid important jobs being delayed. What do you think?'

CLOSING

□□□ **Understanding**   Check that the nurse has understood what you have said.

□□□ **Questions**   Encourage the nurse to ask questions and respond to them.

□□□ **Summarise**   Summarise back to the nurse what has been discussed. Jointly agree upon a plan of action (recommending the completion of an incident form to highlight a near miss and put into motion positive changes in practice).

'I am happy that we have had the opportunity to discuss this matter. As we have agreed, we will have two sheets at the front desk to remind each other of outstanding jobs. I hope that this will benefit both the staff and the patients and prevent any mishaps happening in the future.'

COMMUNICATION SKILLS

□□□ **Rapport**   Attempt to establish rapport with the nurse through the use of appropriate eye contact. Maintain appropriate body language and an open posture throughout the interview.

□□□ **Listening**	Demonstrate an interest and concern in what the nurse says. Show active listening and listen empathetically.
□□□ **Pauses**	Pace the information and use appropriate pauses. Allow the nurse to express her feelings freely and without interruption. Do not be dismissive or condescending to the nurse.
□□□ **Verbal Cues**	Use non-verbal and verbal cues, i.e. tone and pace of voice, nodding your head where appropriate.

EXAMINER'S EVALUATION

0 1 2 3 4 5

□□□□□□ Overall assessment of interprofessional negotiation
□□□□□□ Role player's score
Total mark out of 26

COMMUNICATION SKILLS: Negotiation with Patients

INSTRUCTIONS: You are a foundation year doctor in A&E. Miss Edwardo has had lower back pain for the past 2 weeks since a fall. She has already had an X-ray and blood tests, which were normal. The back pain is still present although she has been taking ibuprofen. Miss Edwardo attends today, demanding an MRI.

INTRODUCTION

0 1 2

☐☐☐ **Introduction** Introduce yourself. Confirm the name and occupation of the patient.

☐☐☐ **Ideas** Elicit the patient's ideas and understanding of what is going on.

'I understand that you had a fall 2 weeks ago and the back pain has not resolved. Could you please tell me what you think is going on in relation to your back pain?'

☐☐☐ **Concerns** Encourage the patient to express her concerns and deal with them appropriately. Her concerns include an undetected fracture and need for an MRI.

'I understand that things have been difficult for you with the back pain you have been experiencing. I am here to listen and help you. Is there any specific concern you have that you wish to discuss with me today?'

☐☐☐ **Expectations** Elicit the patient's expectation as to what can be achieved in this consultation.

☐☐☐ **Acknowledge** Acknowledge the patient's emotional state (worried and demanding).

12.4

FOCUSED HISTORY

☐☐☐ **Symptoms** Has there been any change in her symptoms? Has the analgesia been helpful? Establish the presence or absence of red flag symptoms (weight loss, incontinence, numbness, weakness, loss of function).

☐☐☐ **Treatment** What type of analgesia is the patient taking and how often? Are there any other medications which she has been taking?

☐☐☐ **Effect on Life** Elicit the effect of the pain on her daily activities (washing, dressing, cooking, mobilising, etc.) and work (requiring time off) and elicit any negative social and psychological effects on the patient's life.

NEGOTIATION

☐☐☐ **Reassure**

Reassure the patient that her symptoms are unlikely to be serious.

'I appreciate that you are worried about the back pain and it is still troubling you. I would like to reassure you that all your blood tests are completely normal and an X-ray has not shown anything of concern. From what you have told me about your back pain, it appears that your pain is muscular in nature and thankfully it does not display any worrying signs or symptoms.'

☐☐☐ **Own Agenda**

Explain that an MRI scan is not necessary at the moment. Emphasise that it would not change her current management.

'I appreciate that you are concerned that your back pain has not improved as fast as you had hoped and that you feel that an MRI scan would help us do something more. However, I do not think that performing an MRI scan at this stage would change the way we are managing your back pain.'

☐☐☐ **Compromise**

Negotiate an agreed compromise. Offer alternative or additional analgesics

'I appreciate that you feel we could be doing more for your back pain and I am sorry that you are still suffering with it. It appears that you have had a nasty fall and that the painkillers we gave you are not controlling your symptoms effectively. I suggest that we could try a stronger painkiller this time and consider some physiotherapy and see how you respond.'

CLOSING

☐☐☐ **Follow-up**

Arrange an appropriate follow-up.

'If your symptoms worsen at any point or if you experience problems passing urine or opening your bowels or any numbness or weakness in your legs you should urgently seek medical help. Otherwise I would expect your symptoms to improve in the next couple of weeks as long as you take plenty of rest and do not lift or carry anything heavy.'

☐☐☐ **Summarise**

Summarise what has been agreed and come up with an action plan.

COMMUNICATION SKILLS

☐☐☐ **Rapport** Attempt to establish rapport with the patient through the use of appropriate eye contact. Maintain appropriate body language and an open posture throughout the interview.

☐☐☐ **Listening** Demonstrate an interest and concern in what the patient says. Show active listening and listen empathetically.

☐☐☐ **Behaviour** Avoid dismissing her individual fears and concerns. Avoid offering inappropriate reassurance.

☐☐☐ **Verbal Cues** Use non-verbal and verbal cues, i.e. tone and pace of voice, nodding your head where appropriate.

EXAMINER'S EVALUATION

0 1 2 3 4 5

☐☐☐☐☐☐ Overall assessment of negotiation
☐☐☐☐☐☐ Role player's score

Total mark out of 32

Prejudice and Intolerance

INSTRUCTIONS: You are a foundation year House Officer in general medicine. Miss Elaine is a 29-year-old inpatient on your ward. Her female partner came to visit her this morning and the couple have been receiving abusive comments from other patients on the ward. The ward sister has told you that the patient would like to be moved into a side room, but it is not currently available as it is occupied by an MRSA-positive patient. Speak to the patient and her partner and agree upon an acceptable solution. You will be marked on your communication skills and ability to negotiate a suitable outcome.

INTRODUCTION

0 1 2

☐☐☐ **Introduction**   Introduce yourself. Confirm the name of the patient and her partner and confirm their relationship.

☐☐☐ **Ideas**   Elicit the patient's ideas and understanding of what is going on.

'I am one of the doctors looking after this ward. You raised some concerns with the ward sister. Can you please tell me what is going on?'

☐☐☐ **Concerns**   Encourage the patient to express her concerns and deal with them appropriately. Her concerns include discrimination and lack of privacy.

'I am here to listen and help you. Can you please tell me if there are any specific concerns you are worried about?'

☐☐☐ **Expectations**   Elicit the patient's expectation (transfer to side room).

☐☐☐ **Acknowledge**   Acknowledge the patient's emotional state (worried and demanding).

12.5

NEGOTIATION

☐☐☐ **Response**   Recognise that the couple are upset by the comments they have received and show empathy by agreeing that they are unacceptable and hurtful.

☐☐☐ **Own Agenda**   Explain that side rooms are normally reserved for patients with specific illnesses which require isolation, or for patients who are dying.

☐☐☐ **Confidentiality**   If asked the reasons why a patient is in the side room, do not disclose the reason and explain that you cannot breach confidentiality.

'I would like to reiterate that the hurtful comments you received are totally unacceptable and I am here to try and resolve this problem for you. I understand that you have asked to be moved to a side room for privacy. Unfortunately I have to inform you that all the side rooms are occupied. However, even if one were to be made available, they cannot be used for this purpose. Side rooms are reserved for patients with specific illnesses which require isolation. We also use these rooms for patients who are very sick and are likely to die.'

☐☐☐ **Compromise**　　Tell the couple that you will speak to the nurse in charge and ask if there is a possibility that the patient can be moved to another bed. Explain that due to the nature of hospitals with busy staff and low availability of spare beds, this is not guaranteed and may not be possible immediately.

Curtains　　Suggest to the couple that they keep the curtains drawn around the bed to ensure privacy during visits.

'I am sorry that you are upset that you could not be moved to a side room. However, I can suggest a number of ways that may help and rectify your problem. I will ask the bed managers to try and transfer you to another ward. However, as you may appreciate, the hospital is quite busy and this may take a few days to organise. In the meantime I suggest that when your partner visits you should draw your curtain around your bed to maintain your privacy and stop unwanted intrusions.'

☐☐☐ **Patients**　　Explain to the couple that you or one of the nursing staff will speak with the patients who have been making abusive comments to remind them that such behaviour is unacceptable.

☐☐☐ **Summarise**　　Summarise to the patient what has been agreed.

COMMUNICATION SKILLS

☐☐☐ **Rapport**　　Attempt to establish rapport with the patient and partner through the use of appropriate eye contact. Maintain appropriate body language and an open posture throughout the meeting. Do not be dismissive or discriminatory towards the patient.

☐☐☐ **Questions**　　Encourage and respond to the couple's questions.

☐☐☐ **Listening**　　Demonstrate interest and concern in what the couple say. Listen to them empathetically.

☐☐☐ **Pauses**   Pace your information and use appropriate pauses. Allow the couple to express their feelings freely and without interruption.

☐☐☐ **Verbal Cues**   Use non-verbal and verbal cues, i.e. tone and pace of voice, nodding your head where appropriate.

EXAMINER'S EVALUATION

0 1 2 3 4 5

☐☐☐☐☐☐ Overall assessment of prejudice and intolerance issues

☐☐☐☐☐☐ Role player's score

Total mark out of 29

COMMUNICATION SKILLS: **Ethical Issues**

INSTRUCTIONS: You are a foundation year House Officer in general practice. Mr Johnston has been informed that he is HIV positive and he has come in to discuss this with you. He does not wish his HIV status to be recorded in his practice notes. He has already been counselled at the HIV clinic regarding his diagnosis. Discuss and negotiate an appropriate outcome with Mr Johnston. You will be marked on your communication skills and ability to deliver information and negotiate a suitable solution.

INTRODUCTION

0 1 2

☐☐☐ **Introduction** Introduce yourself. Confirm the patient's name. Establish rapport with him.

☐☐☐ **Ideas** Elicit the patient's reasons for attendance.

☐☐☐ **Concerns** Encourage the patient to express his concerns and deal with them appropriately. Elicit the patient's wish to withhold information from the notes and his wife.

☐☐☐ **Acknowledge** Acknowledge the individual's emotional state (recognise that he is fearful, anxious and worried).

'I understand that you have recently been diagnosed with HIV and are concerned that your diagnosis will be recorded in your medical file which may be accessed by your wife. I appreciate your request and would like to discuss this further with you today.'

EXPLORATION

NOTE: Your exploration should be centred on two themes: confidentiality (not divulging or discussing any patient's sensitive information) and transmission risk (to his wife).

☐☐☐ **Negotiate** Explain to the patient the need to document his HIV status in the notes.

☐☐☐ **Confidentiality** Reassure him that all members of the team are under a strict code of confidentiality.

'I appreciate your concerns and I am fully aware that you would not like anyone to know about your HIV status. However, I would like to stress that by having your HIV status documented in your notes this will help all the health professionals to provide you with the best help and care available.

'It is also important to record your HIV status since HIV can present in a number of ways. Without this information you may be misdiagnosed and receive inappropriate treatment. Also if you are to be started on treatment for HIV, these drugs may interact with other medications that you may be prescribed, hence it is important to know what you are taking.

'I would like to stress that anyone who has access to your medical notes abides by a strict code of confidentiality. This means that our staff cannot discuss or disclose your condition to anyone else without your consent.'

☐☐☐ **Transmission**　Inform the patient that HIV can be transmitted sexually and that his wife has a high risk of contracting the disease.

'I understand that you do not want your wife to be informed about your condition. Do you know how HIV is passed or transmitted to another person? HIV can be passed on by unprotected sex or through blood contamination.

'I appreciate that you are in a very difficult position and that you are worried about the potential effect on your relationship with your wife if she found out. However, by not telling her you are putting her at risk of contracting HIV.'

☐☐☐ **Understanding**　Check that the patient understands what has been explained.

☐☐☐ **Decision**　Find out if the patient is prepared to have his HIV status documented in his notes and whether he will disclose it to his wife.

'I am glad that you have agreed to have your HIV status documented in the notes and that you would like some more time to deliberate about informing your wife. I believe that it is extremely important to inform your wife as soon as possible to prevent any harm from reaching her. I appreciate your need to think about this further and my advice would be to use protection in the form of condoms in the meantime.'

Ethical Issue

Inform his GP	If, despite your negotiations, the patient is persistent in his refusal to allow you to inform other healthcare workers, you should respect his wish.
Inform his wife	If the patient refuses to inform his wife (who is exposed to risk or has already been infected) then it is appropriate to disclose information to such individuals (against the wishes of the patient) in order to protect them from risk of serious harm or death. The patient should be informed of your intention to do so.

☐☐☐ **Reassure**   Inform the patient that you will not disclose any information to other relatives or people whom you do not believe are at risk.

☐☐☐ **Follow-up**   Offer the patient a follow-up appointment in 4 weeks.

Breaching Confidentiality

A rough guide to breaching confidentiality

It is good medical practice to contact your medico-legal representatives (MDU, MPS) or the General Medical Council (GMC) for further advice and clarity on when to breach confidentiality

Breach	You are notifying a birth or death of a patient
	A court order has been passed obliging you to do so
	A search warrant has been issued by a judge, which requires you to
	The police have asked for the personal details (name and address) of one of your patients who has committed an offence (no clinical details)
	The patient has a notifiable disease (HIV/AIDS is *not* notifiable)
	You are notifying the termination of a pregnancy
Discretion req.	A third party (e.g. a relative, a partner of an HIV+ patient) is at high risk of harm
	Patients who are medically unfit to drive continue to do so
	You want to share information with other healthcare members
	You are assisting in the detection and prevention of serious crime
Do not breach	The patient has committed a minor crime (e.g. burglary, vandalism)
	You want to prevent minor harm to someone else (e.g. verbal abuse)
	You have not obtained consent from a patient before informing a third party (employer, insurer, etc.)
	Such a disclosure is for mere amusement (e.g. in conversations, etc.)

COMMUNICATION SKILLS

☐☐☐ **Rapport**   Attempt to establish rapport with the patient through the use of appropriate eye contact. Maintain appropriate body language and an open posture throughout.

☐☐☐ **Questions**   Encourage the patient to ask questions.

☐☐☐ **Listening** Demonstrate an interest and concern in what the patient says. Show active listening and listen empathetically.

☐☐☐ **Summarise** Summarise the consultation and check the patient understands what has been said.

0 1 2 3 4 5

☐☐☐☐☐☐ Overall assessment of ethical issues

☐☐☐☐☐☐ Role player's score

Total mark out of 29

COMMUNICATION SKILLS: **English as a Foreign Language**

INSTRUCTIONS: You are a foundation year House Officer in general practice. Mrs Rosa Prelavic is a 28-year-old woman from Bulgaria who has come to the practice to see a doctor. She came to the UK just 6 months ago and speaks very little English. Appropriately explore her reasons for attendance. You will be marked on your communication skills and ability to formulate an appropriate management plan.

INTRODUCTION

0 1 2

□□□ **Introduction** Introduce yourself. Confirm the patient's name, age and occupation. Use appropriate words and body language, such as pointing to yourself to make it clear to the patient who you are.

□□□ **Language** Confirm where the patient is from, what her first language is and if she can speak English.

□□□ **Interpreter** State that you would normally ask for an interpreter or someone in the practice who may also speak the same language as the patient.

□□□ **Equipment** Utilise the equipment made available to you, when necessary, such as a pen, paper, clock and calendar.

HISTORY

□□□ **Elicit** Elicit the main problems and concerns of the patient. Use appropriate short sentences and words to enable the patient to understand. Point to parts to the body, such as head, neck, chest and abdomen, so that the patient can confirm which part of the anatomy is of concern to her.

□□□ **Mime** Use appropriate body language and facial expressions to indicate symptoms, such as pain, fever, shivers, coughing, sneezing and vomiting, so that the patient can agree when the correct symptom is given. This will enable you to get closer to a likely diagnosis, for example a common cold.

□□□ **Timing** Use a calendar or the pen and paper to find out how long this problem (e.g. a sore throat) has been going on for.

12.7

☐☐☐ **Assoc. History** Attempt to ascertain what medications the patient is taking, i.e. the pill, and whether she smokes cigarettes or drinks alcohol. Mime each item as appropriate.

☐☐☐ **Expectations** Establish what the patient would expect from the consultation, i.e. the patient may ask for antibiotics stating 'penicillin'.

☐☐☐ **Summarise** Summarise back to the patient your key findings using simple and understandable terms to check if your history is correct.

MANAGEMENT

☐☐☐ **Treatment** Explain to the patient that she does not need antibiotics for the time being and that at the moment she needs regular paracetamol and fluids. You should use verbal and non-verbal means of explaining *'no need antibiotic'* and use diagrams to indicate paracetamol use. The diagram should include a clock or numerical timings to explain four times daily usage of two tablets with a drink.

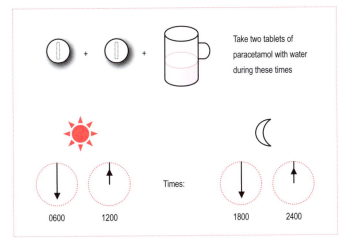

Suggested diagram to draw when trying to explain paracetamol use to a patient with English as a foreign language

☐☐☐ **Understanding** Check the understanding of the patient by asking her verbally and using non-verbal cues after showing her the written instructions. The non-verbal cue can take the form of thumbs up and at the same time asking if the patient understands.

□□□ **Follow-up**   An appropriate follow-up should be arranged.
This should be explained verbally and by using the
calendar or written cues. You should also write down
clearly the details of the treatment, instructions you
have given and follow-up arrangements (such as
returning in a week if symptoms have not resolved)
and hand this to the patient. Explain to the patient
that she should show these details to an English-
speaking friend or acquaintance who should translate
them to her in her own language.

Reception   Explain to the examiner that you would request the
receptionist to book an interpreter with the patient
or arrange for language line assistance on their next
appointment.

COMMUNICATION SKILLS

□□□ **Rapport**   Attempt to establish rapport with the patient
through the use of appropriate eye contact. Maintain
appropriate body language and an open posture
throughout the meeting.

□□□ **Rephrasing**   Rephrase questions and statements as appropriate to
help the patient understand what you are saying.

□□□ **Cues/Aids**   Use verbal and non-verbal cues and aids (writing,
drawing, pointing) to help communication.

□□□ **Style**   Maintain a positive approach that avoids being
patronising to the patient. Do not be abrupt,
dismissive, condescending or judgemental to the
patient.

EXAMINER'S EVALUATION

0 1 2 3 4 5

□□□□□□ Overall assessment of dealing with a foreign patient
□□□□□□ Role player's score
Total mark out of 32

404

Discharging Patients

DISCHARGING PATIENTS: **Myocardial Infarction**

INSTRUCTIONS: You are a foundation year House Officer in cardiology. Mr Chany has been in hospital for 10 days after an anterior myocardial infarction. He will be discharged in the next day or two with cholesterol lowering medication, aspirin, clopidogrel, ramipril and GTN spray (prn). Find out what the patient understands about his discharge and give him any appropriate advice.

INTRODUCTION

0 1 2

☐☐☐ **Introduction**   Introduce yourself. Confirm the patient's name and age.

☐☐☐ **Purpose**   Mention the purpose of the consultation.

'I understand that you are soon to be discharged home from the ward. The team has been discussing your progress and we are all happy to see that you are doing so much better. How do you feel about this?'

★ Explore the Patient's . . .

☐☐☐ **Understanding**   Find out what the patient understands about his planned discharge. What has he already been told?

☐☐☐ **Concerns**   Do you have any particular concerns with your illness or with going home?

☐☐☐ **Home Situation**   Do you live in a house or a flat? Do you have any stairs?

☐☐☐ **Social Support**   Do you live alone or with anyone? Do you have any support from your family? Did you have any services in place prior to coming into hospital?

☐☐☐ **Medication**   Establish from the patient what treatments he is taking.

★ Medication Advice

13.1

☐☐☐ **Anticoagulant**   Advise him of the importance of taking aspirin and clopidogrel 75 mg daily because it helps to thin his blood and reduces the risk of a second heart attack.

☐☐☐ **GTN Spray**   Advise to take two puffs of the spray if he experiences chest pain. He can repeat it after 10 minutes but after that should seek medical help if the pain is still present.

☐☐☐ **Statin**   Advise him on the need to reduce cholesterol and tell him that the statin should be taken at night.

☐☐☐ **ACE Inhib.** Advise him that the ACE inhibitor provides good BP control and protects against a further MI.

☐☐☐ **Concordance** Mention to him the importance of taking the medications regularly as advised.

'You have done very well after your heart attack and have made a good recovery. To reduce the risk of having another heart attack we strongly recommend that you continue to take the medications we started you on whilst in hospital. It is important to take them on time and regularly. You were started on aspirin and clopidogrel, which work to thin the blood and reduce the risk of suffering another heart attack. Simvastatin, the tablet you take at night, helps to reduce the level of cholesterol in your blood. Ramipril has been shown to reduce death from cardiac events by up to 20%. You will also be given a GTN spray device. You should spray two puffs of this spray underneath your tongue if you experience any chest pain.'

✶ Additional Points

☐☐☐ **Employment** If patient is in employment he should try and return to work after two months. If he has a job lifting heavy objects or doing manual work he should change to lighter employment.

☐☐☐ **Exercise/Sex** Advise to exercise lightly but regularly. He should abstain from sex for up to one month.

☐☐☐ **Lifestyle** Advise him on the importance of eating fruit, vegetables and fibre and reducing red meat and fried food. He should stop smoking and reduce his alcohol intake.

Travel He should avoid driving for 4–6 weeks and avoid flying for up to 2 months.

Chest Pain Inform the patient that he should seek immediate medical advice if he experiences chest pain similar to his MI or experiences chest tightness radiating to his jaw or left arm.

'In addition to the medication, there are a few general measures I need to inform you about. Firstly, I understand that you work as an IT executive in a stressful job. Unfortunately, because of your heart attack it is important that you take a break from any occupation for around 2 months. This should provide enough time for your body to readjust and return to near normal daily function. If your job is particularly stressful, it is important to consider the possibility of reducing the stress or if need be, changing jobs for the sake of your health. Exercise is important, but you should exercise lightly initially, perhaps for a few months. Things like sexual relations should be avoided for at least a month, simply because it causes additional strain on the body and the heart. If you are not doing so already, it is important to cut down on fatty foods and dairy products. You should also stop smoking and reduce your alcohol level to a minimum. In relation to travelling, the general advice is to take a break from driving for up to 6 weeks and not to fly for 2 months.'

CLOSING

☐☐☐ **Follow-up**   Organise a follow-up appointment in 2 months' time.

☐☐☐ **Understanding**   Check that the patient understands the information provided.

Questions   Encourage the patient to ask questions and respond to them.

☐☐☐ **Summarise**   Give a brief summary to the patient about what has been discussed. Jointly agree on an action plan and conclude the interview.

Secondary Prevention for Myocardial Infarction

Mnemonic for secondary prevention of MI: 'ABCDE'
Aspirin, **A**ntiplatelet drug (clopidogrel), **A**CE inhibitor, **B**-blocker, **B**P control, **C**holesterol-lowering drug (statin), **D**iet, **D**iabetic control, **D**on't smoke, **E**xercise

Medication	All patients with a confirmed acute MI should be started on aspirin (indefinitely), ACE inhibitor, statin and beta blocker
NSTEMI	Clopidogrel should be combined with low dose aspirin (75 mg) for 12 months, thereafter clopidogrel should be stopped
STEMI	Clopidogrel should be combined with low dose aspirin, started during the first 24 hours of diagnosis and continued for 4 months. Thereafter, the clopidogrel should be stopped
+ HF	Patients diagnosed with HF and left ventricular systolic dysfunction should be started on an aldosterone antagonist (spironolactone) within 3–14 days post MI (preferably after the ACE inhibitor)
Exercise	20–30 minutes of physical exercise a day to the point of slight breathlessness is recommended
Diet	A Mediterranean diet including fruit, vegetables, fish and bread is recommended. Reduce meat and

	replace cheese and butter with vegetable and plant oils
Smoking	Patients are advised to stop smoking. Offer smoking cessation advice
Sexual Activity	Patients can resume normal sexual activity after 4 weeks
General Advice	Patients can consider air travel 2 months after an MI. Should avoid driving for 1 month (group 1 – cars, motorbike)

COMMUNICATION SKILLS

☐☐☐ **Rapport**   Establish rapport with the patient and maintain it throughout the interview.

☐☐☐ **Listening**   Demonstrate interest and concern in what the patient says. Show active listening and listen empathetically.

☐☐☐ **Pauses**   Pace the information and use appropriate pauses. Allow the patient to speak his feelings freely and without interruption.

☐☐☐ **Verbal Cues**   Use non-verbal and verbal cues, i.e. tone and pace of voice, nodding your head where appropriate.

Sequence of Elevated Enzymes after MI
Mnemonic: 'Time to **CALL 4** help'
The order of enzyme raising post MI: **T**roponin, **C**K-MB, **A**ST, LDH

EXAMINER'S EVALUATION

0 1 2 3 4 5
☐☐☐☐☐☐ Overall assessment of discharging patient (MI)
☐☐☐☐☐☐ Role player's score
Total mark out of 33

DISCHARGING PATIENTS: **COPD**

INSTRUCTIONS: Mr Miah, a 53-year-old chef, was admitted into hospital following an acute infective exacerbation of COPD and is now ready for discharge with home oxygen and antibiotics. You have been asked to discuss these discharge arrangements with him. You will be marked on the information you provide and your communication skills.

INTRODUCTION

0 1 2

☐☐☐ **Introduction** — Introduce yourself. Confirm the patient's name and age.

☐☐☐ **Purpose** — Mention the purpose of the consultation.

'I understand that you are soon to be discharged home from the ward. The team has been discussing your progress and we are all happy to see that you are doing so much better. How do you feel about this?'

★ Explore the Patient's . . .

☐☐☐ **Understanding** — Establish what the patient understands of his planned discharge. What has he already been told?

☐☐☐ **Concerns** — Do you have any particular concerns with your illness or with going home?

☐☐☐ **Home Situation** — Do you live in a house or a flat? Are there any stairs to climb?

☐☐☐ **Social Support** — Do you live alone or with anyone? Do you have any support from your family? Did you have any services in place prior to coming into hospital?

☐☐☐ *Smoking* — *Have you stopped smoking? Does anyone else in your household smoke?*

☐☐☐ **Medication** — Establish from the patient what treatments he is taking.

★ Medical Advice

☐☐☐ **Antibiotics** — Advise him of the importance of completing the full course of antibiotics (7 days).

☐☐☐ **Inhalers** — Advise the patient to take his usual inhalers salmeterol (long-acting beta blocker and steroids 2 × puffs bd) and ipratropium bromide (anticholinergic, 2 × puffs qds).

13.2

☐ ☐ ☐ **Prednisolone** Advise the patient to take prednisolone to reduce the symptoms of COPD. The patient should continue taking 30 mg of prednisolone for the next 7–14 days.

☐ ☐ ☐ **Home Oxygen** Inform the patient that in order to get the full benefits of the therapy he will need to be on supplemental oxygen for at least 15 hours a day.

Oxygen Therapy in COPD Patients

Long-term oxygen therapy has been shown to reduce mortality in COPD. Patients with COPD who are being considered for long-term oxygen therapy should first be assessed by a specialist (respiratory team, respiratory nurse). They must also stop smoking to reduce the risk of fire hazards (burns, fire) and be on oxygen therapy for at least 15 hours a day to see any medical benefit. It is best delivered with a concentrator, via nasal prongs at 2–4 L/min (depending on the patient's clinical presentation and ABGs).

Indications for Initiating Oxygen Therapy

Patients with COPD should be initiated on oxygen therapy if they have an abnormal ABG (pO_2 <7.3 kPa when stable or pO_2 of 7.3–8.0 kPa when stable with other features including secondary polycythaemia, nocturnal hypoxaemia, peripheral oedema or pulmonary hypertension). It should be considered with an abnormal spirometer test (severe airflow obstruction with FEV1 of <30% of predicted or moderate airflow obstruction FEV1 30–49% predicted), O_2 sat. <92% on air, evidence of cyanosis, polycythaemia, raised JVP or peripheral oedema.

☐ ☐ ☐ **Concordance** Mention the importance of taking medications regularly as advised.

'You have done very well after your recent exacerbation of COPD and have made a good recovery. In order to reduce the risk of having further exacerbations we strongly recommend that you continue to take the medications we started you on in hospital in addition to your regular inhalers. It is important to take them on time and regularly. You were started on a weeks' course of antibiotics and it is important to complete the course. You have also been started on a 2-week course of steroid (prednisolone) which works to reduce the inflammation in your lungs. Finally, you will now have home oxygen therapy. It is important to take 15 hours of oxygen a day to achieve maximal benefits.'

★ Additional Points

☐ ☐ ☐ **Smoking** Stress the importance of stopping smoking and explain how it is contraindicated with home oxygen (fire hazard).

Travel	Advise the patient to seek medical advice before planning any air travel.	

Long-Term Oxygen Therapy and Air Travel

Patients with COPD on long-term oxygen or have a FEV1 <50% of predicted should consult a doctor and be fully assessed before considering or embarking on any flight abroad. Commercial airplanes fly at altitudes of up to 12 500 metres and require the cabin to be pressurised. This can reduce the pO_2 levels on aircraft and can drop a healthy person's oxygen saturation from 97% to 93%. As a result there is risk of increasing hypoxia in an already hypoxic patient especially in COPD patients. Patients with pO_2 of less than 9.3 kPa at sea level should consult the airline company and receive supplemental oxygen while travelling, while patients with significant hypoxia (<6.7 kPa) or hypercapnia are advised not to fly. Patients with bullous disease should be informed of the potential risk of developing a pneumothorax while on their journey

---

Spirometer

Advise the patient he will require a spirometer test prior to discharge.

☐☐☐ **Vaccines**

Inform the patient that he should have a yearly flu vaccine and check that he has had the pneumococcal vaccine (once in a lifetime).

'In addition to the medication, there are a few general measures I need to inform you about. Firstly, the home oxygen therapy that you will be discharged with can be a fire hazard. It is essential that no one smokes in your house. If you are planning any air travel it is important to seek medical advice before booking your ticket. You may require a formal assessment to determine whether you can fly or not. Finally, you should take a yearly flu jab at your GP to reduce the exacerbations you suffer and check that you have had a pneumococcal vaccine which is necessary only once in your life.'

CLOSING

☐☐☐ **Follow-up**

Arrange for the patient to be seen in outpatients in 2 months' time and inform him that a respiratory nurse may visit him at home in the coming days to assess him.

☐☐☐ **Understanding**

Check that the patient understands the information provided.

☐☐☐ **Questions**

Encourage the patient to ask questions and respond to them.

☐☐☐ **Summarise**   Give a brief summary back to the patient about what
                           has been discussed. Jointly agree on an action plan
                           and conclude the interview.

COMMUNICATION SKILLS

☐☐☐ **Rapport**   Establish and maintain rapport throughout the
                           interview.

☐☐☐ **Listening**   Demonstrate an interest and concern in what
                           the patient says. Show active listening and listen
                           empathetically.

☐☐☐ **Pauses**   Pace the information and use appropriate pauses.
                           Allow the patient to speak his feelings freely and
                           without interruption.

☐☐☐ **Verbal Cues**   Use non-verbal and verbal cues, i.e. tone and pace of
                           voice, nodding head where appropriate.

EXAMINER'S EVALUATION

0 1 2 3 4 5

☐ ☐ ☐ ☐ ☐ ☐ Overall assessment of discharging patient (COPD)

☐ ☐ ☐ ☐ ☐ ☐ Role player's score

Total mark out of 37

INSTRUCTIONS: Mr Jacksonion is a 37-year-old builder who has been admitted into hospital following a seizure at work while on a ladder. This is his third attendance at hospital with a similar problem in recent months. All investigations are normal, he has been diagnosed with epilepsy and the patient has been informed. You have been asked to discuss discharge arrangements with him and identify any needs he may have. You will be marked on the information you provide and your communication skills.

INTRODUCTION

0 1 2

☐ ☐ ☐ **Introduction**   Introduce yourself. Confirm the patient's name and age.

☐ ☐ ☐ **Purpose**   Mention the purpose of consultation.

'I understand that you are soon to be discharged home from the ward. Since all the tests have come back normal, you have been told that you suffer from epilepsy. I would like to discuss a number of issues surrounding epilepsy, prior to your discharge.'

★ Explore the Patient's . . .

☐ ☐ ☐ **Understanding**   Find out what the patient understands of his planned discharge. What has he already been told?

☐ ☐ ☐ **Concerns**   Do you have any particular concerns with your illness or with going home?

☐ ☐ ☐ **Medication**   Establish from the patient what treatment he is taking.

★ Medical Advice

☐ ☐ ☐ **Concordance**   Mention the importance of taking medications regularly as advised, keeping up to date with repeat medications and not running out of tablets.

13.3

☐ ☐ ☐ **Interactions**   Advise the patient not to consume alcohol whilst on medication due to possible interactions. The patient should inform any health professional that he is on antiepileptic medication before taking any other tablets (antibiotics, warfarin, OCP, TB medication).

☐ ☐ ☐ **Blood Tests**   Advise the patient about the need for regular blood tests to check for compliance and dosage of anticonvulsants.

'You have told me you have been started on carbamazepine, two tablets twice a day. It is important that you take your medication as directed, on time and regularly. You should get your repeat prescriptions in plenty of time from your GP and you should never run out. Because of the way these tablets work, they interact with a number of medications which can alter their effectiveness. Therefore, you should inform any health professional (pharmacist, nurse, doctor) before taking any other medication. Similarly, alcohol affects the performance of this medication and should be avoided. Your GP will be sending you for regular blood tests to check the medication levels in your system to ensure you are taking the medication correctly.'

★ Additional Points

▢▢▢ Employment — Advise the patient that they must inform their employers about their diagnosis. Any jobs that require working at heights, driving or dangerous machinery must be avoided.

▢▢▢ Driving — Enquire about transport arrangements for discharge home. Tell the patient that he must stop driving and notify both the DVLA and his car insurance company of the diagnosis.

The DVLA Rulings and Restrictions on Common Medical Conditions

Condition	Group 1 (Cars, Motorcycles)	Group 2 (LGV, PCV)
MI	No driving for 1 month. Does not need to notify the DVLA	6 week disqualification with exercise/functional test requirements prior to relicensing
1st Seizure	Multiple seizures within 24 hrs are considered a single event. No driving for 1 year with medical review before restarting (even if associated with drugs and alcohol). Must be notified*	10-year ban if unprovoked or 5 years if associated with drugs or alcohol
Epilepsy	Three-yearly reissues required. Full licence if seizure free (on medication) for 7 yrs	Full licence if seizure free for >10 yrs without anticonvulsant medication
Stroke	No driving for 1 month and may resume if clinical recovery is satisfactory (absence of visual field, cognitive, limb function impairment). Must be notified	Refusal and revocation of licence for at least 1 year pending subsequent medical review (ECG)

*Special consideration may be given with clearly identified non-recurring provoking causes

☐☐☐ **Bathing** Stress the importance of leaving the door open when having a bath or shower. If he goes swimming, he should always inform the lifeguard that he is epileptic.

☐☐☐ **Withdrawing** Advise the patient that he must be seizure free for at least 2 years before withdrawal or tapering down anticonvulsants can be considered.

'In addition to the medication there are a few general measures I need to inform you about. Firstly, you should inform your employers about your diagnosis and avoid any jobs that involve working at heights or on dangerous machinery. You must also stop driving and notify the DVLA about your diagnosis. When taking a bath, it is advisable to leave the door open in case of an emergency. If you go swimming, do inform the lifeguard about your epilepsy. Before we can consider reducing or stopping your medication, you must be seizure free for at least two years on your tablets. I am sure that this is a lot of information to take in. Feel free to contact us again if you require more information.'

CLOSING

☐☐☐ **Follow-up** Inform the patient that he will be reviewed by a specialist in 2 months' time in outpatients.

☐☐☐ **Understanding** Check that the patient understands the information provided.

Questions Encourage the patient to ask questions and respond to them.

☐☐☐ **Summarise** Give a brief summary back to the patient about what has been discussed. Jointly agree on an action plan and conclude the interview.

COMMUNICATION SKILLS

☐☐☐ **Rapport** Establish and maintain rapport throughout the interview.

☐☐☐ **Listening** Demonstrate interest and concern in what the patient says. Show active listening and listen empathetically.

☐☐☐ **Pauses** Pace information and use appropriate pauses. Allow the patient to express his feelings freely and without interruption.

☐☐☐ **Verbal Cues** Use non-verbal and verbal cues, i.e. tone and pace of voice, nodding your head where appropriate.

0 1 2 3 4 5

☐ ☐ ☐ ☐ ☐ ☐ Overall assessment of discharging patient (seizure)

☐ ☐ ☐ ☐ ☐ ☐ Role player's score

Total mark out of 30

DISCHARGING PATIENTS: **Wound Infection**

INSTRUCTIONS: Mr Kruger is a 58-year-old part-time gardener who suffers from diabetes. He sustained a foot injury whilst working. His wound has been cleaned and debrided, and he is now ready to be discharged on a course of co-amoxiclav. You have been asked to discuss discharge arrangements with him. You will be marked on the information you provide and your communication skills.

INTRODUCTION

0 1 2

☐☐☐ **Introduction**   Introduce yourself. Confirm the patient's name and age.

☐☐☐ **Purpose**   Mention the purpose of the consultation.

'I understand that you are soon to be discharged home from the ward. The team has been discussing your progress and we are all happy to see that you are doing so much better. How do you feel about this?'

★ Explore the Patient's . . .

☐☐☐ **Understanding**   Find out what the patient understands about his planned discharge. What has he already been told?

☐☐☐ **Concerns**   Do you have any particular concerns with your illness or with going home?

☐☐☐ **Home Situation**   Do you live in a house or a flat? Do you need to use any stairs?

☐☐☐ **Social Support**   Do you live alone or with anyone? Do you have any support from your family? Did you have any services in place prior to coming into hospital?

☐☐☐ **Medication**   Establish from patient what treatments he is taking.

★ Medical Advice

☐☐☐ **Antibiotics**   Advise the patient of the importance of completing a full course of antibiotics of co-amoxiclav, three times a day for one week. Warn him about possible side effects, such as nausea, vomiting, diarrhoea and thrush (women).

☐☐☐ **Analgesia**   Advise the patient about taking his analgesia (paracetamol, co-dydramol) regularly to relieve the pain.

☐☐☐ **DM control**   Ask the patient to monitor closely his BM levels to achieve ideal glucose control.

13.4

□□□ **Concordance** Mention the importance of taking the medications regularly as advised.

'You have done very well after your small operation on your leg and have made a good recovery. It is important to take your antibiotics (co-amoxiclav) regularly three times a day, and complete a full course for 7 days. This will help clear any infections from the wound and allow it to heal smoothly. It is also important to take your diabetic medication regularly and to keep your diabetes under tight control. Infections in diabetics are more common and tend to last longer in people with poor control. Your wound will continue to be sore for some time. It is important to take simple analgesia for pain control as and when you need it (maximum four times a day).'

★ **Additional Points**

□□□ **Dressing** Stress the importance of wound care management by having his dressing changed by his practice nurse.

□□□ **Elevating Foot** Advise the patient to rest his leg, keep it elevated above heart level and avoid excessive standing on it.

□□□ **Discharge** Advise the patient to seek medical help if the wound becomes painful or emits a foul-smelling discharge.

□□□ **Employment** Recommend the patient to take time off work (2 weeks).

'In addition to the medication, there are a few general measures I need to inform you about. At the moment your wound is healing and will require regular changes of the dressing which can be done by your GP practice nurse. This will allow us to monitor its progress as well as ensuring it is clean and healing well. We recommend that when you rest keep your foot elevated above the level of your heart to prevent swelling developing in your leg. You can do this by resting your leg on a chair with two pillows beneath it. If your wound becomes more painful or starts to discharge again I advise you to seek medical advice. I also recommend that you take a couple of weeks off work as your form of employment requires long periods of standing which could affect the wound.'

CLOSING

□□□ **Follow-up** Arrange for the patient to be seen in outpatients in 2 months' time.

□□□ **Understanding** Check the patient understands the information provided.

Questions	Encourage the patient to ask questions and respond to them.
□□□ **Summarise**	Give a brief summary to the patient about what has been discussed. Jointly agree on an action plan and conclude the interview.

COMMUNICATION SKILLS

□□□ **Rapport**	Establish rapport with the patient and maintain it throughout the interview.
□□□ **Listening**	Demonstrate an interest and concern in what the patient says. Show active listening and listen empathetically.
□□□ **Pauses**	Pace the information and use appropriate pauses. Allow the patient to speak his feelings freely and without being interrupted.
□□□ **Verbal Cues**	Use non-verbal and verbal cues, i.e. tone and pace of voice, nodding head where appropriate.

EXAMINER'S EVALUATION

0 1 2 3 4 5
□ □ □ □ □ □ Overall assessment of discharging patient (wound)
□ □ □ □ □ □ Role player's score
Total mark out of 34